Clinical Uses of Prism

A Spectrum of Applications

Clinical Uses of Prism

A Spectrum of Applications

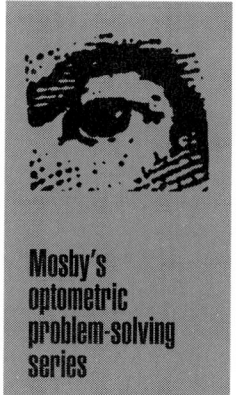

Mosby's
optometric
problem-solving
series

Edited by

Susan A. Cotter, O.D., F.A.A.O., F.C.O.V.D.

Diplomate in Binocular Vision and Perception;
Associate Professor,
Department of Clinical Education,
Illinois College of Optometry,
Chicago, Illinois

Series Editor

Richard London, M.A., O.D., F.A.A.O.

Diplomate in Binocular Vision and Perception;
Pediatric and Rehabilitative Optometry,
Oakland, California

with 113 *illustrations*

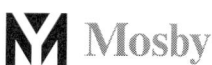 Mosby

St. Louis Baltimore Boston Carlsbad Chicago Naples New York Philadelphia Portland
London Madrid Mexico City Singapore Sydney Tokyo Toronto Wiesbaden

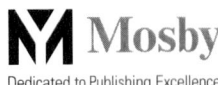

Mosby
Dedicated to Publishing Excellence

A Times Mirror
Company

Executive Editor: Martha Sasser
Associate Developmental Editor: Kellie F. White
Project Manager: John Rogers
Production Editor: George B. Stericker, Jr.
Series Design: Jeanne Wolfgeher
Manufacturing Supervisor: Tim Stringham

Printed in the United States of America
Composition by Carlisle Communications, Ltd.
Printing/binding by Plus Communications

Mosby–Year Book, Inc.
11830 Westline Industrial Drive
St. Louis, Missouri 63146

Library of Congress Cataloging-in-Publication Data
Clinical uses of prism / edited by Susan A. Cotter.
          p. cm. — (Mosby's optometric problem-solving series)
     Includes bibliographical references and index.
     ISBN 0-8151-1810-4
     1. Prisms (Ophthalmology) I. Cotter, Susan A. II. Series.
     [DNLM: 1. Vision Disorders—therapy. 2. Optics—instrumentation.
     WW 140 C6418 1995]
     RE780.C56   1995
     617.7′5—dc20
     DNLM/DLC   94-36459

95 96 97 98 99 / 9 8 7 6 5 4 3 2 1

Contributors

William L. Brown, O.D., Ph.D., F.A.A.O.

Diplomate in Low Vision;
Associate Professor of Optometry,
Department of Clinical Education,
Illinois College of Optometry,
Chicago, Illinois;
Private Practice,
Winamac, Indiana

Elizabeth E. Caloroso, O.D., M.Opt., F.A.A.O.

Professor,
Coordinator, Pediatrics/Disability
  Service,
Coordinator, Pediatric Optometry and
  Vision Therapy Residency,
Optometric Center of Fullerton,
Southern California College of
  Optometry,
Fullerton, California

Susan A. Cotter, O.D., F.A.A.O., F.C.O.V.D.

Diplomate in Binocular Vision and
  Perception;
Associate Professor,
Department of Clinical Education,
Illinois College of Optometry,
Chicago, Illinois;
Private Practice,
Olympia Fields, Illinois

Kelly A. Frantz, O.D., F.A.A.O., F.C.O.V.D.

Diplomate in Binocular Vision and
  Perception;
Associate Professor,
Department of Clinical Education,
Illinois College of Optometry,
Chicago, Illinois

David B. Henson, Ph.D., M.Sc.

Department of Optometry and Vision
  Sciences,
University of Wales,
College of Cardiff,
Cardiff, Wales,
United Kingdom

David G. Kirschen, O.D., Ph.D., F.A.A.O.

Chief of Binocular Vision/
  Orthoptics,
Doris Stein Eye Research Center,
UCLA School of Medicine,
Los Angeles, California;
Associate Professor of Visual Science
  and Optometry,
Southern California College
  of Optometry,
Fullerton, California;
Private Practice,
Brea, California

Rachel V. North, Ph.D., M.Sc.

Department of Optometry and Vision
  Sciences,
University of Wales,
College of Cardiff,
Cardiff, Wales,
United Kingdom

Michael W. Rouse, O.D., M.S.Ed., F.A.A.O.

Diplomate in Binocular Vision and
  Perception;
Professor,
Chief, Vision Therapy Services,
Optometric Center of Fullerton,
Southern California College of
  Optometry,
Fullerton, California

J. James Saladin, O.D., Ph.D., F.A.A.O.

Professor,
College of Optometry,
Ferris State University,
Big Rapids, Michigan

Selwyn Super, Dip. Optom., M.Ed. (Psych), D.Ed., F.A.A.O.

Diplomate in Binocular Vision and
  Perception;
Professor Emeritus,
Department of Optometry,
Rand Afrikaans University;
Private Practice,
Johannesburg, South Africa

Norman J. Weiss, O.D., F.A.A.O.

Diplomate in Low Vision;
Executive Director and Chief of Clinical
  Services,
Western New York Center for the
  Visually Impaired;
Director, Low Vision Clinic,
Erie County Medical Center;
Private Practice,
Buffalo, New York

Bruce Wick, O.D., Ph.D., F.A.A.O.

Diplomate in Binocular Vision and
  Perception;
Associate Professor,
College of Optometry,
University of Houston;
Private Practice,
Houston, Texas

To Betty Caloroso—
who taught me that "prisms are not poison."
And of course to Lou and the kids
(Katie, Peter, Danny, Minnie, Earl, and Angie).

Preface

Personal Note

In 1983 I interviewed for a residency position at the State University of New York (SUNY) College of Optometry. One of the interviewers, Dr. Rick London, asked me, "Have you ever prescribed prism for a patient?" When I answered that I had not, he asked me why. I explained that my instructors had never suggested that we prescribe prism for a patient and, in fact, had given me the impression that we should not prescribe prism at all. I remembered scary stories of patients "eating prism"—coming back year after year and requiring greater and greater magnitudes as time went on. I clearly recall becoming very uncomfortable as I explained my anti-prism position because I realized then that I had no substantial basis (either from research studies or from personal clinical experience) for what I was saying. I remember Rick nodding his head in an understanding way, as if he had heard this story before, and I just knew that I was either misinformed or wrong.

Well, I didn't do the residency at SUNY. Instead, I went to Southern California College of Optometry (SCCO), where I did a residency in children's vision. There I had the privilege of working with Dr. Betty Caloroso, who promptly alleviated my fears and rectified my misconceptions about prescribing prism. She taught me that "prism is not poison" (only sometimes) and that it can be safely prescribed provided one makes an accurate diagnosis and follows certain guidelines. During my year at SCCO I learned that prism is an indispensable tool for managing binocular vision disorders (especially strabismus), and I probably prescribed more prism in that year than many practitioners do in their whole career!

Ironically, 8 years after my SUNY residency interview (and hundreds of prism diopters later), Rick London approached me about editing a textbook on the clinical applications of prism. It was not until I started working on the project that I recalled our discussion about the supposed evils of prescribing prism. Rick says he doesn't remember our conversation during that interview. I suspect that perhaps it was a subconscious thing. It's way too coincidental!

•   •   •

Prisms are a powerful therapeutic tool and have been used in ophthalmic corrections for more than a century; yet, a literature search on this topic is disappointing. Yes, there are textbooks that contain information about the properties and optics of ophthalmic prisms; but little has been written about how to actually prescribe prism (i.e., when and when not to, how much, and in what form). I find it odd that there are any number of texts giving guidelines on the prescribing of glaucoma medication but not any with guidelines on the prescribing of prism—which could be part of the reason why many practitioners avoid prism. This book has been compiled to fill that void.

Its purpose is to provide both practitioners and students with a comprehensive guide to the different clinical applications of prism. It is intended to serve as a useful resource for authoritative clinical information. Each of the 11 chapters pertains to a separate area. First is Bill Brown's thorough review of the optical principles of prism. Then Kelly Frantz and I address (in Chapter 2) the idiosyncrasies of measuring ocular deviations with prism, which may affect the accuracy of deviation measurements that we use to write prescriptions, and (in Chapter 3) the practical issues of implementing prescribed prism. Rachel North and David Henson's comprehensive literature review and discussion of prism adaptation in heterophoric patients follow—providing insight as to why some practitioners may have been unsuccessful in prescribing prism. Jim Saladin and Bruce Wick have excellent chapters (5 and 6) with very specific clinical guidelines on prescribing prism for horizontal and vertical heterophoria patients. David Kirschen's chapter (7) summarizes the results of a nationwide clinical trial investigating the Prism Adaptation Test in surgically managing acquired esotropia and provides additional support of the notion that normal sensory fusion is important in the treatment of strabismus. When and how to prescribe prism for patients with different types of strabismus and at varying ages are thoroughly addressed by Betty Caloroso and me (in Chapter 8), with illustrative case reports to document points made. In Chapter 9 Mike Rouse presents a specific treatment protocol and an impressive case report illustrating how to prescribe overcorrecting prism to eliminate anomalous correspondence in constant esotropes. Selwyn Super presents (in Chapter 10) a behavioral optometry interpretation of how to use prism for vision therapy purposes. Finally, Bill Brown joins Norm Weiss (in Chapter 11) to discuss the various uses of prism in low vision.

The text is written for practicing clinicians. Although most of the contributors have academic credentials, nearly all are clinicians and provide direct patient care. All have been chosen to present material in areas in which they possess considerable expertise. They have been generous in sharing their clinical pearls so that we might provide better care for patients who seek our services. Regardless of whether the reader is a novice or a seasoned prescriber of prism, I guarantee that sufficient information will be found herein to incorporate new techniques and strategies into his or her ongoing practice.

Acknowledgments

First, I would like to extend my gratitude to three people who have had a strong influence on my career path. Betty Caloroso, an outstanding clinician, fostered my interest in the area of strabismus and amblyopia and served as an exemplary role model in the clinic. Watching Betty diagnose and treat strabismic preschoolers is an experience that everyone should have. Mike Rouse, an excellent optometric educator and clinician, taught me how to teach and inspired me to pursue a career in optometric education. He has been a great friend and mentor, and has been immensely supportive of my career. Lou Hoffman, a remarkable person and an insightful clinician, provided guidance and support during my residency and has always been generous in sharing his considerable clinical wisdom and experience (as well as his dirty jokes).

In addition, I'd like to acknowledge the help and support of the following people: Rick London, the series editor, for his conception of the idea, persistence in making the series a reality, and guidance along the way; Kelly Frantz, for her advice, friendship, moral support, and willingness to lend a sympathetic ear; and Sue Mirman, for her significant assistance in the initial stages of this project, in particular for her thoughtful reviews of several chapters and for chasing down and verifying references, as well as for her friendship and support. Thanks go to Al Pouch, who created the photograph for the book cover, Karl Frantz and the ICO classes of 1995 and 1996, who provided ideas and input on the book title; and Alan French and Kathy Niemann, for their tedious reference work.

Finally, I wish to thank the authors for their time and efforts (a special thanks to Bill Brown for his assistance in helping meet the last deadline), and I'd like to express my appreciation to the editorial and production staff at Mosby, in particular Kellie White and production editor George Stericker—a "master wordsmith."

                                                                    Susan A. Cotter

Contents

1

Optical Principles of Prism

William L. Brown

Key Terms

minimum angle of deviation	deviation	vergence
	prism diopter	prism effectivity
Prentice's rule	duction	aberration
decentration	version	image displacement

Prism is a seemingly simple optical element that can produce powerful visual effects. Its performance, however, is affected by many variables, and these must not be overlooked if the anticipated effect for the patient is to be obtained.

Definitions

A prism causes light to be changed in direction. The change is termed *deviation,* and the amount of deviation prism is denoted by the deviating or prism *power.*

A *plano prism* has deviating power but no refracting power. It consists of two flat refractive surfaces joined at an angle (Fig. 1-1). The line of intersection between the surfaces is the *apical (dihedral* or

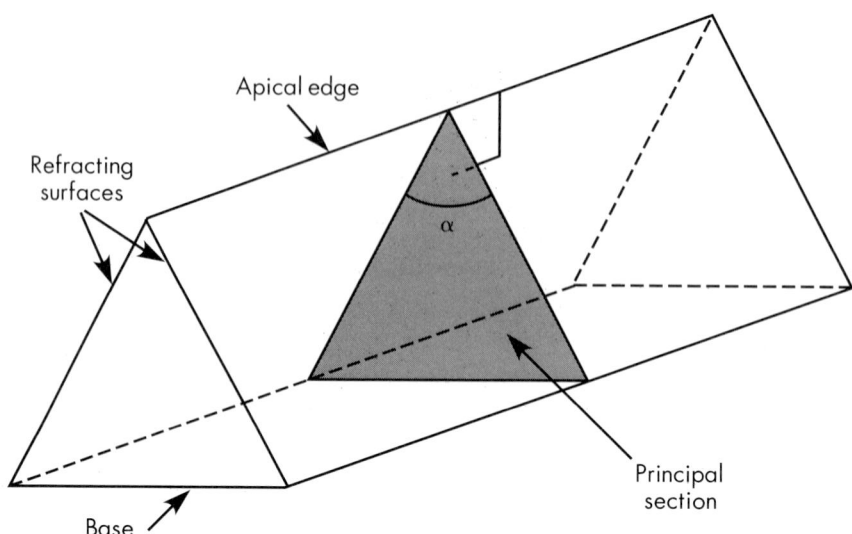

FIGURE 1-1 A refracting prism consists of two refractive surfaces joined at the apical angle (α), with the base situated opposite the apical angle. A principal section is perpendicular to the apical edge.

refracting) edge of the prism. A *principal section* lies in a plane perpendicular to the apical edge. The angle α between the two surfaces in a principal section is the *apical* (dihedral, refracting) *angle.*

The base of the prism is the side opposite the apical angle.

Prism Deviation

When a ray of light is incident in a plane perpendicular to the apical edge, it will remain in that plane when it emerges from the second surface (Fig. 1-2). Incident on the first surface at an angle of i_1 (from the normal to the surface), the ray is refracted at the first surface, passes to the second surface where it is refracted again, and emerges at an angle of refraction i'_2. Both refractions obey Snell's law of refraction.

The index of refraction of the prism is denoted by n'. In this chapter it will be assumed that the prism is surrounded by air (index of refraction, 1.0).

When a prism is surrounded by air, the emerging ray is deviated toward the base. The angle between the emergent ray and the incident ray is the angle of deviation (δ) (Fig. 1-2). The angle of deviation for any plano prism is

$$\delta = i + i'_2 - \alpha. \tag{1}$$

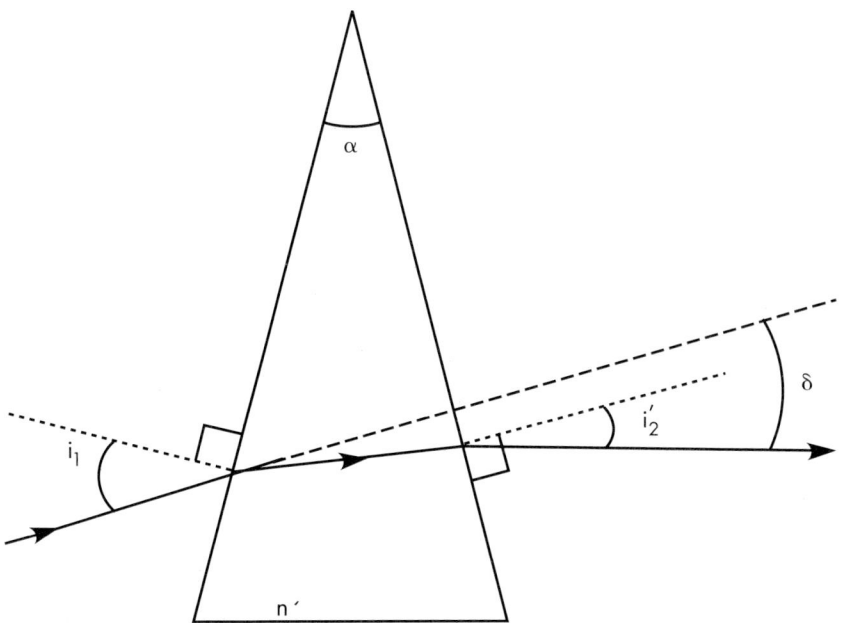

FIGURE 1-2 A principal section of a prism made of material with an index of refraction (n') illustrating the angle of incidence (i'_1) at the first surface, the angle of refraction (i'_2) at the second surface, and the angle of deviation (δ).

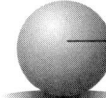

CLINICAL PEARL

When a prism is held in front of the eye, the prismatic effect on the eye may be different from the labeled power if the prism orientation is not carefully controlled.

The angle of deviation is not constant for a prism but varies according to the angle of incidence. Thus when a prism is held in front of the eye, the prismatic effect on the eye may be different from the labeled power if the prism orientation is not carefully controlled. The smallest angle of deviation occurs when the ray of light traverses the prism symmetrically, so that $i_1 = i'_2$ (Fig. 1-3). This *minimum angle of deviation* (δ_{min}) satisfies the following expression:

$$n' = \frac{\sin[(\alpha + \delta_{min})/2]}{\sin (\alpha/2)} \tag{2}$$

Since the ray is deviated only by the two refracting surfaces, the base of the prism has no effect. The base of the prism is important

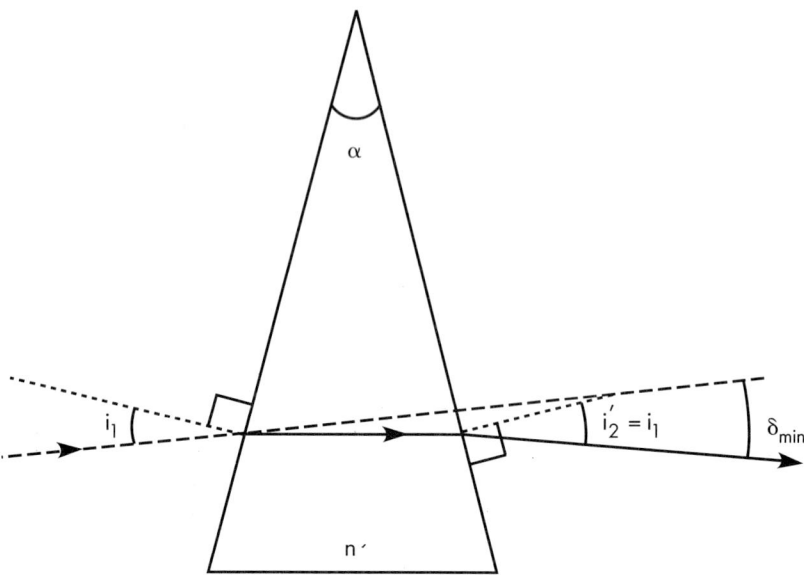

FIGURE 1-3 The minimum angle of deviation (δ_{min}) occurs when a ray of light traverses the prism symmetrically (so that $i_1 = i'_2$).

only for internal reflection. If the angle of incidence on the second surface is too large, the ray will be internally reflected toward the base, where it may be internally reflected again. This effect occurs with smaller angles of incidence on the second surface for the small percentage of light that is reflected when refraction also occurs. Such multiple reflections are often disturbing to the patient.

Ophthalmic Prism

Prisms used in vision applications are termed *ophthalmic* prisms. These frequently have an apical angle less than 10°, in which case they can be considered thin. When a thin prism is held so light enters nearly perpendicular to the first surface, the angle of incidence is small, as are the angles of refraction at the surfaces and the angle of deviation for the prism. For small angles, expressed in radians, the sine of the angle is approximately equal to the angle itself. Applying this small angle approximation to each of the sines in Equation 2 yields a much simpler expression:

$$\delta = (n' - 1)\alpha \qquad\qquad (3)$$

As long as light enters the prism nearly perpendicular to the first surface (angle of incidence close to zero, or "normal incidence"), Equation 3 states the angle of deviation for a thin prism quite accurately. For instance, if a plastic prism (n'= 1.50) has an apical angle of 5°, the angle of deviation for a ray incident close to normal to the first surface is δ = (1.50 − 1)(5°) = 2.5°. The unit for δ is the same as that used for α.

Units of Deviation

The deviating power (angle of deviation) is the most important attribute of an ophthalmic prism. As noted earlier, the deviating power (δ) is dependent not only on the apical angle and index of refraction of the prism but also on the angle of incidence. For light incident close to normal on the first surface of a thin prism, however, the angle of deviation as expressed in Equation 3 is independent of the angle of incidence. This is one reason that the power of an ophthalmic prism is defined as the angle of deviation when the incident ray is normal to the front surface of the prism. Another important reason is that this represents the orientation of the front surface of many prisms when mounted in trial lens rings for clinical testing.

Although the angle of deviation could be designated in degrees, the unit most commonly used is the prism diopter, first introduced by Prentice.[1] The magnitude of an angle in prism diopters (denoted by Δ) is 100 times its tangent (Fig. 1-4):

$$\delta(\Delta) = 100 \tan \delta \tag{4}$$

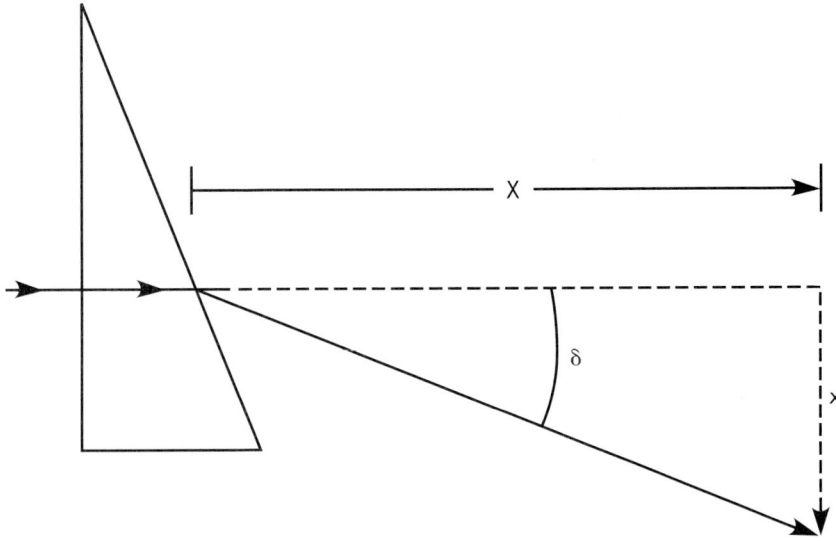

FIGURE 1-4 The angle of deviation (w) in prism diopters is defined as 100 tan δ and equals x(cm)/X(m).

The equivalent of 1° in prism diopters is (100)(tan 1°) = 1.75 Δ; an angle of one prism diopter is 0.57 degree. Since the angle in prism diopters is proportional to the tangent of the angle, it is not linearly proportional to the angle in degrees. For example, the prism diopter equivalent of 20° is not twenty times the number of prism diopters in 1° (that is, not 20(1.75) = 35 Δ), but rather 100 tan 20° = 36.4 Δ.

The tangent function in the definition of prism diopter emphasizes the displacement (x) of the ray at a distance (X) from the prism (Fig. 1-4): tan δ = x/X. If x and X are in meters, then 100(x) gives x in cm and Equation 4 becomes

$$\delta(\Delta) = 100 \tan \delta = 100x(m)/X(m) = x(cm)/X(m) \qquad (5)$$

The displacement (x) is measured perpendicular to the incident ray. For a particular angle of deviation, x is proportional to the distance X. If the angle of deviation is 2 Δ, for example, the displacement (x) is 2 cm at 1 m. If the distance is doubled (to 2 m), the displacement also is doubled (to 4 cm).

Displacement of Images

When a real object is viewed through a prism, each of the diverging rays is deviated toward the base of the prism (Fig. 1-5, A). The image point from which the diverging rays appear to come is displaced toward the apex. Since this is the most common situation in which prisms are used (that is, looking at real objects from which rays diverge), it is commonly stated that rays are deviated toward the base of a prism while the image is displaced toward the apex.

However, this is not true if the rays entering the prism converge toward a *virtual* object point on the other side of the prism (Fig. 1-5, B). Whereas each ray is deviated toward the base of the prism, the image is also displaced toward the base. Certain ophthalmic instruments, such as the lensometer, are designed with prisms positioned to cause this type of displacement. When a prism is measured through the lensometer, the target image is displaced toward the base of the prism.

Prism Orientation

It is not sufficient to use the power alone to describe a prism and its effect. The power must be accompanied by the direction of the base. The coordinate system used to identify the meridian of the prism base is the same as the one used for cylinder lenses, with zero to the observer's right (the patient's left) and with angles increasing counterclockwise (Fig. 1-6).

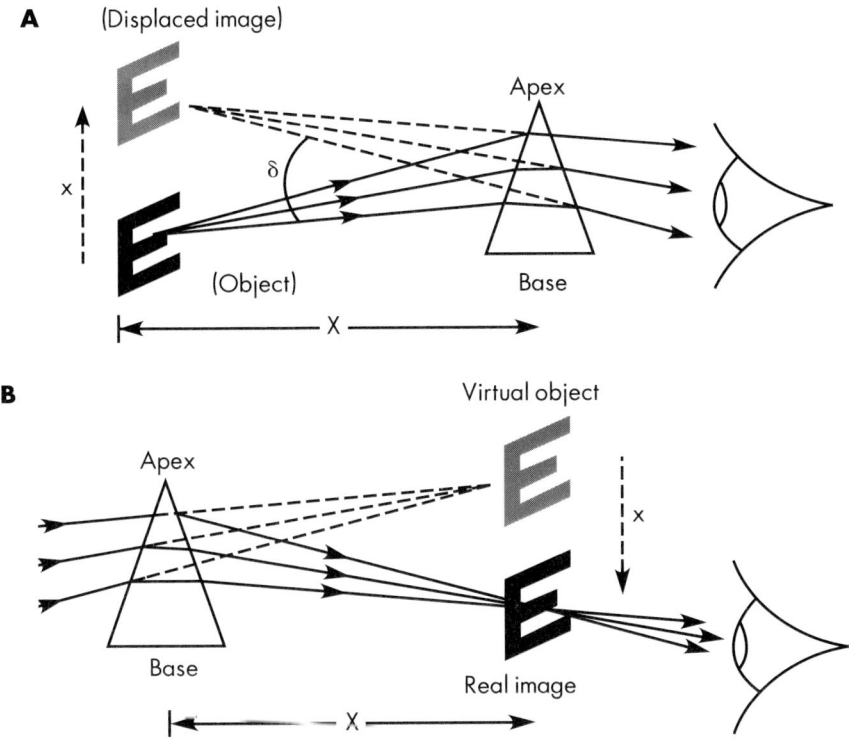

FIGURE 1-5 A, An image formed by diverging rays is displaced toward the apex of the prism. **B,** An image formed by converging rays is displaced toward the prism base.

Prism with its base upward in the vertical meridian is termed *base-up* (BU) prism but prism with its base downward in the vertical meridian is termed *base-down* (BD). Since "up" and "down" are used to denote vertical directions, it might be expected that "left" and "right" would be used for horizontal prism. However, the nose is used as a reference point instead. Prism along the horizontal meridian is termed *base-out* (BO) if the base is away from the patient's nose, and *base-in* (BI) if the base is toward the nose.

For vertical prism, if the same direction label is used the direction of the base is the same for each eye; that is, BU means the base is up regardless of which eye is used. For horizontal prism, however, the same label means the *opposite* "left-right" directions for the two eyes. BO prism in front of the right eye, for example, means the base is to the right but in front of the left eye means its base is to the left. Similarly, the base for BI prism is to the left for the right eye and to the right for the left eye.

Prism with its base in oblique meridians can be identified in several ways. Most commonly it is specified as a horizontal component (BI or

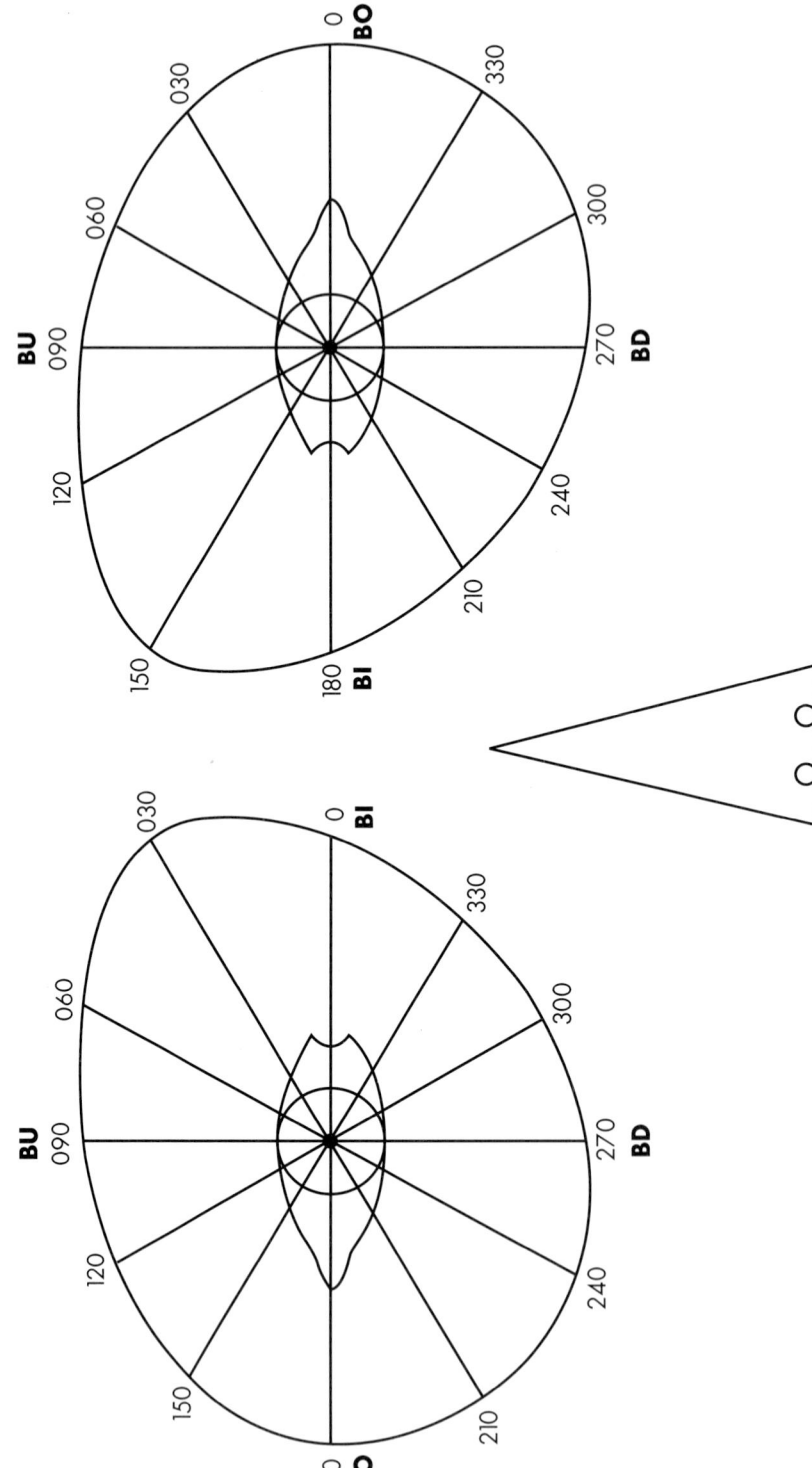

FIGURE 1-6 The direction of the base of a prism is specified using angles in a coordinate system having 0 to the observer's right (patient's left). Angles increase counterclockwise.

BO) together with a vertical component (BU or BD). It can also be denoted as a single prism magnitude, however, with its base in a particular meridian. The base of the single prism is in an oblique meridian if it has both horizontal and vertical components.

If angles from 0 to 180 are used to identify the meridian, an extra description is needed to specify in which of the two possible directions within that meridian the base is pointed. For instance, in Figure 1-7 the base of the prism before the right eye is in meridian 060 (using a 0-180 system) but is down and out in 060, not up and in, which would be the other possibility. In this case if the prism has a power of 5 Δ, it would be specified as 5 Δ BD & BO @ 060.

Alternatively, the meridian can be specified using a 360° system, in which the prism base direction is denoted unequivocably using an angle from 0 to 360. The prism in Figure 1-7 would be totally described as 5 Δ base @ 240.

Monocular Prism Effects

When one eye is covered and a prism is held in front of the other, the eye rotates toward the apex of the prism to view the displaced image. These monocular movements of the eye are termed *ductions*. When the eye looks through BD prism, it rotates upward, undergoing *sursumduction* (or supraduction). With BU prism the eye rotates downward, undergoing *infraduction*. BO prism induces *adduction* (movement toward the nose), and BI prism *abduction* (movement away from the nose).

Binocular Prism Effects

Prism causes a change in the relative directions of the lines of sight of the two eyes. These changes can have a profound effect on the patient's visual comfort and binocularity.

When both eyes view a distant object, the lines of sight are parallel. If the eyes rotate equal amounts, keeping the angles between the lines of sight unchanged, the eye movements are termed *versions* or *conjugate eye movements*. If BO prism, for example, is held in front of the right eye and an equal amount of BI prism is held in front of the left eye, both eyes will rotate to the left through equal angles and will remain parallel. The eyes will also remain parallel and rotate to the right if BI prism is held in front of the right eye and an equal amount of BO prism is in front of the left eye. Likewise, the eyes undergo conjugate movements if equal amounts of BU prism or BD prism are held in front of each eye.

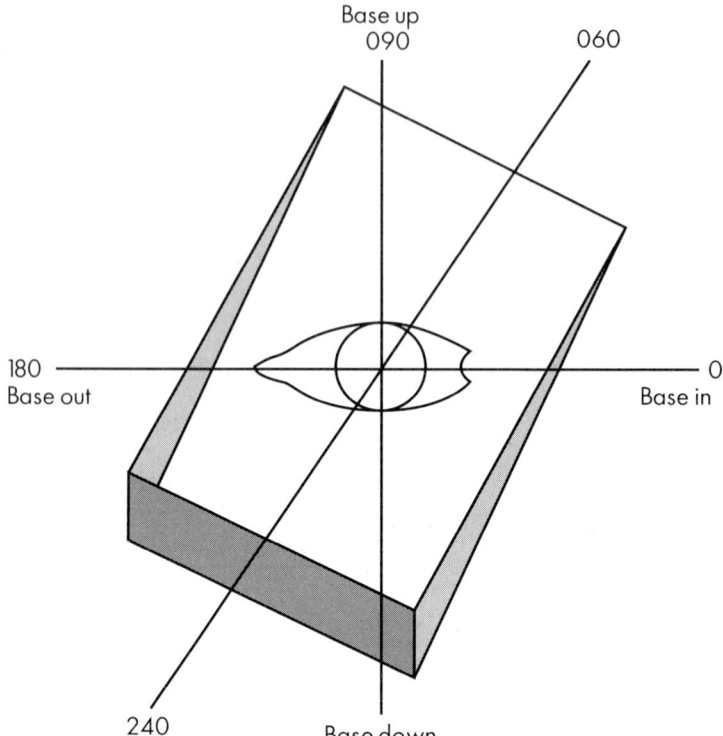

FIGURE 1-7 The direction of the base of this prism held in front of the patient's right eye could be specified as either base @ 240 (based on a 360° system) or BD & BO @ 060 (based on a 180° system).

Eye movements that change the angle between the lines of sight are termed *disjunctive* or *vergence* movements. If small amounts of BO prism are held in front of each eye, both eyes will rotate inward toward one another, a movement termed *convergence*. Small amounts of BI prism before each eye cause the eyes to turn outward away from each other, a movement termed *divergence*.

Resultant prism effect is the net amount of prism that causes the angle between the two lines of sight to change. When prism held in front of the eyes causes only conjugate eye movements, the angle between the lines of sight remains constant and the resultant prism effect is zero.

For example, if 3 Δ BO is held in front of right eye and 3 Δ BI in front of the left, both eyes rotate 3 Δ to the left, leaving the angle between the lines of sight unchanged so the resultant prism effect is zero. If the prism in front of the right eye is changed to 4 Δ BO, the right eye will turn 4 Δ to the left while the left turns only 3 Δ to the left. The net resultant prism is 1 Δ BO, which causes a net convergence between the two eyes.

If 3 Δ BO is held in front of the right eye and 2 Δ BO in front of the left, the net resultant prism is 5 Δ BO. The same net increase in convergence of 5 Δ is caused by any combinations of prisms yielding a resultant prism effect of 5 Δ BO. For instance, 5 Δ BO right eye and 0 Δ left eye or 0 Δ right eye and 5 Δ BO left eye both yield the same net 5 Δ increase in convergence between the lines of sight.

Lateral prisms having the same direction (that is, both BO or both BI) in front of the two eyes produce a net resultant prism that can be found by adding the two powers together. If the prisms have different directions, they are subtracted to find the net resultant prism; the direction of the resultant prism is that of the larger of the two prisms. It is not necessary to specify an eye for the resultant horizontal prism, since the same prism direction will cause the same net convergence or divergence whether it is placed before the right eye or the left eye.

For vertical prisms the net resultant prism is found by adding the prism powers if the prism directions are different (one BU and the other BD) and subtracting them if the directions are the same (both BU or both BD). For example, the net resultant prism for a combination of 1 Δ BDOD and 3 Δ BDOS is 2 Δ BDOS. The resultant prism for the combination of 1 Δ BDOD and 2 Δ BUOS is 3 Δ BDOD. Vertical prism of 3 Δ BDOD is equivalent to 3 Δ BUOS.

The eye must be specified for resultant vertical prism. Whereas 2 Δ BDOD causes the right eye to rotate 2 Δ upward relative to the left, 2 Δ BDOS causes the left eye to rotate 2 Δ upward relative to the right. These are different positions between the lines of sight, so describing a vertical prism as 2 Δ BD without specifying the eye is insufficient.

Prentice's Rule

Ophthalmic lenses change the direction of rays that pass through them in much the same way as prisms do. However, the prismatic effect for lenses increases with distance from the optic axis of the lens. Figure 1-8 shows two rays entering a lens parallel to and above the optic axis. The lens deviates the first ray (labeled *1* and located a distance of d_1 from the axis) through an angle of deviation (δ_1). The second ray (which lies farther from the axis, at a distance of d_2) is deviated through a larger angle (δ_2). It is clear from the diagram that as ray *1* travels the distance f' from the lens it is deviated through a distance d_1. From the definition of prism diopter, the angle of deviation (δ_1) is expressed by $\delta_1 (\Delta) = d_1 \text{ (cm)}/f' \text{ (m)}$. But $1/f' = F$, the refracting power

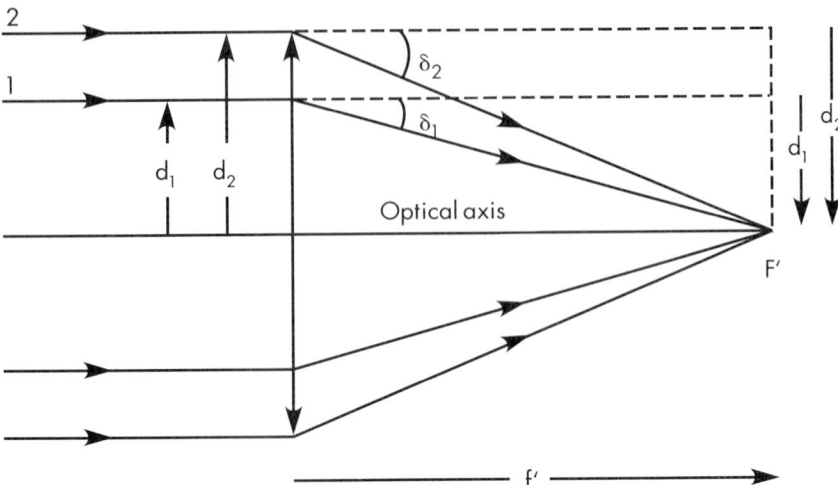

FIGURE 1-8 Rays parallel to the axis are deviated by varying amounts of prism power, depending on the distance (d) from the axis, to cross at F' (the secondary focal point). From the diagram and the definition of a prism diopter ($\delta = d[cm]/f'$ [m]) Prentice's rule is derived, $\delta = dF$.

of the lens. Therefore the angle of deviation can be expressed as $\delta_1(\Delta)$ = d_1 F. The same definition can be applied to ray 2.

In general, the angle of deviation in prism diopters, which represents the prism power (P) produced by the lens, is given by *Prentice's rule:*

$$P = \delta = dF \qquad\qquad (6)$$

where d is the distance (in centimeters) from the optical axis to the point on the lens where the prism is produced and F is the power of the lens (in diopters) in the meridian containing the point.

According to Prentice's rule, the amount of prismatic effect produced through a lens increases as the distance from the optical axis increases. The direction of the base of the prism depends on whether the power of the lens is plus or minus. Figure 1-8 illustrates the effect of a plus lens, through which the ray is deviated toward the optical axis. Recall that rays of light are deviated toward the base of a prism. Therefore the deviation of rays produced by a plus lens brings to mind a prism having its base toward the axis. A plus lens can be pictured as a series of prisms whose bases are toward the axis, with the power of the prisms increasing as the distance from the axis increases. Likewise, a minus lens can be conceptualized as a series of prisms with their bases away from the axis.

It is convenient to remember this principle by illustrating a plus lens as two prisms base to base (Fig. 1-9, *A*) and a minus lens as two

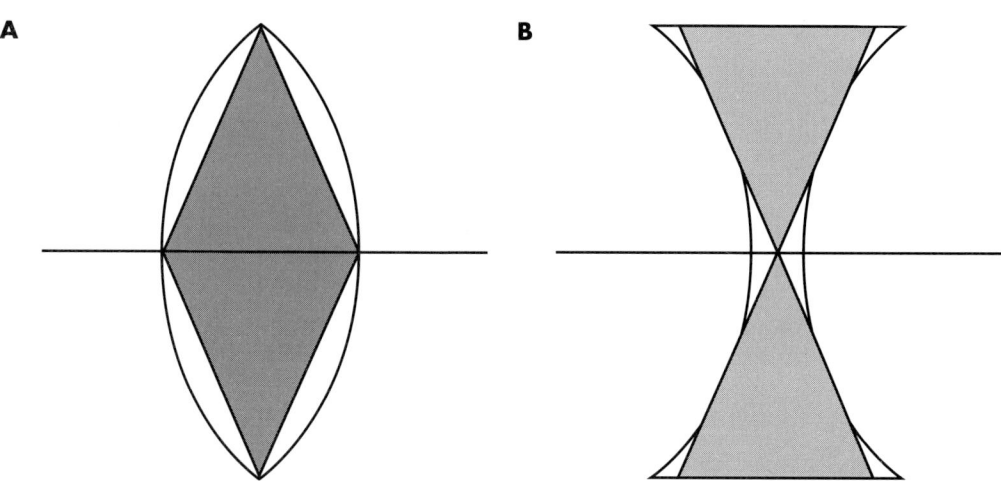

FIGURE 1-9 The direction of the base of the prism induced as a ray passes through a lens can be determined by representing the plus lens as a series of prism elements with bases toward the axis, **A,** and a minus lens as prism elements with bases away from the axis, **B.**

prisms apex to apex (Fig. 1-9, *B*). This is simply a convenience for remembering base direction; one must remember that prism power in a lens is not constant but gradually increases with distance from the axis.

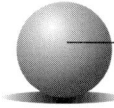

CLINICAL PEARL

The amount of prismatic effect through a lens is not constant but gradually increases as the distance from the optical axis increases.

Lateral and Vertical Components of a Prism

Although a prism can be described using a single power and the direction of its base, it is more commonly denoted clinically by identifying a horizontal meridian and vertical component. When combined, these two prism components produce the same effect on the eye as the single prism that could have been used.

One reason for employing horizontal and vertical components is that clinical testing evaluates horizontal and vertical function separately. For example, lateral phoria and vergence testing may reveal that horizontal prism is indicated whereas vertical phoria and vergence testing may indicate a need for vertical prism.

Another reason for employing horizontal and vertical components is that when prism is prescribed, the laboratory that fabricates the lens is accustomed to manipulating the lens to produce horizontal and vertical prism rather than a single prism power at an oblique angle.

An instance in which clinical testing does not give horizontal and/or vertical prism amounts directly is the prism scanning technique sometimes used in low vision patients with eccentric viewing. A prism is rotated in front of the eye to find the meridian of optimal effect. The meridian is often oblique. When the prism is ordered from the laboratory, it is helpful to provide the horizontal and vertical components of the prism as usual. The division of a prism into the two components is the topic of this section.

The results of combining prisms can be determined graphically or mathematically by representing each prism as a vector with proper length and direction. In Figure 1-10 a prism is represented on a coordinate system as a vector. The length of the vector represents the prism power (P), and the angle (θ) between the positive direction of the x axis and the vector is the direction of the base of the prism. The vector points in the direction of the base of the prism.

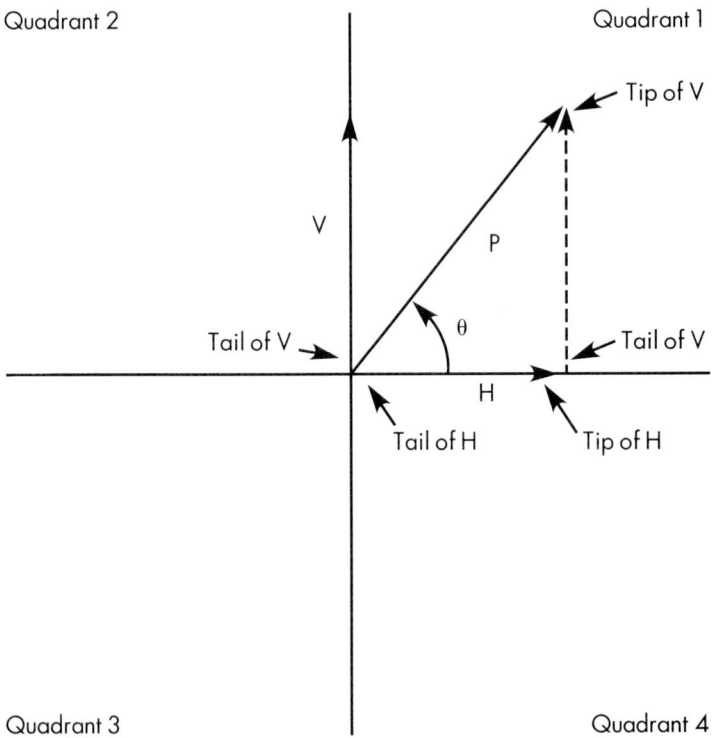

FIGURE 1-10   A prism having a power (P) with its base at an angle (θ) can be resolved into horizontal (H) and vertical (V) components.

In Figure 1-10 the horizontal component is labeled *H* and the vertical component *V*. When H and V are added vectorially, they sum to *P*; P is the power of the single prism that has the same prismatic effect as the combination of H and V. The magnitudes of the horizontal and vertical components are found from the following relationships, which can be easily derived from the trigonometry of the right triangles in Figure 1-10:

$$H = P\cos\theta \tag{7}$$

$$V = P\sin\theta \tag{8}$$

For example, suppose a 3 Δ BU & BI @ 060 prism is held in front of the right eye. The horizontal and vertical components of the prism are

$$H = 3\ \Delta \cos 60 = +1.5\ \Delta\ (\text{BI for the right eye})$$

$$V = 3\ \Delta \sin 60 = +2.6\ \Delta\ (\text{BU})$$

This means that if a 1.5 Δ BI prism and a 2.6 Δ BU prism are held in front of the right eye the same prismatic effect will be produced as when a 3 Δ prism is held with a BU & BI @ 060 orientation.

Superposition of a Horizontal and a Vertical Prism

Just as a single prism can be divided into horizontal and vertical components, a horizontal prism and a vertical prism can be combined (superimposed) to produce an effect equivalent to that of a single prism power. For example, assume that testing shows a patient could benefit from 1.5 Δ BI and 2.6 Δ BUOD prism. (Although prism is usually prescribed in 0.5 Δ steps clinically, the same values from the example above will be used to show the relationship between the procedures.) It is decided to use a temporary Fresnel prism to test the patient's acceptance before permanently incorporating the prism into the lenses. It is possible to use two separate Fresnel prisms, 1.5 Δ BI on the left lens and 2.5 Δ (close to 2.6) BU on the right lens. However, it is also possible to economize and use a single Fresnel prism to produce both the horizontal and the vertical component.

The single power (*P*) is found by adding the horizontal and vertical powers vectorially. Figure 1-10 shows the coordinate system, with *H* and *V* representing the horizontal and vertical prisms respectively from the observer's viewpoint. H and V are added vectorially by placing the tip of one to the tail of the other. The tip of each vector shows the direction of the base of the prism. In this case *V* has been moved from its position on the vertical axis (*solid line*) to place its tail on the tip of *H*, keeping the length and direction of V (*dashed line*) the same as in its original position. As the diagram shows, the resultant prism will have its base in the first quadrant, with a direction angle (θ)

between 0 and 090. If the diagram is made accurately to scale, the power can be found by measuring the length of the resultant vector (P) and the angle (θ) can be measured with a protractor.

More commonly, however, P is calculated by applying the pythagorean theorem to the right triangle:

$$P = \sqrt{H^2 + V^2} \tag{9}$$

The angle θ for the direction of the base can be determined using the tangent:

$$\tan \theta = V/H \tag{10}$$

In our example the resultant prism parameters are

$$P = \sqrt{(1.5)^2 + (2.6)^2} = \sqrt{9} = 3\ \Delta$$

$$\tan \theta = +2.6\ \Delta/+1.5\ \Delta = 1.73$$

$$\theta = 60°$$

A single 3 Δ Fresnel prism BU & BI @ 060 on the right lens produces the same effect as the 1.5 Δ BI and 2.6 Δ BUOD prisms.

If the proper quadrant for the resultant prism is to be found from the calculations rather than from the diagram, it is important to keep track of signs when θ is calculated. This is discussed further in Appendix A.

Superposition of Two Oblique Prisms

Just as a single prism can be found to replace a horizontal and a vertical prism, so a single prism power can be found to replace any combination of two or more prisms held in front of one eye regardless of orientation. The resultant prism power is found by adding the prisms vectorially. This can be done graphically by adding vector representations of the prisms on an accurately scaled diagram or mathematically. Further discussion appears in Appendix B.

Decentration

The location of the optical center (OC) in a spectacle lens is specified by its distance from the geometrical center (GC) of the lens. The distance from the GC to the OC is termed decentration. Decentration is "in" when the OC is moved from the GC toward the nose and "out" when it is moved away from the nose.

Most lens prescriptions call for zero prism, in which case the OCs are placed in front of the pupil centers. The amount of decentration to place the OCs at the pupil centers is given by the following two relationships, one for each eye:

$$RDec = FPD/2 - RPD \tag{11}$$

$$LDec = FPD/2 - LPD \tag{12}$$

RDec and *LDec* are the decentrations for the right and left lenses respectively. *FPD* is the frame PD, which is the distance between the geometrical centers of the two lenses. The frame PD is the sum of the horizontal width of the lens (the A dimension in the boxing system) and the distance between the two points on the lenses that are closest together (the DBL in the boxing system). *RPD* and *LPD* are the right and left monocular PDs respectively of the patient.

One way of producing prism is to decenter the OC away from the eye. The amount of prism induced is given by Prentice's rule. The total decentration is the sum of the decentration to place the OC at the eye plus the decentration to move the OC away from the eye to achieve the desired prism.

For a plus lens, decentering from the eye is in the same direction as the base of the prism to be produced. (A plus lens is decentered *in* to produce BI prism.) For a minus lens, decentering from the eye is in the *opposite* direction from the base of the prism to be produced.

CLINICAL PEARL

For a plus lens, the lens is decentered in the same direction as the base of the prism to be produced; for a minus lens, the lens is decentered in the opposite direction from the base of the prism to be produced.

Simple, or plano, cylinders have zero refracting power in the axis meridian. The base of all prism in a simple cylinder is oriented perpendicular to the axis meridian. Consider a simple cylinder for the left eye having a power of -2.00 DC $\times$ 030 (Fig. 1-11). The base of the prism at all points off the axis is in meridian 120. For instance, at point *A* in Figure 1-11 the prism is BU and BI @ 120. For point B on the axis, the prism is zero; there is zero power from the cylinder in the axis meridian and the distance from the axis is zero, so application of Prentice's rule gives zero.

For example, suppose the patient's prescription is OD $+5.00 - 1.00 \times$ 090, OS $+3.00 - 1.00 \times 180$ with 2 Δ BI. The frame PD is 70 and the patient's right and left monocular PDs are 32 and 31 respectively. The prism is to be provided equally in the two lenses. Decentrations to move the OCs to the eyes are

$$RDec = FPD/2 - RPD = 70/2 - 32 = 3 \text{ mm in}$$

$$LDec = FPD/2 - LPD = 70/2 - 31 = 4 \text{ mm in}$$

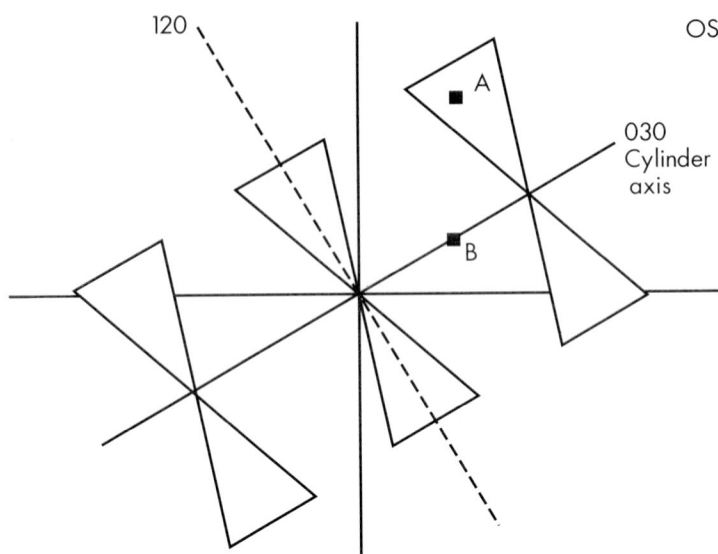

FIGURE 1-11 A simple cylinder −2.00 × 030 is diagrammed with several prism elements showing that the direction of the base of the prism is always perpendicular to the axis. At point *A* the prism is base-up and base-in @ 120; at point *B*, on the axis, it is zero (0).

The next step is to determine how far and in which direction the OC must be moved from the eye to produce the desired prismatic effect at the eye. The magnitude of this second element of decentration is calculated from Prentice's rule. For lateral prism the power of each lens in the horizontal meridian is used, which is +4.00 D for the right eye and + 3.00 D for the left.

Right eye: $d = \delta/F = 1\ \Delta/4\ D = 0.25\ cm = 2.5\ mm\ in$
Left eye: $d = \delta/F = 1\ \Delta/3\ D = 0.33\ cm = 3.3\ mm\ in$

The direction of this decentration is inward for both eyes since the OC of a plus lens must be decentered inwardly to produce BI prism. Total decentration to produce the 1 Δ BI in each eye are

Right eye: 3 mm in + 2.5 mm in = 5.5 mm in

Left eye: 4 mm in + 3.3 mm in = 7.3 mm in

Vertical prism can be produced in similar fashion through decentration in the vertical meridian. Assume that the patient's prescription is OD −4.00 − 1.00 × 090, OS −3.00 − 1.00 × 180 with 1 Δ BUOS. The vertical dimension of the frame (B dimension) is 44, and the patient's pupil is 24 mm above the lower edge of the lens. It is decided to provide all of the prism in the right lens. Since BUOS is equivalent to BDOD, 1 Δ BDOD must be provided in the right lens.

The vertical center of the lens is (44/2) 22 mm above the lower edge. The eye is therefore 2 mm above the center of the lens, and the lens would be decentered 2 mm up to place the OC in front of the eye. The power in the vertical meridian of the right lens is −4.00 D. According to Prentice's rule, the OC must be moved d = δ/F = 1 Δ/4 D = 0.25 cm = 2.5 mm from the eye for the vertical prism. To obtain BDOD with minus power, the lens must be decentered in a direction opposite the necessary base, so the OC must be moved up 2.5 mm. The total decentration vertically is (2 mm + 2.5 mm) 4.5 mm up. The OC must be located (22 mm + 4.5 mm) 26.5 mm above the lower edge of the lens.

Cylinders with Oblique Axes

When the eye looks through a spherocylinder lens having an oblique axis, the calculation for the induced horizontal and vertical prism components is more complicated. The prism contributed by the sphere is the same as in the previous example, but the contribution by the cylinder is more complex. The problem is that the base of the prism produced by the cylinder is always perpendicular to the axis.

The procedure for finding the prism components of the cylinder involves finding the length (d) along the perpendicular from the viewing point (E) to the axis (Fig. 1-12).

Example

A patient's prescription is OD −3.00 −2.00 × 060. While reading he or she views 2 mm in (x) and 10 mm down (y) from the OC of the lens. Through how much lateral and vertical prism does the patient view?

Horizontal Spherical Component

H_s = xF_s = (0.2 cm) (3.00 D) = 0.60 Δ BI

Vertical Spherical Component

V_s = yF_s = (1.0 cm) (3.00 D) = 3.0 Δ BDOD

Horizontal and Vertical Cylinder Components

The graphical solution involves making a scale drawing of the vertical and horizontal meridians and the axis meridian.

1. Place the viewing point (E) for the eye at the proper displacement (x and y) from the OC and drop a perpendicular from the viewing point to the axis.
2. Note from the diagram that for a minus cylinder the prism components at E will have BI and BD directions in this example.

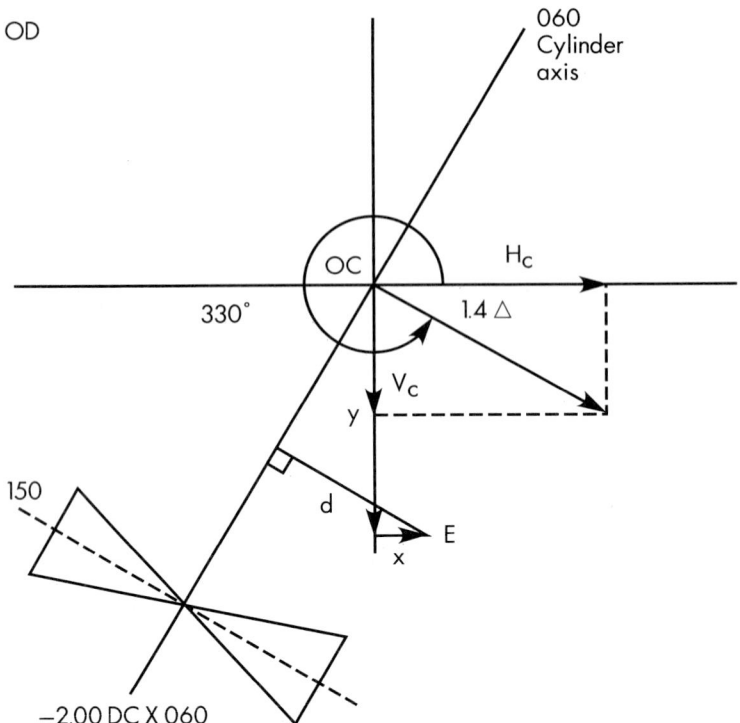

FIGURE 1-12 The eye looks through a −2.00 DC × 060 at a viewing point (*E*) that is *x* cm nasal and *y* cm below the optical center (*OC*). The prism at *E* from the cylinder has its base along 150, perpendicular to the axis. The perpendicular distance (*d*) from the axis to *E* is used in Prentice's rule to find the prism amount (1.4 Δ). The right part of the diagram shows the resultant prism vector (1.4 Δ) resolved into the horizontal (*H*$_c$) and vertical (*V*$_c$) components.

3. Measure the length (d) of the perpendicular from E to the axis, which in this example is (0.7 cm) 7 mm (once the scale of the diagram is taken into account).
4. Determine the prism at E from the cylinder using the cylinder power F$_c$ in Prentice's rule: δ = dF$_c$ = (0.7 cm)(2.00 D) = 1.4 Δ BD & BI @ 150.
5. Determine the horizontal and vertical components of the prism by constructing a vector 1.4 units long in meridian 150 (middle right in Fig. 1-12). Drop a perpendicular to the horizontal meridian to find the horizontal component (H$_c$) and a perpendicular to the vertical meridian to find the vertical component (V$_c$). Measure the lengths of the components to find the horizontal and vertical prism, which in this case are (H$_c$) 1.2 Δ BI and (V$_c$) 0.7 Δ BDOD.

Total Horizontal and Vertical Components

The total horizontal and vertical prism is the sum of the horizontal and vertical contributions respectively from both the sphere and the cylinder:

$$H = H_s + H_c = 0.6 \;\Delta\; BI + 1.2 \;\Delta\; BI = 1.8 \;\Delta\; BI$$
$$V = V_s + V_c = 3.0 \;\Delta\; BDOD + 0.7 \;\Delta\; BDOD = 3.7 \;\Delta\; BDOD$$

The total horizontal and vertical prismatic effects induced by looking away from the OC of a spherocylinder lens can also be calculated mathematically. This method is described in Appendix C.

Decentration for Cylinders with Oblique Axes

In the previous discussion the horizontal and vertical prismatic effects were calculated for a known viewing point located at specific horizontal and vertical distances from the OC. These methods do not help, however, when it is the decentration to produce desired prismatic effects that must be determined.

For example, if the prescription is $+6.00 - 2.00 \times 035$ and $1.0 \;\Delta\;$ BO is needed, the horizontal and vertical decentrations must be calculated. Appendix D lists the equations that can be used for this purpose.

Prism by Surface Fabrication

An alternative to decentering the lens to produce prism is for the laboratory to add prism when the second surface of the lens is finished. If the ophthalmic lens is tilted in the surface generator while the second surface is fabricated, an angle is produced between the two surfaces that results in prism. Although the amount of prism obtainable from decentration is low for normal lens powers, amounts of 10 to 15 Δ can be obtained through surface fabrication.

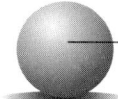

CLINICAL PEARL

Although the amount of prism obtainable from decentration is low for normal lens powers, amounts of 10 to 15 Δ can be obtained through surface fabrication.

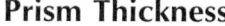

Prism Thickness

Figure 1-13 shows a cross section of a flat plano prism with a truncated apical edge. The thickness at the apex is t_A, the thickness at

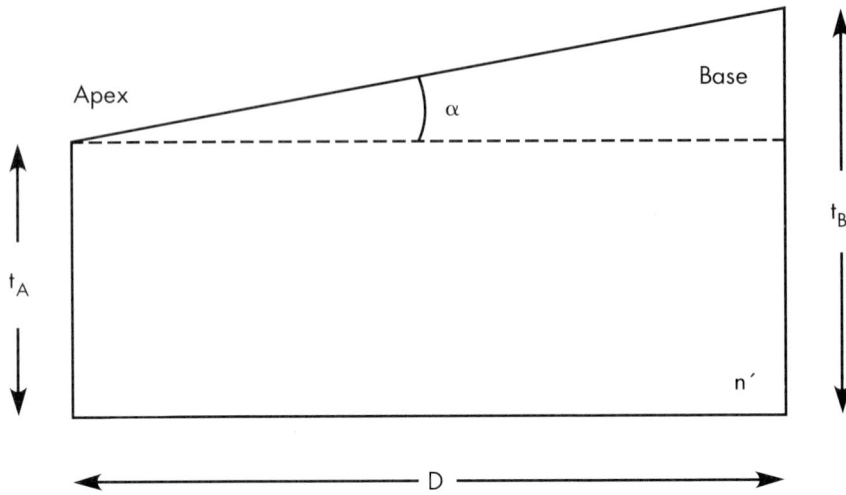

FIGURE 1-13 A truncated flat plano prism of diameter D has an apical thickness (t_A), a base thickness (t_B), which is greater than t_A, an index of refraction (n'), and an apical angle (α).

the base is t_B, the distance from apex to base is D, and the index of the prism is n'. When Equation 3 relating the apical angle and the angle of deviation for a thin prism, Equation 4 for changing degrees to prism diopters, and the tangent of angle α from the triangle in Figure 1-15 are used, it can be shown[2] that:

$$t_B = t_A + D\delta/(100[n'-1]) \tag{13}$$

The distances t_B, t_A, and D have the same units, and the prism power δ is in prism diopters. For prism ground on a 50 mm diameter lens made of ophthalmic crown glass, the thickness of the base is approximately 1 mm per prism diopter greater than that of the apex.

Lens and Prism Thickness

When the OC of the lens is at the GC, the variation in thickness between the GC and the edge of the lens will be dependent on the lens power, the index of refraction, and the distance from the GC to the edge. When prism is present at the GC, whether from decentration or from surface fabrication, it contributes to the variation in thickness according to Equation 13.

Figure 1-14, A, shows a plus lens decentered so its OC is nasal to the GC, and Figure 1-14, B, the same lens divided into two parts: a

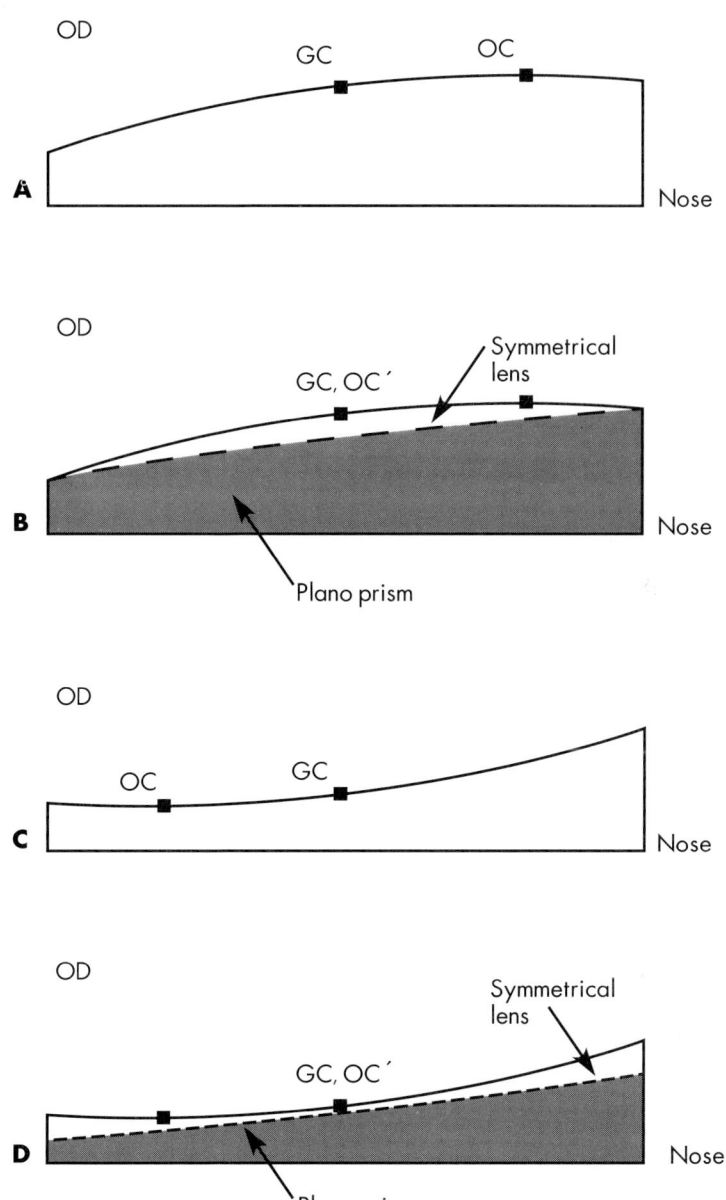

FIGURE 1-14 **A,** A plus lens with the optical center (*OC*) moved nasally from the geometrical center (*GC*). **B,** The decentered plus lens diagrammed as a plano prism and a symmetrical lens with its optical center (*OC′*) at the *GC*. **C,** A minus lens with the *OC* moved temporally from the *GC*. **D,** The decentered minus lens diagrammed as a plano prism and a symmetrical lens having its *OC′* at the *GC*.

centered lens and a plano prism. The centered lens component has its OC labeled *OC'*. A minus lens, decentered out, is shown similarly in Figure 1-14, *C* and *D*.

When a plus lens is decentered, the edge toward which it is decentered (the nasal edge in Figure 1-14, *A*) is thicker than the other edge. When a minus lens is decentered, the edge toward which it is decentered (the temporal edge in Figure 1-14, *C*) is thinner than the other edge.

Figure 1-14, *B* and *D*, illustrates the factors that determine whether the relative thickness at the edge of a lens is greater or less than that at the GC of the lens. For the plus lens with BI prism (Fig. 1-14, *B*) the thickness at the temporal edge will always be less than at the GC, regardless of the power of the prism or lens, because both the prism and the symmetrical lens have less thickness at that edge. The nasal edge, however, may be thinner, thicker, or the same as the GC depending on how much BI prism is at the GC and how much plus power is in the lens. The prism adds thickness while the symmetrical lens subtracts thickness at the edge. For BO prism, the thickness of a plus lens at the nasal edge will always be less than at the GC but the temporal edge thickness will vary in its relative magnitude.

For a minus lens with BI prism (Fig. 1-14, *D*) the thickness at the nasal edge will always be greater than at the GC because both the prism and the symmetrical lens add thickness at the edge. The relative thickness of the temporal edge depends on the magnitudes of the two components. The opposite relationships are true for BO prism.

Prism Effectivity

The angle through which the eye rotates while viewing an object through a prism is not always equal to the angle of deviation of the prism. In Figure 1-15, *A*, the object at *M* is located a distance (*l*) in front of the prism; the prism is distance *z* in front of the center of rotation (*CR*) of the eye. The image (*M'*) of the object viewed through the prism is displaced angle δ, the deviating angle of the prism. However, the angle of rotation of the eye ($δ_e$) is smaller than the angle of deviation of the prism.

$$δ_e = (δl)/(l + z) \tag{14}$$

The angle of rotation is the effective power of the prism. In Equation 14, either of two conditions will make the angle of rotation equal to the prism angle δ. If the object distance (l) is infinite or the

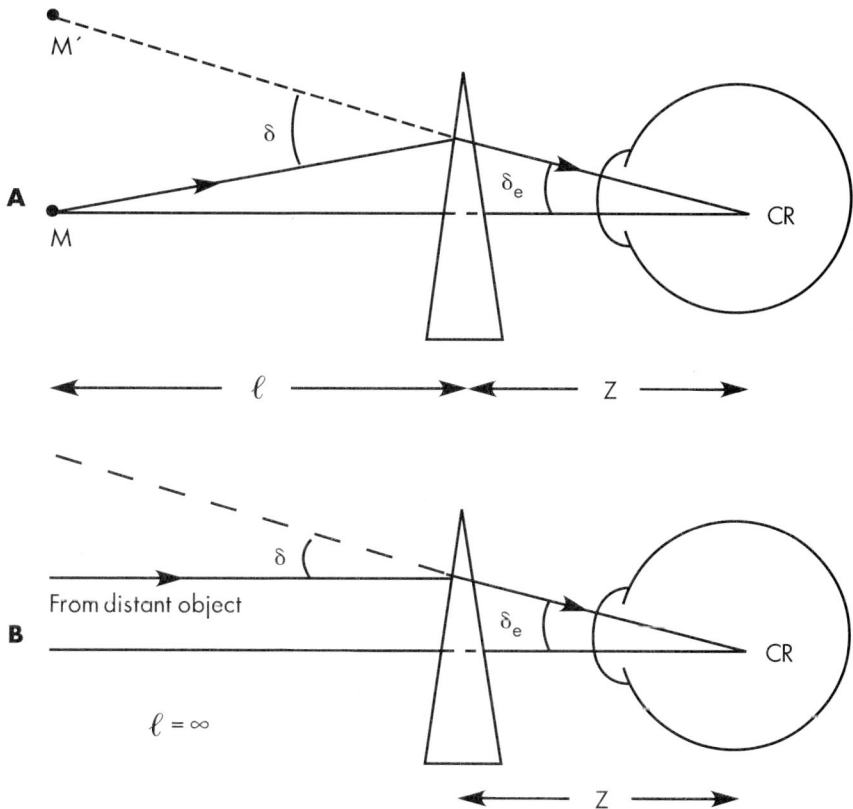

FIGURE 1-15 The effective power (δ_e) of a prism having a power δ is the angle of rotation of the eye caused by the prism. For a near object, **A,** δ_e is less than δ whereas for a distant object, **B,** it equals δ. *CR,* Center of rotation.

prism is placed at the center of rotation (z = 0), then $\delta_e = \delta$. The first situation is illustrated in Figure 1-15, *B*. The second situation is unrealistic since the prism cannot be placed at the center of rotation.

For a near object, the eye does not rotate as much as the prism power implies and the angle of rotation decreases as the prism is held farther from the eye. This shows why it is clinically important to consistently hold a prism in the same plane during near testing. Failure to do so will lead to different rotation demands on the eye (see Chapter 2). Since prescribed prism will be placed in the spectacle plane, the test prism should be held in that plane. For distant objects the effective prism power is the same as the prism power regardless of prism position.

Aberrations

Images through prisms are degraded by the same aberrations as lenses, including spherical aberration, oblique astigmatism, and curvature of the field. Chromatic aberration is especially noticeable (Fig. 1-16). The angle of deviation for the blue end of the spectrum (δ_b) is larger than for the yellow end (δ_y), which in turn is larger than for the red (δ_r). If a white object against a black background is viewed through a BD prism (Fig. 1-16), white light from each of the points in the white object is spread into a spectrum with blue above and red below. The upper edge of the image will have a bluish fringe, and the lower edge a reddish fringe. If viewed through BU prism, the fringes will be reversed. If a black object is viewed on a white background, the fringes will also be reversed.

Because of the change in angle of deviation from base to apex, distortion is very prominent in prisms. The following distortions in the image are evident[3-5] (Fig. 1-17): (1) a nonuniform increase in angular magnification from base to apex; (2) a curving of lines perpendicular to the base-apex line such that the ends of the lines point toward the apex of the prism; (3) a slanting of lines parallel to

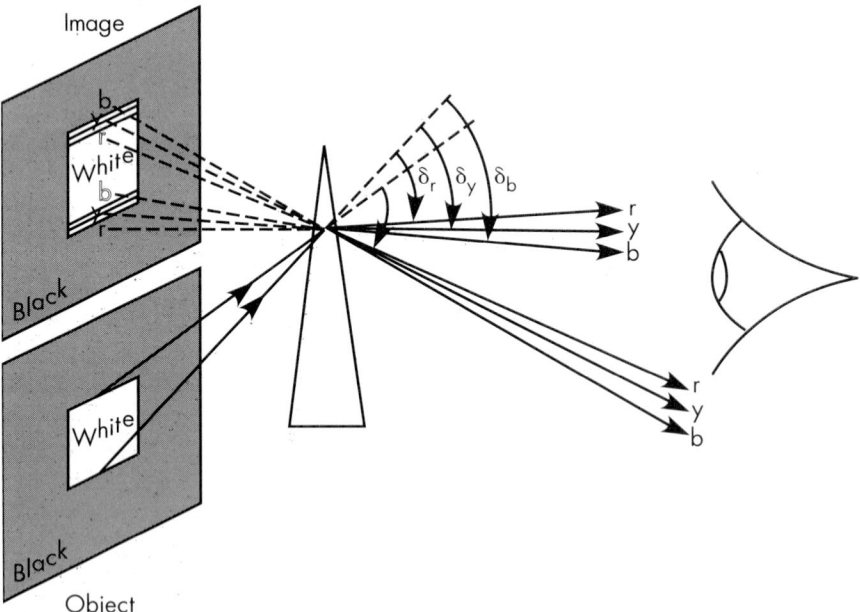

FIGURE 1-16 Chromatic aberration in a prism. A white square on a black background viewed through a base-down prism is displaced upward; due to chromatic aberration, it has a bluish fringe on top and a reddish fringe on the bottom.

the base-apex line; and (4) different magnifications in the planes parallel and perpendicular to the base-apex line.

With BO prism before each eye, vertical lines (perpendicular to the base-apex line) appear convex toward the base of each prism. The binocular image of a vertical line will appear concave toward the observer because of crossed disparity. A vertical line viewed through

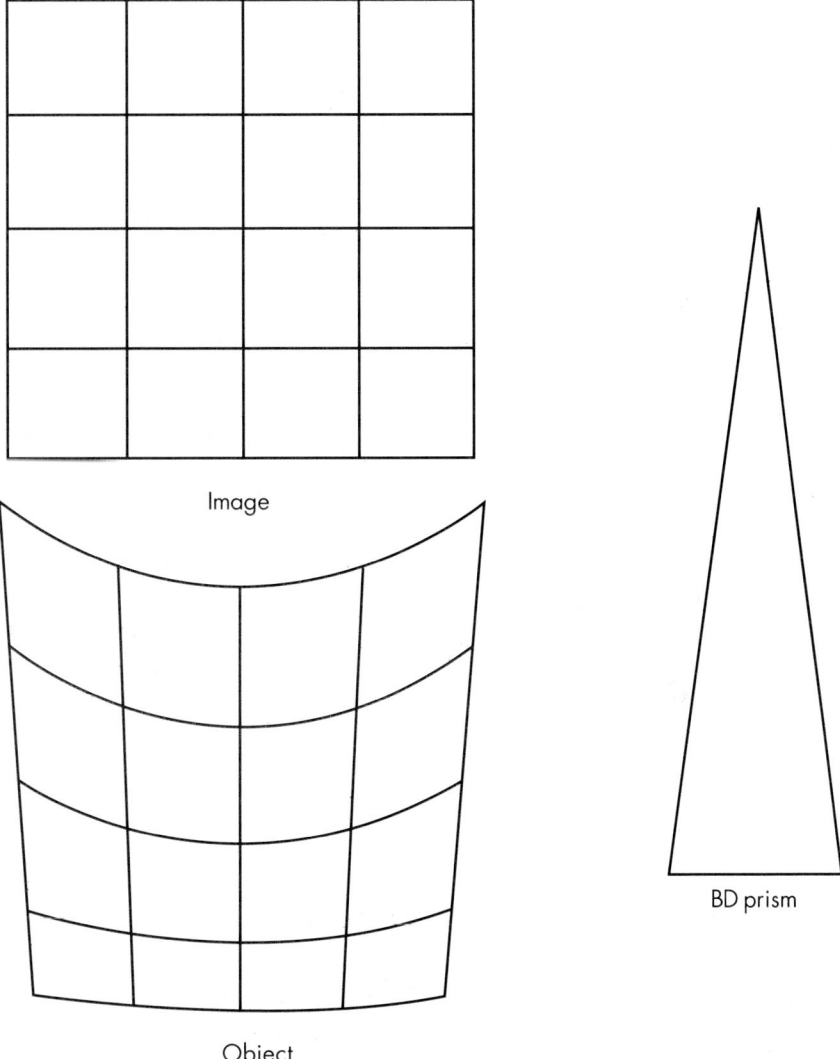

Image

Object

BD prism

FIGURE 1-17 Distortions through a prism. A square grid viewed through a base-down prism is displaced upward and distorted, as shown by the diagram of the image.

BI prisms will appear convex toward the observer because of un-crossed disparity.

For flat prisms the components of distortion depend on the prism power, the apical angle, and the index of refraction. They do not depend on the distance between the eye and the prism or on the prism thickness.

For prism in a lens the curvature of lines perpendicular to the base-apex line cannot be eliminated by changing the base curve of the lens. However, it can be minimized by using very steep front curves (greater than +12.00 D). The asymmetrical magnification along the base-apex meridian can be eliminated with steep front curves near +9.00 to +12.00 D. When the front surface is flat, the change in angular magnification of lines parallel to the base as the eye scans along the base apex line is zero.

Prisms also produce internal reflections, which cause concentric rings toward the base of the prism. These can be essentially eliminated with an antireflection coating.

Since the various components of distortion and internal reflection increase with prism power, it is preferable to split prism powers greater than 3 Δ between the eyes.

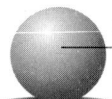

CLINICAL PEARL

Because distortion and internal reflection increase with prism power, it is preferable to split prism powers greater than 3 Δ between the eyes.

Fresnel Prism

Fresnel press-on prisms (developed by the Optical Sciences Group) are thin plastic prisms made of polyvinyl chloride. They consist of a series of tiny prism elements aligned with their bases in the same direction. The thickness of each tiny element is small, which keeps the thickness and weight of the whole to a minimum. The prism adheres to the rear surface of an ophthalmic lens. Powers from 0.5 to 30 Δ are available. (See chapter 3 for additional information.)

Adams et al.[6] found that Fresnel prisms (base horizontal) produce less overall horizontal and vertical magnification than conventional prisms do but more asymmetrical horizontal magnification and more change in vertical magnification with horizontal gaze. The grooves between the base of one element and the apex of the adjacent element cause light scatter and increased diffraction with decreasing element width. Both factors decrease visual acuity.

Measuring Prism

The power of an unknown plano prism can be determined by measuring the deviation. A meter stick is placed a convenient distance away (say, at 2 m), its "0" mark at one of the vertical lines. The prism is held in front of the eye with its base apex line horizontal so the top edge of the prism will split the pupil; the eye looks over the top as well as through the prism. A second vertical marker is moved (by an assistant) so that, when the eye views it above the pupil (unaffected by the prism), it lines up with the displaced image of the first marker seen through the prism. As illustrated in Figure 1-4, the distance between the two vertical markers is the displacement (x) and the power can be calculated:

$$\delta(\Delta) = x(cm)/X(m)$$

Prism in an ophthalmic lens is measured by means of a lensometer. First, the position of the major reference point (MRP) is marked on each lens with a marking pen. For verification of a newly ordered lens the MRP is marked at the PDs as specified; if the prism is to be measured in glasses that the patient is wearing, the pupillary centers serve as the MRPs and should be marked on the lenses. Then, with the rear surface against the lens stop, the mark on the right lens is centered over the lens stop of the lensometer. If there is prism at the MRP, the lensometer target is displaced from the center of the reticle (crosshair) in the direction of the base of the prism. Figure 1-18 shows the target for the right eye displaced up and in; therefore the prism is BU and BI. Finally, a perpendicular is mentally dropped from the center of the target to the horizontal meridian to get the horizontal component of the prism (2 Δ BI in this case). A perpendicular is mentally dropped also from the center of the target to the vertical meridian to get the vertical component of the prism (3 Δ BUOD). The mark on the left lens is centered on the lens stop, and the horizontal and vertical components found: 2.5 Δ BI and 2 Δ BDOS. The total prismatic effect is 4.5 Δ BI and 5 Δ BUOD (or BDOS).

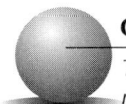

CLINICAL PEARL

The position of the major reference point (MRP) is marked on each lens when measuring prism by means of a lensometer. For verfication of a newly ordered lens, the MRP is marked at the PDs as specified; if the prism is to be measured in glasses that the patient is wearing, the pupillary centers serve as the MRPs and should be marked on the lenses.

If the prism power exceeds the range of the reticle so the mire (target) is displaced out of view, an auxiliary horizontal and/or vertical prism (trial prism or loose prism) is placed on the surface of the lens to bring the target into view so it can be measured on the reticle. The results are modified by the power of the auxiliary prism(s). For example, if a 5 Δ BO prism were held in front of the right lens (Fig. 1-18), and the mires showed the same lateral displacement, the total horizontal prism in the right lens would be (2 Δ BI + 5 Δ BI) = 7 Δ BI. The BO auxiliary prism would compensate for BI prism in the lens.

Some lensometers have special "prism compensator" attachments for measuring prisms up to 15 Δ.

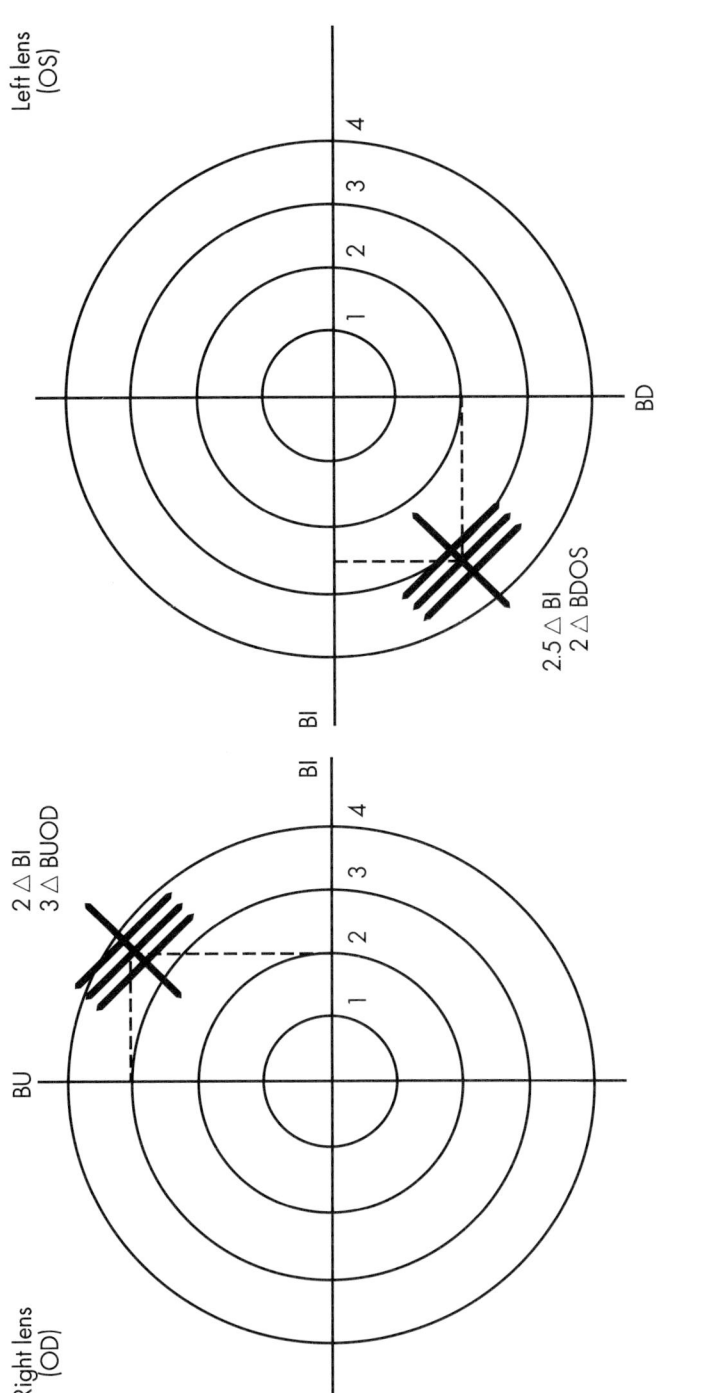

FIGURE 1-18 Prism measurement by lensometry. The lensometer target is displaced upward and inward for the right eye, downward and inward for the left. The direction of displacement is the direction of the prism base. Each *circle* on the reticle is 1 Δ. Perpendiculars to the horizontal and vertical meridians give the horizontal and vertical components of the prism powers, which are added to obtain the total prismatic effect.

Appendix A: Determining the Quadrant for Resultant Prism

When the quadrant for the resultant prism is to be found using tan θ = V/H (Equation 10) rather than a diagram, a sign must be accurately assigned to both the horizontal prism (H) and the vertical prism (V). Horizontal distances measured to the right are positive; distances to the left are negative. Vertical distances upward are positive, and distances downward are negative. For the right eye the base of BI prism (to the right from the observer's viewpoint) is in the positive (x) direction so it is assigned a plus sign whereas BO is assigned a minus sign. For the left eye BI is assigned a minus sign and BO a plus sign. For both eyes BU is positive and BD is negative.

Attention to detail is needed particularly when the resultant prism is in the second or third quadrant. Figure 1-10 shows the upper right quadrant designated 1, the upper left 2, the lower left 3, and the lower right 4. The tangent (Equation 10) is positive when both V or H are either positive or negative. This occurs in the first and third quadrants. In either case, when the inverse tangent is taken to find θ, the calculator will return a positive angle in the first quadrant (less than or equal to 90°).

For example, suppose a 3 Δ BI prism and a 1 Δ BD prism are combined in front of the left eye (Fig. 1-19). The diagram makes it clear that the resultant should lie in the third quadrant. The calculations are

$$P = \sqrt{(1)^2 + (3)^2} = \sqrt{10} = 3.2 \ \Delta$$

$$\tan \theta = -1/-3 = +0.333$$

$$\theta_c = +18°$$

where θ_c is the angle provided by the calculator. Obviously +18° does not move the prism base into the third quadrant as expected. This is because the calculator is quite ignorant; it knows only about quadrants 1 and 4 and nothing about 2 and 3. However, both H (−1) and V (−3) are negative, which occurs only in the third quadrant, just as the diagram predicts. Therefore 180° must be added to obtain the correct answer:

$$\theta = \theta + 180 \ \text{(for third quandrant)}$$

$$\theta = 18 + 180 = 198°$$

The same analysis must be made to distinguish quandrants 2 and 4. The tangent is negative in these since either H or V (but not both) is negative. The angle provided by the calculator for the inverse tangent will be negative, in the fourth quandrant. If an angle in the second quandrant is required, 180° is added. This occurs when H is negative and V is positive.

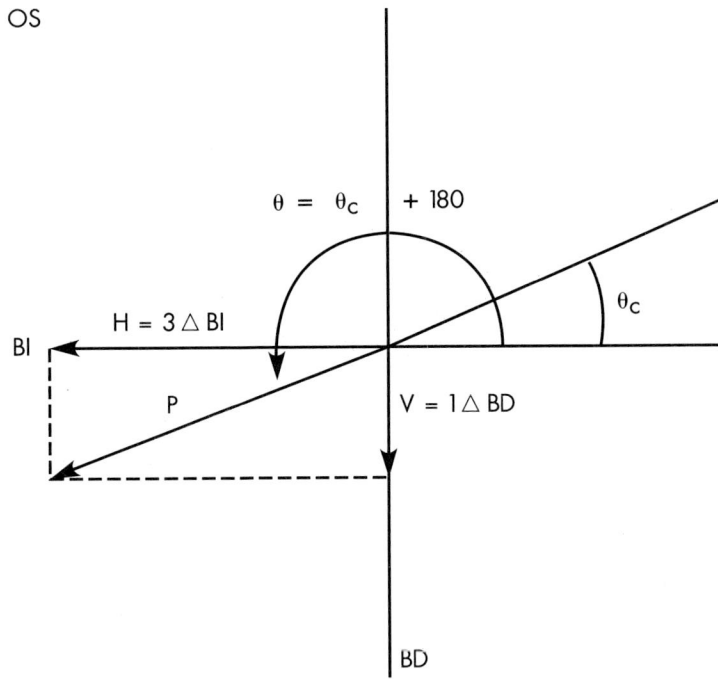

FIGURE 1-19 The combination of a 3 Λ base-in and a 1 Δ base-down prism over the left eye yields a single resultant prism of power P with its base at angle θ. Note that the resultant prism has its base-in the third quadrant; thus the angle read from the calculator (θ_c) must be modified by 180°.

Appendix B: Mathematical Method for Resultant Prism— Oblique Prisms

The single prism that replaces two oblique prisms can be calculated mathematically. First, the vectors representing each prism are divided into horizontal and vertical components. Next, all horizontal components and all vertical components are added together. Finally, the resultant horizontal and vertical vectors are combined to find the single resultant vector.

Figure 1-20, A, illustrates two prisms (P_1 and P_2) represented by two vectors. The length of the vector represents the magnitude of the prism power whereas angles θ_1 and θ_2 represent the orientation of the bases. H_1 and V_1 represent the horizontal and vertical vector components of prism P_1 and H_2 and V_2 the horizontal and vertical vector components of prism P_2. Applying Equations 7 and 8 to each prism:

$$H_1 = P_1 \cos \theta_1 \tag{15}$$

$$V_1 = P_1 \sin \theta_1 \tag{16}$$

$$H_2 = P_2 \cos \theta_2 \tag{17}$$

$$V_2 = P_2 \sin \theta_2 \tag{18}$$

For example, suppose the 3 Δ BU & BI @ 060 prism used earlier is combined with a 2.5 Δ BD & BI prism @ 150 in front of the right eye. The horizontal and vertical components for the first prism as found earlier are

$$H_1 = 3 \ \Delta \cos 60 = +1.5 \ \Delta \ (\text{BI for the right eye})$$

$$V_1 = 3 \ \Delta \sin \ 60 = +2.6 \ \Delta \ (\text{BU})$$

For the second prism the direction of the base is in the fourth quadrant (BD and BI for the right eye). The base direction in the 360° coordinate system used for vectors is (150 + 180) 330°. The components of the second prism are

$$H_2 = 2.5 \ \Delta \cos 330 = +2.2 \ \Delta$$

$$V_2 = 2.5 \ \Delta \sin \ 330 = -1.2 \ \Delta$$

The total horizontal component (H) of the two prisms is the sum of H_1 and H_2 whereas the total vertical component (V) is the sum of V_1 and V_2:

$$H = H_1 + H_2$$

$$V = V_1 + V_2$$

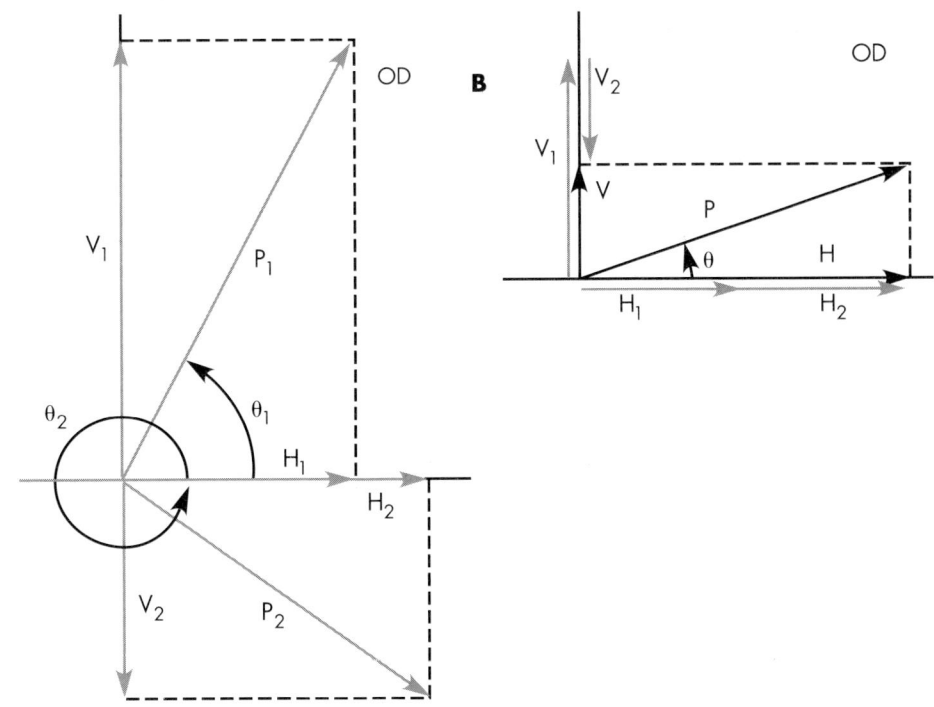

FIGURE 1-20 A, Two prisms (P_1 and P_2) are combined by first resolving each into its horizontal (H_1 and H_2) and vertical (V_1 and V_2) components. **B,** The total horizontal component (H) and total vertical component (V) are then combined to find the resultant prism (P), with its base at θ.

In the example the resultant horizontal and vertical components are

$$H = +1.5\ \Delta + (+2.2\ \Delta) = +3.7\ \Delta\ (BI)$$

$$V = +2.6\ \Delta + (-1.2\ \Delta) = +1.4\ \Delta\ (BU)$$

In other words, a 3.7 Δ BI and a 1.4 Δ BU prism held in front of the right eye have the same effect as the two original prisms. In most clinical situations this would be an acceptable representation of the resultant prismatic effect, since prism powers are most often denoted as horizontal and vertical components.

The magnitude of the single prism that would replace the original prisms is found by vectorially adding the resultant horizontal and vertical components (Fig. 1-20, *B*). The magnitude (P) of the resultant prism and the angle (θ) is found using Equations 9 and 10:

$$P = \sqrt{H^2 + V^2}$$

$$P = \sqrt{(+3.7)^2 + (+1.4)^2} = \sqrt{15.6} = 4.0\ \Delta$$

$\tan \theta = V/H$

$\tan \theta = +1.4\ \Delta/+3.7\ \Delta = +0.378$

$\theta = +21°$

A 4 Δ prism with its base at 21° (or BU & BI @ 021) has the same effect as the original two prisms. A Fresnel prism could be positioned this way.

Appendix C: Mathematical Method to Find the Horizontal and Vertical Prism Induced Away from the OC of a Spherocylinder

Each of the steps in the graphical procedure to find prism away from the OC of a spherocyclinder with an oblique axis can be expressed mathematically, resulting in a solution totally by calculation. To determine the direction of the resultant prism components, however, a special coordinate system must be used that utilizes symmetry relative to the nose. The reason for this unique coordinate system is that horizontal prism is labeled with the same direction relative to the nose when the physical directions are different. For instance, the direction of the base for BO prism is to the right for the right eye and to the left for the left eye.

The following convention is used for the coordinate system[7]:

1. Position of the Viewing Point E
The horizontal distance (x) and the vertical distance (y) from the OC to the viewing point are assigned signs as follows:

E nasal to OC: x positive

E temporal to OC: x negative

E above OC: y positive

E below OC: y negative

2. Cylinder Axis Direction
The angle for the cylinder axis of the left lens is the axis in the standard spherocylinder notation. The axis of the right lens is 180 minus the axis in the standard notation.

3. Trigonometric Relationships
$$d = x \sin \theta + y \cos \theta \qquad (19)$$

Prism effect at E from cylinder:

$$\delta = F_c d = F_c(x \sin \theta + y \cos \theta) \qquad (20)$$

Horizontal prism component from cylinder:

$$H_c = F_c(x \sin \theta + y \cos \theta)\sin \theta \qquad (21)$$

Vertical prism component from cylinder:

$$V_c = F_c(x \sin \theta + y \cos \theta)\cos \theta \qquad (22)$$

Horizontal component from sphere:

$$H_s = xF_s \qquad (23)$$

Vertical component from sphere:

$$V_s = yF_s \qquad (24)$$

4. Base Directions

H positive: BO

H negative: BI

V positive: BD

V negative: BU

5. Total Prismatic Effect at E from Both Sphere and Cylinder:

$$H = H_s + H_c = xF_s + F_c(x \sin \theta + y \cos \theta)\sin \theta \qquad (25)$$

$$V = V_s + V_c = yF_s + F_c(x \sin \theta + y \cos \theta)\cos \theta$$

Appendix D: Decentration of a Spherocylinder to Produce Prism

The horizontal and vertical decentrations (x and y) necessary to produce a horizontal (H) and a vertical (V) prismatic effect can be calculated from the following equations.

If Equations 23 and 24 are rearranged algebraically, one can solve for x and y:

$$x = (DH - BV)/(F_s[F_s + F_c]) \tag{26}$$

$$y = (-BH + AV)/(F_s[F_s + F_c]) \tag{27}$$

where $D = F_s + F_c \cos^2 \theta$, $B = F_c \sin \theta \cos \theta$, and $A = F_s + F_c \sin^2 \theta$.

The equations for *x* and *y* can be used to determine the necessary horizontal and vertical decentrations to obtain horizontal and vertical prism by decentration.

References

1. Prentice CF: A metric system of numbering and measuring prisms, *Arch Ophthalmol* 19:64-75, 128-135, 1890.
2. Fannin TE, Grosvenor T: *Clinical optics*, Boston, 1987, Butterworths, p 108.
3. Morgan MW: Distortions of ophthalmic prisms, *Am J Optom Arch Am Acad Optom* 40:344-350, 1963.
4. Ogle KN: Distortion of the image by ophthalmic prisms, *AMA Arch Ophthalmol* 47:121-131, 1952.
5. Ogle KN: *Researches in binocular vision*, New York, 1972, Hafner Publishing, pp 130-132.
6. Adams AJ, Kapash RJ, Barkan E: Visual performance and optical properties of Fresnel membrane prisms, *Am J Optom Arch Am Acad Optom* 48:289-297, 1971.
7. Bennett AG: *Emsley and Swaine's ophthalmic lenses*, London, 1968, Hatton Press, pp 128-130.

Self-Assessment Questions

1. A patient presents with a 4 Δ Fresnel prism on the left eye, its base at up and out 30°. How much lateral prism effect is the patient receiving?
   a. 0.5 Δ
   b. 2.0 Δ
   c. 3.0 Δ
   d. 3.5 Δ

2. While prism in a right ophthalmic lens is being measured using a lensometer with an 8 Δ BI auxiliary prism in front of the lens, the mire is displaced nasally to the third ring of the reticle. How much lateral prism is present?
   a. 5 Δ BI
   b. 5 Δ BO
   c. 11 Δ BI
   d. 11 Δ BO

3. While viewing through 3 Δ BO in front of each eye, a patient sees a vertical line. Which of the following describes the most likely appearance of this line?
   a. concave toward the patient
   b. convex toward the patient
   c. convex to the right
   d. convex to the left

4. A patient requires 2 Δ BIOS. The prescription is −5.00 DS. The decentration necessary to place the optical center at the eye is 3 mm in. What is the total decentration necessary to produce the required prism?
   a. 1 mm out
   b. 2 mm in
   c. 4 mm out
   d. 7 mm in

Answers: 1. d.   2. b.   3. a.   4. a.

2

Idiosyncrasies of Measuring with Prism

Kelly A. Frantz
Susan A. Cotter

Key Terms

Prentice position	primary angle of	measurement errors
frontal plane	deviation	Hering's law
position	secondary angle	prism effectivity
minimum deviation	of deviation	spectacle-induced
position	polarization	prism

Many clinicians take for granted that objective measurements (in other words, cover testing) of ocular deviations will be accurate, provided the patient can adequately follow instructions such as maintaining fixation on a target. On the other hand, clinicians may be less certain regarding the reliability of subjective measurements (for example, fixation disparity curves), which require critical observations by the patient. In fact, both types of measurements are influenced by factors that may not be widely known.

Objective measurements are influenced by positioning of prisms and prism bars; one must hold them differently for primary gaze as

We wish to thank Susan Mirman, O.D., for her assistance.

opposed to secondary and tertiary gaze positions and for distance versus near fixation. In addition, measurement of the primary and secondary angles of deviation in noncomitant strabismus requires positioning the prism over a specific eye. Problems arise when two prisms are stacked together to measure an angle for which a single prism will not suffice, or when a deviation is measured over spectacles with attached Fresnel prism. In either case the prism powers do not add algebraically. Furthermore, spectacle-induced artifacts may result in erroneous measurements if the spectacles are of sufficient power or the ocular deviation is large.

Subjective procedures such as measuring stereopsis through prism that neutralizes an ocular deviation, or fixation disparity testing through loose prisms, may be adversely affected by polarization properties of some plastic prisms. In addition, neutralization of phorias can be influenced by prism position, reflections, and chromatic dispersion. The purpose of this chapter is to acquaint the reader with potential problems encountered when using prism to measure ocular deviations and to provide suggestions for increasing accuracy of prism measurements.

Objective Measurements

Primary Gaze with Distance Fixation

Cover testing commonly employs loose prisms or prism bars for neutralization of a strabismic or phoric deviation. Among the possible ways to hold prisms for this measurement are the three shown in Figure 2-1.[1] The Prentice position (Fig. 2-1, A), in which the ocular surface of the prism is perpendicular to the line of sight of the deviating eye, is the correct position for glass prisms. Clinically, however, it is common to use plastic prisms held in the frontal plane position (Fig. 2-1, B), with the ocular surface in the frontoparallel plane and perpendicular to the direction of the fixated target.[2] Individual plastic prisms actually are calibrated to be held in the minimum deviation position (Fig. 2-1, C), in which light is deviated equally at each surface of the prism. This position requires a slight angling of the prism base away from the patient's face, compared to the frontal plane position. Plastic prism bars, both horizontal and vertical, are calibrated for the minimum deviation position as well.* Use the frontal plane position (that is, the ocular surface of the prism perpendicular to the direction of the fixated target) to obtain accurate measurements with plastic prisms in primary and nonprimary posi-

---

*Richard Daley, Astron International, Mt Dora, Fla, 1992.

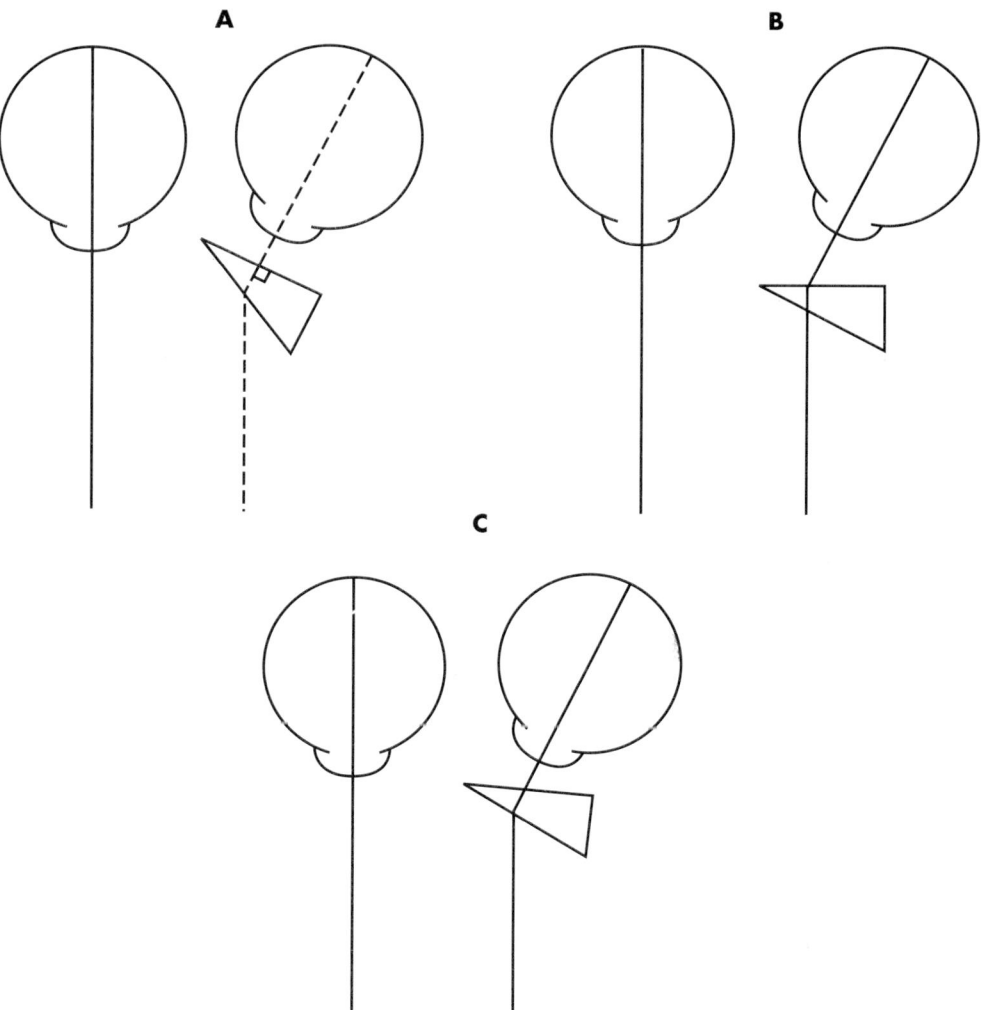

FIGURE 2-1 Prisms in the, **A,** Prentice position (recommended for use with glass prisms), **B,** frontal plane position (recommended for use with plastic prisms), and, **C,** minimum-deviation position. The last is the position for which plastic prisms are actually calibrated.

tions of gaze. Thompson and Guyton[1] have concluded that there is no clinically significant difference with loose plastic prisms between measurements in the frontal plane position and measurements in the minimum deviation position. They therefore recommend the frontal plane position for both loose plastic prisms and plastic prism bars, because it is a much easier position to achieve accurately. However, the Prentice position should be avoided when using plastic prisms (particularly with large prism powers); a 40 Δ plastic prism held in the Prentice position has an actual power of 72 Δ.

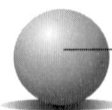

CLINICAL PEARL

Use the frontal plane position (that is, the ocular surface of the prism perpen-dicular to the direction of the fixated target) to obtain accurate measurments with plastic prisms in primary and nonprimary positions of gaze.

Nonprimary Gaze

To obtain accurate measurements with plastic prisms in nonprimary positions of gaze, the frontal plane position should be used (that is, with the ocular surface of the prism *perpendicular* to the direction of the fixated target).[2,3] For example, Figure 2-2, *A*, depicts the proper position of a base-out prism before the abducting right eye (*solid line*) for measuring an esodeviation in right gaze. Note that the ocular surface of the prism is perpendicular to the direction of the target (located to the patient's right). The common error made in this situation is keeping the prism's ocular surface in the frontal plane while the eyes move into right gaze, or rotating the prism in the same direction as the head if right gaze is achieved by having the patient turn his/her head to the left. Figure 2-2, *B*, shows the correct and incorrect prism positions for a similar measurement with prism before the adducting left eye. Likewise, measurements in upward and downward gazes require tilting of the front surface of the prism in the same direction as the fixation target. Alternatively, the prism should be kept in the original primary gaze position if the head is turned up or down to achieve vertical gaze positions. Errors of prism placement in nonprimary gaze positions may either mask or create a false impression of noncomitance. This, in turn, may result in under- or overreferrals for neurological testing, or incorrect choice of an ex-traocular muscle surgical technique. Discrepancies between labeled prism power and actual power become significant for prisms of 25 Δ or greater with a rotation error of only 10° away from the correct position. The resulting errors in measurement increase dramatically for larger powers and greater errors of rotation.[3]

Noncomitant Deviations

Noncomitant deviations vary in magnitude from one field of gaze to another, and with one eye fixating as opposed to the other, due to under- and overactions of the extraocular muscles. These deviations can have a paretic, myogenic, or structural cause. The primary angle of deviation is that measured with the unaffected eye fixating; by

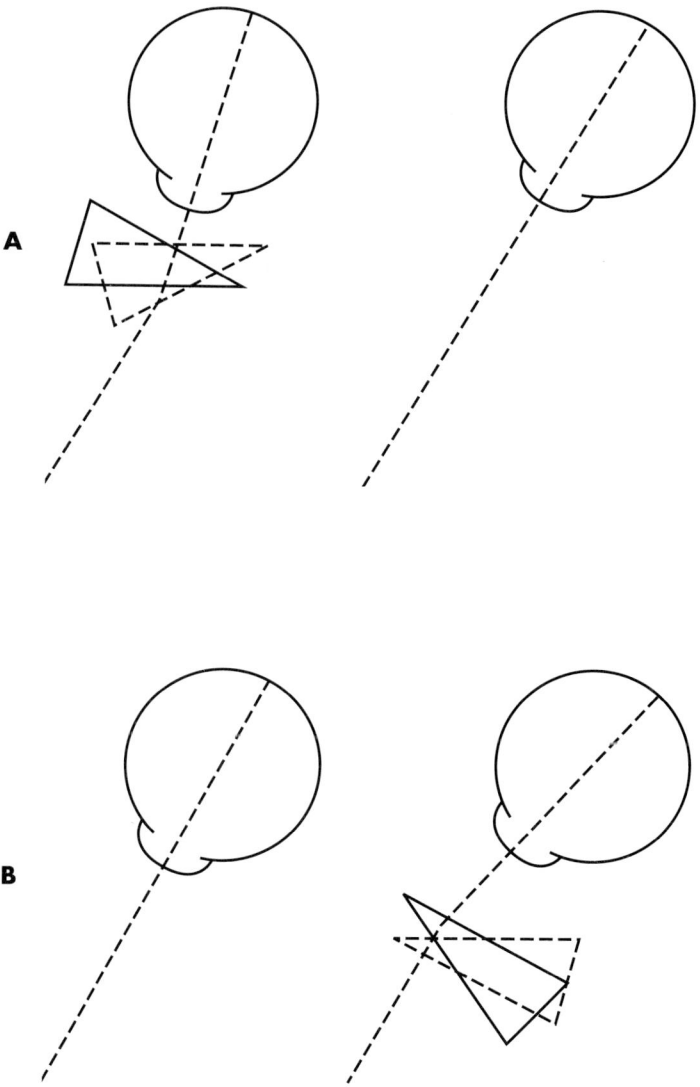

FIGURE 2-2 A, Neutralization of an esodeviation at distance in right gaze. The *solid-line* prism is positioned correctly over the abducted right eye, with its ocular surface perpendicular to the direction of the target held to the patient's right. The *dashed-line* prism is placed incorrectly in the patient's frontal plane. **B,** Same esodeviation being neutralized at distance in right gaze, with the *solid-line* prism now positioned correctly before the adducted eye. The *dashed-line* prism is placed incorrectly in the patient's frontal plane.

definition it is smaller than the secondary angle, which results when the affected eye is fixating. To measure the primary angle of deviation, it is necessary to place the prism before the affected eye, allowing the unaffected eye to fixate the target directly.[4] Because less innervation is required for the sound eye to fixate, the smaller angle will be measured in this situation. The sound eye is considered to be "fixating" throughout the alternate cover test regardless of which eye is occluded at a given moment because only the sound eye views the target from a physically straight position. Meanwhile, the fellow eye is aimed in another direction and the appropriate measuring prism compensates for this deviation. The examiner may watch only the eye behind the prism, although the correct measuring prism will neutralize the movement of both eyes whether the deviation is comitant or noncomitant. (Residual movement of one eye would result from a dissociated deviation, not from incomitance.)[4]

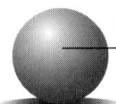

CLINICAL PEARL

To measure the primary angle of deviation, it is necessary to place the prism before the affected eye, allowing the unaffected eye to fixate the target directly. Conversely, when measuring the secondary angle of deviation, it is necessary to place the prism before the unaffected eye to allow the affected eye to assume a straight-ahead position of fixation.

In contrast, when the affected eye must fixate the target, more innervation to the underacting muscle is needed to move the eye into a fixating position. Because of Hering's law, excessive innervation thus flows to the yoke muscle of the unaffected eye. The result is an overaction of the sound eye and a larger angle of deviation. To measure this angle, the prism must be placed before the unaffected eye so the affected eye will assume a straight-ahead position of fixation. The eye behind the prism will thus be allowed to deviate to the position resulting from the excessive innervation it receives, and the proper prism will place the target's image on its fovea.[4]

Near Fixation

If a prism is not properly positioned, measurement errors can arise when deviations are neutralized by cover testing with near fixation. Because it is necessary to keep the ocular surface of the prism perpendicular to the direction of the fixation target (to avoid measurement error), the prism must be rotated slightly inward when the target is at near point; this will allow for convergence of the patient's lines of sight.[2]

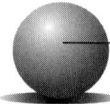

CLINICAL PEARL

Because it is necessary to keep the ocular surface of the prism perpendicular to the direction of the fixation target (so measurement error will be avoided), the prism must be rotated slightly inward when the target is at near point.

Another consideration when cover testing is performed at near point is prism effectivity. With a near target, a prism's effective power decreases as it is moved away from the eye (closer to the target).[2,5] This reduction may be calculated using the following formula:

$$E = P - (d/h \times P)$$

where *E* is the effective power (in Δ), *P* is the labeled prism power, *d* is the distance (in mm) from the center of rotation of the eye to the prism, and *h* is the distance (in mm) from the prism to the fixation target. It is common to hold the prism approximately 25 mm from the ocular center of rotation; for a target at a distance (h) of 40 cm, the quantity (*d/h*) becomes 6.25%. This is the percentage reduction in effective power for any prism held in this location.[5] As a result more prism power will be required to neutralize a given deviation, the farther the prism is held from the eye.[2] Thompson and Guyton[2] recommend that, to avoid significant measurement errors, prisms be held no more than 2 cm from the center of rotation (approximately 1 cm from the cornea). They also offer a formula[2] for calculating the required prism power when greater distances from the eye are used.

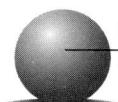

CLINICAL PEARL

To avoid significant measurement errors with near fixation, prisms should be held no more than 2 cm from the center of rotation (approximately 1 cm from the cornea).

Adding Prisms Together

When measuring the size of a deviation that falls between two available prism powers, the examiner may be inclined to hold two prisms together in an attempt to create the desired power. However, the total power of two prisms held surface to surface is always *greater* than the sum of the two labeled powers, whether the measurement is made with distance or near fixation.[1,2] The reason for this is that only one of the prisms can be positioned properly (in the frontal plane for plastic prisms) while the other's position is governed by the angle of the front surface of the first prism.[1] Table 2-1 gives the total power

TABLE 2-1

Deviation for the Addition of Two Plastic Prisms Stacked Together, with the Posterior in the Frontal Plane Position

Added Prism (Δ)	Initial Prism (Δ)											
	10	12	14	16	18	20	25	30	35	40	45	50
1	11	13	15	17	19	21	27	32	37	43	48	54
2	12	14	16	18	20	23	28	33	39	45	50	56
3	13	15	17	19	22	24	29	35	40	46	52	58
4	14	16	18	21	23	25	30	36	42	48	54	61
5	15	17	20	22	24	26	32	38	44	50	56	63
6	16	19	21	23	25	27	33	39	45	52	59	66
7	17	20	22	24	26	29	35	41	47	54	61	68
8	19	21	23	25	28	30	36	42	49	56	63	71
9	20	22	24	27	29	31	37	44	51	58	66	74
10	21	23	25	28	30	33	39	46	53	60	68	77
12	23	25	28	30	33	35	42	49	57	65	74	84
14	25	28	30	33	35	38	45	53	61	70	80	91
16	28	30	33	36	38	41	49	57	66	76	87	100
18	30	33	35	38	41	44	52	61	71	82	95	110
20	33	35	38	41	44	47	56	66	76	89	104	122
25	39	42	45	49	52	56	66	78	93	110	133	165
30	46	49	53	57	61	66	78	94	114	141	183	264
35	53	57	61	66	71	76	93	114	144	195	315	—
40	60	65	70	76	82	89	110	141	195	339	—	—
45	68	74	80	87	95	104	133	183	315	—	—	—
50	77	84	91	100	110	122	165	265	—	—	—	—

From Thompson JT, Guyton DL: *Ophthalmology* 90:204-210, 1983.

produced by adding two plastic prisms. Notice that very large errors would be made if the examiner were to assume that prisms, especially of high power, can be added arithmetically. The situation at near is complicated by the fact that combinations, just as in single prisms, lose effectivity with increasing distance from the eye.[2] Remember: It is vital to hold the prisms as close to the eye as possible if two must be combined. In contrast to the above discussion concerning horizontal prism combinations, combining a horizontal with a vertical prism causes no changes in the labeled powers.[1]

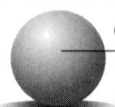

CLINICAL PEARL

The total power of two prisms held surface to surface is always greater than the sum of the two labeled powers, except when a horizontal prism is being combined with a vertical one.

Combining a measuring prism with a Fresnel prism attached to the patient's spectacles also produces a total power greater than the sum of the prisms' labeled powers. Although it is possible to determine the resultant power using a complex equation, it is recommended[2] that examiners not attempt to measure ocular deviations through Fresnel prisms.

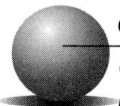

CLINICAL PEARL

Combining a measuring prism with a Fresnel prism attached to spectacles produces a total power greater than the sum of the prisms' labeled powers.

An alternative to stacking prisms together to measure a deviation larger than the available prism powers is to place one prism before each eye. Here again, however, two horizontal prism powers do not add predictably, as shown in Table 2-2. A disadvantage of this method is that with a prism before each eye, neither eye is truly fixating the target directly; a correct measurement of the angle of deviation can result only if the deviation is comitant.[1]

Measurements over Spectacle Lenses

Spectacle lenses of high power can induce a substantial prismatic effect when an eye's line of sight does not pass through the optical

TABLE 2-2

Deviation for the Addition of Two Prisms (Glass or Plastic) with One Held in Front of Each Eye

Left Eye Prism (Δ)	Right Eye Prism (Δ)											
	10	12	14	16	18	20	25	30	35	40	45	50
10	20	22	24	26	29	31	36	41	47	52	58	63
12	22	24	26	29	31	33	38	44	49	55	60	66
14	24	26	29	31	33	35	40	46	52	57	63	69
16	26	29	31	33	35	37	43	48	54	60	66	72
18	29	31	33	35	37	39	45	51	57	63	69	75
20	31	33	35	37	39	42	47	53	59	65	71	78
25	36	38	40	43	45	47	53	59	66	72	79	86
30	41	44	46	48	51	53	59	66	73	80	87	94
35	47	49	52	54	57	59	66	73	80	87	95	103
40	52	55	57	60	63	65	72	80	87	95	104	113
45	58	60	63	66	69	71	79	87	95	104	113	123
50	63	66	69	72	75	78	86	94	103	113	123	133

From Thompson JT, Guyton DL: *Ophthalmology* 90:204-210, 1983.

center of the lens. If the optical centers are correctly positioned for each eye in primary gaze, a strabismic patient's nonfixating eye will view through induced prism during measurement of the deviation. Because plus lenses create a base-in effect for an exotropic eye and a base-out effect for an esotropic eye, in either case the measured strabismic angle will be smaller than it would be without the spectacle-induced prism[6] (Fig. 2-3, A). It will therefore take less measuring prism to neutralize any strabismic deviation (including vertical deviations) when the patient is corrected with plus lenses in spectacle form. Conversely, minus spectacle lenses create base-out prism for an exotropic eye and base-in for an esotropic eye; thus deviations will be larger when measured through minus spectacles than they would be without the spectacle-induced prism (Fig. 2-3, B). The differing measurements become significant with lens powers greater than 5 D,[6] as shown in Tables 2-3 and 2-4. If the patient's spectacles contain a cylindrical correction, the power in the horizontal meridian influences horizontal strabismic angles (eso and exo); likewise, the vertical meridian's power must be considered when one desires to determine the spectacles' effect on vertical strabismus.

CLINICAL PEARL

It will take less measuring prism to neutralize any strabismic deviation when the patient is corrected with plus lenses (>5.0 D) in spectacle form; conversely, deviations will be larger when measured through minus lenses (>5.0 D) than they would be if the patient were wearing contact lenses.

There are several ways to deal with the problem of spectacle-induced prism interference in the measurement of ocular deviations. Tables 2-3 and 2-4 can be used to obtain the true angle of deviation based on lens power and measured angle. Alternatively, if the patient is wearing contact lenses for the measurements, the induced prismatic effect can be eliminated.[7] In addition, an ingenious method described by Archer[8] involves placing the patient's prescription lenses in a trial frame, with the fixating eye's lens centered over its pupil, and marking the optical center of the deviating eye's lens with a felt-tipped pen. Then, with the patient continuing to fixate with the dominant eye, a penlight is directed at the deviating eye through its trial lens. The examiner sights monocularly over the light and moves laterally (or vertically if there is a vertical deviation) until the corneal reflex appears in the same position as it would for an angle kappa measurement. The examiner adjusts this eye's lens so the mark on the lens is aligned with the corneal reflex. Measuring prism may then be placed before this eye for cover testing and the eye, despite being deviated, will view through the optical center of its lens.

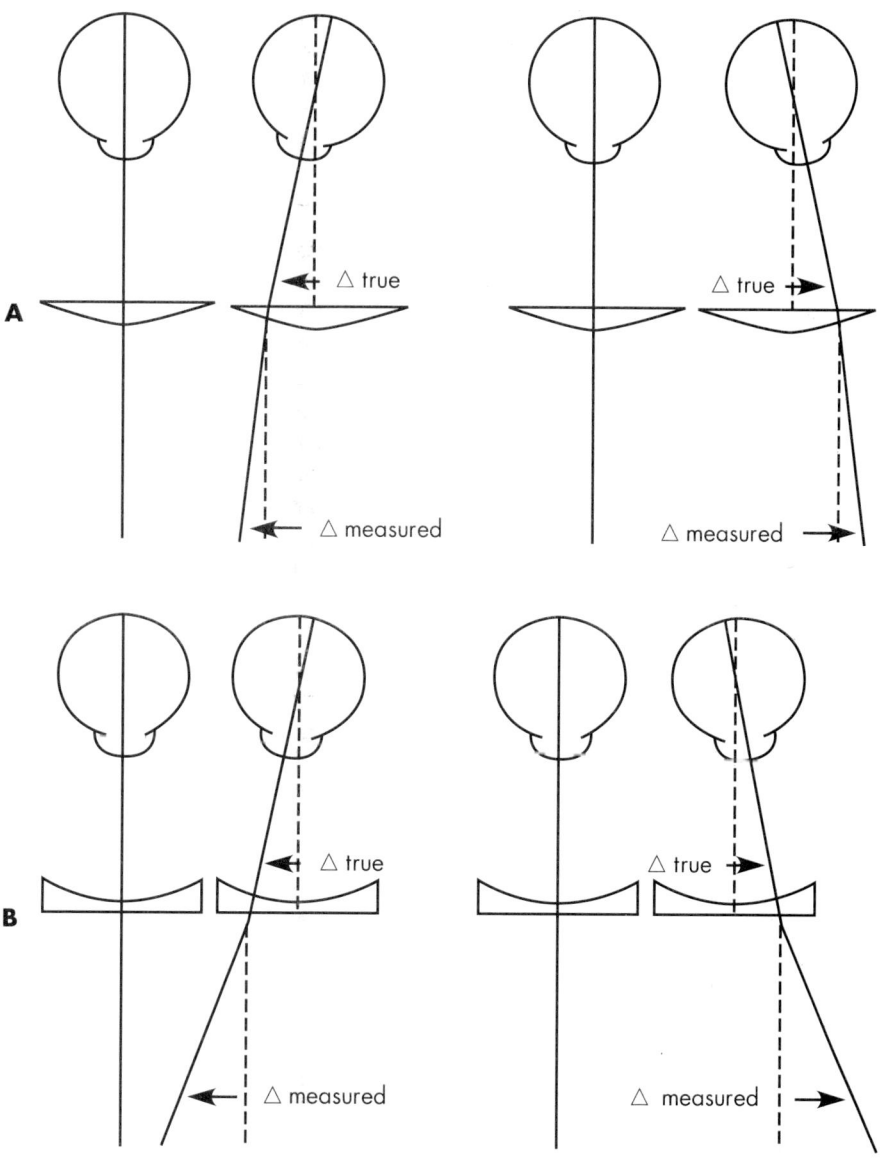

FIGURE 2-3 A, Deviations, whether eso or exo, measured through plus lenses will appear smaller than they actually are because the esodeviation is being measured through a base-out effect and the exodeviation is measured through a base-in effect. In both cases the spectacle-induced prism partially neutralizes the deviation. **B,** The opposite situation exists for deviations neutralized through minus lenses. The spectacle-induced prism makes the measured deviation larger than the actual deviation because the measuring prism must offset the power of the induced prism.

TABLE 2-3
Conversion of Measured Deviation to True Deviation (in Δ) for Hyperopes Wearing Spectacles

Measured Deviation (Δ)	Hyperopic Spectacle Power (D)													
	+1	+2	+3	+4	+5	+6	+7	+8	+9	+10	+12	+15	+20	+30
5	5	5	5	6	6	6	6	6	6	7	7	8	10	20
10	10	11	11	11	11	12	12	13	13	13	14	16	20	40
15	15	16	16	16	17	18	18	19	19	20	21	24	30	60
20	21	21	22	22	23	24	24	25	26	27	29	32	40	80
25	26	26	27	28	29	29	30	31	32	33	36	40	50	100
30	31	32	32	33	34	35	36	38	39	40	43	48	60	120
35	36	37	38	39	40	41	42	44	45	47	50	56	70	140
40	41	42	43	44	46	47	48	50	52	53	57	64	80	160
45	46	47	49	50	51	53	55	56	58	60	64	72	90	180
50	51	53	54	56	57	59	61	63	65	67	71	80	100	200
60	62	63	65	67	69	71	73	75	77	80	87	96	120	240
70	72	74	76	78	80	82	85	88	90	93	100	112	140	280

Find the spectacle power across the top, and the deviation measured along the side; the resultant number is the *true* deviation, whether eso, exo, or hyper.
Modified from Hansen VC: *Am Orthopt J* 39:3-11, 1989.

TABLE 2-4
Conversion of Measured Deviation to True Deviation (in Δ) for Myopes Wearing Spectacles

Measured Deviation (Δ)	Myopic Spectacle Power (D)													
	−1	−2	−3	−4	−5	−6	−7	−8	−9	−10	−12	−15	−20	−30
5	5	5	5	5	4	4	4	4	4	4	4	4	3	3
10	10	10	9	9	9	9	9	8	8	8	8	7	7	6
15	15	14	14	14	13	13	13	12	12	12	12	11	10	9
20	20	19	19	18	18	17	17	17	16	16	15	15	13	11
25	24	24	23	23	22	22	21	21	20	20	19	18	17	14
30	29	29	28	27	27	26	26	25	24	24	23	22	20	17
35	34	33	33	32	31	30	30	30	29	28	27	25	23	20
40	39	38	37	36	36	35	34	33	33	32	31	29	26	23
45	44	43	42	41	40	39	38	37	37	36	35	33	30	26
50	49	48	47	45	44	43	43	42	41	40	38	36	33	29
60	59	57	56	55	53	52	51	50	49	48	46	44	40	34
70	68	67	65	64	62	61	60	58	57	56	54	51	46	40

Find the spectacle power across the top, and the deviation measured along the side; the resultant number is the *true* deviation, whether eso, exo, or hyper.
Modified from Hansen VC: *Am Orthopt J* 39:3-11, 1989.

Measurements with the Head Tilted

If cover testing with prism neutralization is performed with the head tilted as in the Parks Three-Step Test,[9] the examiner might believe the prism should remain in the same position as for testing with the head straight (that is, with its base perpendicular to the floor). If the prism is held in this manner, however, it will no longer move the retinal image in a purely horizontal (or vertical) direction with respect to the retina but will create an oblique movement of the image.[10] The reason for this is that, as the head is tilted, the eyes undergo a slight torsional movement that does not nearly compensate for the head tilt. Thus, the eyes may be considered essentially to tilt with the head and prisms used to measure a deviation must be placed at approximately the same angle as the tilt. The result is a required prism orientation in which the base (if one desires base in or base out) is perpendicular to the orbital floor of the patient rather than the floor of the room. A vertical prism would have its base parallel to the orbital floor.

Subjective Measurements

In general, subjective measurements can be adversely affected by reflections from overhead lights, which may distract the patient. The chromatic dispersion fringes resulting from some prisms may also bother the patient, although these usually can be ignored. One should personally check, in the examining room, the quality of views through the instruments to determine whether lighting conditions might interfere with the measurements and then make any adjustments possible.

Phorias and Subjective Angles of Strabismus

Subjective measurements of a deviation may be made using a Maddox rod or red lens in combination with loose plastic prisms or a rotating plastic prism attached to the Maddox rod (such as the Monocular Maddox Phoria Measure*). Once again, it is important to keep the prisms in the frontal plane position, whether measurements are made in a primary or nonprimary position of gaze. In addition, for measurements with near fixation, it is vital to keep the prism as close to the eye as possible (because of effectivity concerns) and to angle the prism inward to compensate for ocular convergence. Furthermore, remember that high minus spectacle power will increase the apparent angle, and high plus power will decrease it, for moderate to large subjective angles. Tables 2-3 and 2-4 can be applied to both subjective and objective measurements.

---

*Astron International, 1123 Robie Ave, Mt Dora, FL, 32757.

Prism Bar Vergence Ranges

For best clinical accuracy, plastic prism bars should be held in the patient's frontal plane,[2] as previously discussed. For measurements at near point, the bar should be angled inward so its ocular surface is perpendicular to the target direction. Also, near point vergence ranges require that the prism bar be held as close to the eye as possible; otherwise, the reduced effectivity with increased distance will cause overestimation of the vergence range. In other words, the patient will be able to fuse through a larger prism value merely because the prisms have less effective power than the labels suggest.

Techniques Requiring Polarized Filters

Testing of stereopsis through prism that neutralizes a significant ocular deviation often necessitates use of polarized filters; these must be used for fixation disparity curves and associated phoria measurements as well. Although glass prisms (including the phoropter Risley prism) do not create any interference with polarization, Frantz et al.[11] have reported that many plastic prisms do. They found that the effects of the prism-manufacturing process on the polymer material cause some plastic prisms to exhibit polarizing properties of their own that can reduce or eliminate the unique views of the target intended for each eye. Consequently, a patient without stereopsis may respond correctly to random dot forms or lateral disparity circles because the neutralizing prism is allowing one eye to receive information from both eyes' targets. Conversely, a patient capable of stereopsis may respond incorrectly because the eye behind the prism is seeing only the target intended for the other eye. Fixation disparity testing will also be contaminated if each eye no longer sees its nonius line uniquely.[11] In addition, if vision therapy devices such as vectograms are used with plastic prisms, polarization may be adversely affected. Table 2-5 summarizes the possible effects of certain manufacturers' plastic prisms.

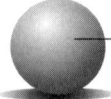

CLINICAL PEARLS

Some plastic prisms exhibit polarizing properties of their own that can reduce or eliminate the unique views of the target intended for each eye. As a result, polarized test results may be adversely affected.

To eliminate this polarization effect, the prism may be placed between the eye and the polarizing filter, although with high-power prisms this is impractical. Therefore it is recommended that prisms be used for polarized testing only if they are known not to interfere. The examiner should check each prism in the set (as well as all prism bars), because the phenomenon is more pronounced with high prism powers. While wearing the polarizing filters and monocularly observing a

TABLE 2-5
Clinical Implications of Combining Plastic Prisms with Polarized Tests*

Strabismic/ suppressing patients may:	Luneau < 25 Δ	Luneau ≥ 25 Δ	Gulden < 25 Δ	Gulden ≥ 25 Δ	Astron < 25 Δ	Astron ≥ 25 Δ
Respond positively to random dot stereopsis	X	X	X	X	X	X
See both eyes' suppression checks	X	X		X		?
Appear to suppress fellow eye instead	X	X				?
Patients with normal binocular vision may:						
Have significantly reduced stereopsis		X		X		
Have slightly reduced stereopsis						X
Respond negatively to random dot stereopsis		X		X		
Appear to suppress	X	X		X		

? means that these effects did not occur for subjects with the 25 Δ Astron prism; however, they might occur with higher powers, which exhibit the polarization phenomenon to a greater degree.
*From Frantz KA, Cotter SA, Brown WL, Motameni M: *J Pediatr Ophthalmol Strabismus* 27:259-264, 1990.

target polarized for the open eye, interpose one prism at a time and view the target through all areas of the prism. If that eye's target remains unchanged, the prism does not exhibit the phenomenon.[11] Fortunately, fixation disparity testing does not frequently require the use of high-powered prisms (most notorious for polarization interference). In addition, if it is necessary to test stereopsis through a large amount of prism, a test that does not need polarizing filters (such as the Lang* or TNO†) may be used.

---

*Clement Clark Inc, 3128 East 17th Ave, Suite D, Columbus, Ohio 43219.
†Alfred P Poll Inc, 900 5th Ave, New York, NY 10021.

Conclusion

It is evident that the examiner must be careful to hold measuring prisms properly for the target position being used, account for significant lens power when deviations are measured through spectacles, not add prism powers together without referring to an appropriate table or formula, and be wary of the polarization effects of certain prisms when performing polarized tests. Improper use of prisms can yield erroneous information; correct use will provide accurate measurements of deviations and fusional abilities necessary for managing ocular deviations with prismatic prescriptions, vision therapy, and strabismus surgery.

References

1. Thompson JT, Guyton DL: Ophthalmic prisms: measurement errors and how to minimize them, *Ophthalmology* 90:204-210, 1983.
2. Thompson JT, Guyton DL: Ophthalmic prisms: deviant behavior at near, *Ophthalmology* 92:684-690, 1985.
3. Repka MX, Arnoldi KA: Lateral incomitance in exotropia: fact or artifact? *J Pediatr Ophthalmol Strabismus* 28:125-128, 1991.
4. Repka MX, Kelman S, Guyton DL: Prism measurement of incomitant strabismus, *Binocular Vis* 1:45-49, 1985.
5. Pascal JI: Effectivity of prisms at near, *Am J Optom Arch Am Acad Optom* 30:84-85, 1953.
6. Scattergood KD, Brown MH, Guyton DL: Artifacts introduced by spectacle lenses in the measurement of strabismic deviations, *Am J Ophthalmol* 96:439-448, 1983.
7. Hansen VC: Common pitfalls in measuring strabismic patients. *Am Orthopt J* 39:3-11, 1989.
8. Archer SM: Direct measurement of strabismic deviation in highly ametropic patients, *Am J Ophthalmol* 98:114, 1984.
9. Griffin JR: *Binocular anomalies: procedures for vision therapy,* ed 2, Chicago, 1982, Professional Press, 11-14.
10. Helveston EM: Prism placement: measurements of horizontal and vertical deviations with the head tilted, *Arch Ophthalmol* 93:483-486, 1975.
11. Frantz KA, Cotter SA, Brown WL, Motameni M: Erroneous findings in polarized testing caused by plastic prisms, *J Pediatr Ophthalmol Strabismus* 27:259-264, 1990.

Self-Assessment Questions

1. The clinically recommended position for holding plastic prisms when measuring the angle of deviation is the
   a. Prentice
   b. frontal plane
   c. minimum deviation
   d. none of these

2. Compared to measurements of strabismus with distance fixation, when a plastic prism is used for near point measurements the best position for it is
   a. rotated slightly inward and held as close as possible to the eye
   b. rotated slightly outward and held as close as possible to the eye
   c. not rotated at all and held as close as possible to the eye
   d. rotated slightly inward and held at least 2 cm from the eye
   e. rotated slightly outward and held at least 2 cm from the eye

3. The prisms most likely to interfere with polarized testing situations are
   a. trial case
   b. glass Risley in the phoropter
   c. low-power plastic
   d. high-power plastic

4. If esotropia is measured through the patient's high minus spectacles, the observed angle will be _____ than the true angle because the patient is receiving a _____ effect from the spectacles.
   a. smaller, base-out
   b. smaller, base-in
   c. larger, base-out
   d. larger, base-in

Answers: 1. b.   2. a.   3. d.   4. d.

3

Practical Considerations in Prism Implementation

Susan A. Cotter
Kelly A. Frantz

Key Terms

decentration	Prentice's rule	ground-in prism
Fresnel	contact lens	clip-on prism
slab-off	sector prism	

Bérard,[1] a proponent of prism use, believed that "the main obstacle in using prisms is their implementation." Determining whether the patient will benefit from prism and exactly how much prism to prescribe is only half the clinical challenge. It must then be decided how the prism should be incorporated into the optical prescription.

The incorporation of prism into an optical prescription can be accomplished in various ways. Horizontal prismatic corrections

We wish to thank Sue Mirman, O.D., for her critical review of the manuscript and assistance with references and Walman Optical for making a duplicate of our patient's prescriptions for Figures 3-5 and 3-8. In addition, we thank Lou Lipschultz, O.D., and Ken Malsch, A.B.O.C. (Family Eyecare Associates, Olympia Fields, Ill), for helping us gather the information for Table 3-2, for supplying frames and lenses for the rest of the photographs, and for lens fabrication (K. Malsch).

(base-in [BI] and base-out [BO]) are limited to spectacle application (versus contact lenses); but they can be supplied as clip-ons, as deliberate decentrations of prescription lenses, as ground-ins, and as Fresnel membranes. When a vertical prismatic correction (base-up [BU] or base-down [BD]) is required, the clinician has the additional options of slab-off prism and in small magnitudes prismatic contact lenses. We will review some of the optical considerations (and limitations) in choosing among these methods of implementing prism. Practical concerns such as availability of base direction, distortion, cosmesis, weight, magnitude limitations, and cost of materials will also be addressed.

Horizontal and Vertical Prism Options

Clip-on Prisms

Although once a common method of compensating for muscle imbalances, clip-on prisms are no longer a popular mode of implementing prism treatment. If used at all, they are generally employed for diagnostic purposes (such as in the clinical trial of a tentative prism prescription). They have lost much of their popularity with the introduction of Fresnel membrane prisms. Standard clip-ons fail to fit well over many frame styles; in addition, they are bulky, heavy, and cosmetically displeasing, and they result in disturbing reflections from the added lens surfaces (Fig. 3-1, A).

The recent popularity of spectacle styles with matching clip-on sunglasses, however, has given the practitioner an additional option. Figure 3-1, B, shows a woman wearing a spectacle frame in which the clip-on sunglass portion has been modified. The sunglass lenses are removed from the clip-on portion and replaced by 5 Δ BO ground-in prism on each spectacle lens. This is ideal for a patient who needs prism for one viewing distance only (such as for driving or for reading) or who needs different amounts of prism for different viewing distances.

CLINICAL PEARL

The lenses from the sunglass portion of a pair of spectacles with matching clip-on sunglasses can be replaced with ground-in prisms for patients who need prism for one viewing distance only or different amounts for different viewing distances.

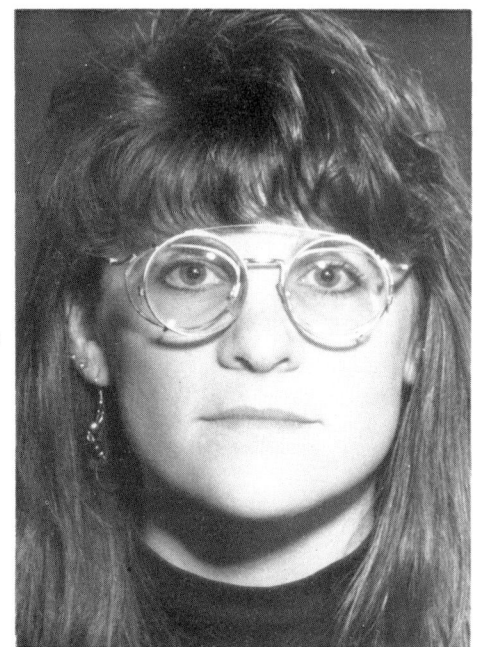

A

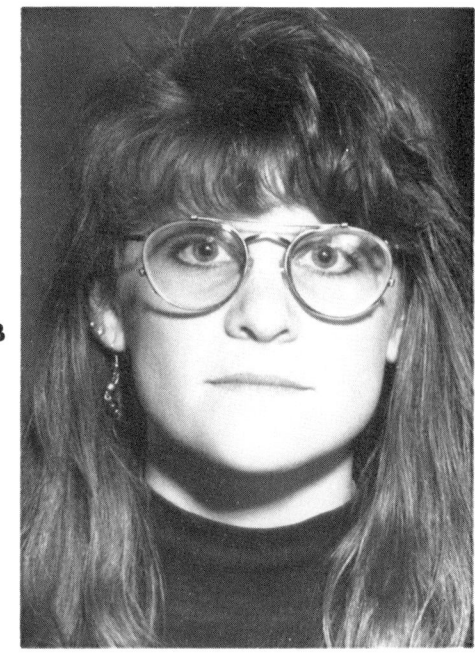

B

FIGURE 3-1 **A,** Standard clip-on prisms of 5 Δ BO over each eye. **B,** Sunglass lenses removed and replaced with 5 Δ BO prisms over each eye in the clip-on portion of a frame that is sold as a set with clip-on sunglasses. (Frame and lenses courtesy Family Eyecare Associates, Olympia Fields, Ill.) Note that the company e clips (Berkeley, Calif) can provide custom clip-ons for any frame.

Decentration of Prescription Lenses

A prismatic effect can be obtained by the decentration of prescription lenses. Displacing the optical centers of the lenses in or out will induce base-in or base-out prism. Likewise, displacing the optical centers of the lenses up or down will induce base-up or base-down prism. The prismatic effect resulting from decentration can be calculated approximately by Prentice's rule (see Chapter 1):

$$P = dF$$

where P is the prismatic power in prism diopters, d is the linear displacement distance in centimeters from the optical center of the spectacle lens to the line of sight, and F is the refracting power of the lens. For example, if a −3.00 diopter (D) spherical lens is decentered 5 mm downward, the decentration induces a prismatic effect of (0.5 × 3.00) or 1.50 prism diopters (Δ). Because the patient is viewing above the optical center of the lens and the lens is minus in power, base-up prism would be induced. Decentration of prescription lenses is most productive when the lenses are of moderate to high power and only a small amount of prismatic effect is needed.

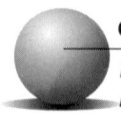

CLINICAL PEARL

Decentration of prescription lenses is most productive when the lenses are of moderate to high power and only a small amount of prismatic effect is needed.

The main advantage of using decentration to produce a prismatic effect is financial; there is no additional laboratory cost for the prism unless a larger blank size is required. Limiting factors include the facts that (1) plano lens blanks cannot be decentered to create prism, (2) available lens blank sizes often are not large enough to create the desired prismatic effect when the prescription lenses are low in power or when large magnitudes of prism are needed, and (3) it is difficult to decenter conventional bifocal lens blanks because of the necessary placement of the bifocal segment.

Ground-in Prism

As an alternative to prism obtained through decentration, prism power may be ground on the spectacle lens by surfacing procedures. (Although the prism power is actually ground onto the surface of the spectacle lens, it is usually referred to as ground-in prism). Unlike prism obtained by decentration, ground-in prism can be incorporated into spectacle lenses that contain little or no lens power. In fact, higher magnitudes of ground-in prism can be incorporated into lower-power lenses because the large thicknesses already present in high-power lenses, especially high minus, can be limiting for ground-in prism. (Using the formula for prismatic power and thickness,[2] you can expect the thickness difference from one edge to the other in a 70 mm Columbia Resin 39 [CR-39] lens blank to change approximately 1.51 mm per prism diopter of power ground into the lens, not counting the thickness due to dioptric power.) The upper limit of prism that can be ground into plastic ophthalmic lenses is approximately 12 Δ per lens for a plano lens and 10 Δ for a −5.00 D lens (assuming the frame does not have a large eye size) before edge thickness becomes too great.

Plastic lenses and a small-size frame are recommended to minimize the weight of the spectacles when a significant amount of ground-in prism is prescribed. Rimless frames should be avoided in these situations because of visibility of the edges. High-index plastic lens material will reduce the thickness of the lens. Generally, ground-in prism is cosmetically superior to Fresnel, except in cases in which there is considerable edge thickness. Special treatments applied to the edges of prismatic spectacle lenses (for example, translucent edge coatings, rolling, and polishing) are effective in maximizing cosmesis when substantial amounts of prism are prescribed. An antireflective coating helps to minimize reflections. Ground-in prism is most appropriate for permanent or long-term use.

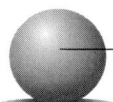

CLINICAL PEARL

Plastic lenses and a small-size frame are recommended to minimize the weight of spectacles when a significant amount of ground-in prism is prescribed.

The practitioner must decide whether to put the prism before one eye or both. There is some disagreement concerning this issue. Sheard[3] recommends that the major portion, if not the total amount, of prism be placed before the nondominant eye whereas Morgan[4] and Fry (cited by Borish)[5] have recommended dividing the prism power between the two eyes, especially if the total power is greater than 3 Δ. Morgan[4] believes that if certain functions of prism (such as the distortions, weight, thickness, and internal reflections) were divided between the eyes the prism prescription would be more acceptable to the patient.

Support for splitting prism equally can be inferred from the work of Adams et al.,[6] who have demonstrated that unequal overall magnification results from a ground-in prismatic correction that has a greater-power prism in one eye than in the other. For example, an induced image size difference of approximately 5% would result from a 15 Δ prism ground into the spectacle lens of one eye only, for a patient wearing spectacle lenses with a 9 D base curve.[6]

In clinical practice, prismatic power is usually split equally between the two eyes unless the amount is less than 2 Δ, and then it is placed before the nondominant eye. If vertical prism is to be ground into one spectacle lens only, a base-up orientation (versus base-down before the other eye) is preferable because distortion is greater toward the base[7] (and patients generally use downward gaze more than upward gaze); also fewer reflections from overhead lights result. Unilateral or asymmetric prism, however, is indicated and often employed in cases of noncomitant deviations because prism is more effective when placed over the affected eye when there is an underacting muscle (see Chapter 8).

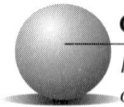

CLINICAL PEARL
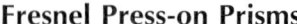

If vertical prism is to be ground into one spectacle lens only, a base-up orientation (versus base-down before the other eye) is preferable because distortion is greater toward the base (and patients generally use downward gaze more than upward); also fewer reflections from overhead lights result.

Fresnel Press-on Prisms

Fresnel Press-on (Fresnel membrane) prisms are a thin flexible plastic material that can be pressed onto conventional ophthalmic lenses. Made of clear optical-grade polyvinyl chloride, they are extremely thin (approximately 1 mm) and have the advantage of conforming and adhering to a smooth surface without adhesive. This permits them to be applied directly to the back surface of a spectacle lens. They are manufactured in circular sheets, and their rather large diameter (67 mm) allows them to be cut to fit almost any frame shape. The membrane is placed with the smooth side against the ocular surface of a spectacle lens, where it adheres securely through surface tension. Fresnel membrane prisms offer a desirable alternative to conventional prisms because their application is quick, their cost is modest, their thickness and weight are negligible, and a wide range of powers is available.

Based on an adaptation of the Fresnel lens principle,[8] plasticized polyvinyl chloride is molded into uniformly thin sheets to produce Fresnel membrane prisms.[9] The Fresnel principle, shown in Figure 3-2, is based on the fact that the refracting power of a prism is determined primarily by the angle between the two refracting surfaces (that is, the apex angle). It is a widely known fact that by reducing the overall size of a lens, one can also reduce the base thickness of a conventional prism. For example, Figure 3-2 shows that reducing the size of the lens (and therefore the base-apex dimension of the prism) from 24 to 12 mm reduces the prism base thickness from 6 mm to 3 mm. A reduction of the base-apex dimension to 4 mm reduces the base thickness to 1 mm, and a further reduction to 2 mm decreases the base thickness to 0.5 mm. As shown in Figure 3-2, the deviating power of the prism remains the same regardless of the base-apex dimension or overall size of the lens. A Fresnel membrane prism, therefore, can be considered a series of identical plastic prisms with their base-apex lines parallel, lying side by side on a thin platform of plastic. This layer of small prisms has the same deviating power as a conventional prism of the same material but is only about 1 mm thick.

Fresnel prisms are ideal for in-office use. Applying them is quite easy. The spectacle lens to which the Fresnel prism is to be affixed is

Fresnel Membrane Prism

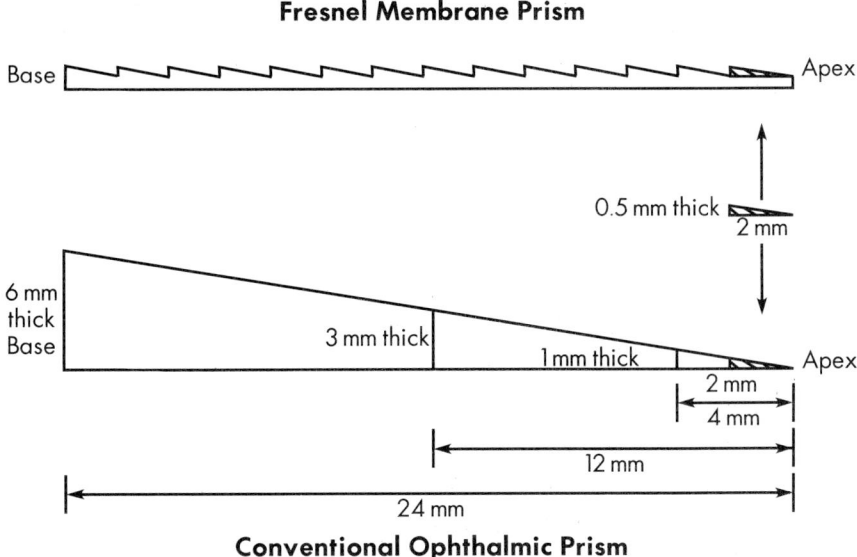

Conventional Ophthalmic Prism

FIGURE 3-2 Much thinner than a conventional prism of the same magnitude, the Fresnel membrane prism is a series of identical prisms (note shaded prism on the right), with their base-apex lines parallel, lying side by side on a thin platform of plastic. Because the deviating power of a prism is determined primarily by the apex angle, it remains the same regardless of the base-apex dimension.

removed from the frame. The smooth surface of the Fresnel prism is placed against the ocular surface of the lens with its base oriented in the desired direction. The prism and lens combination is placed on a flat surface and the shape of the lens is traced on the membrane with a pen. The membrane is then cut by hand with a sharp scissors just inside the tracing mark (Fig. 3-3). The goal is for the membrane to be approximately 1 mm smaller than the ocular surface of the spectacle lens. Once the membrane has been cut, the spectacle lens alone is reinserted into the frame and cleaned. The membrane and spectacle lens are then immersed in a bowl of warm water and with the membrane correctly positioned its smooth surface is slid against the ocular surface of the spectacle lens. The center of the membrane is pressed firmly against the lens, with gradual outward-moving pressure, and any excess water and bubbles are squeezed out with the fingers. At this point, the combination is removed from the water, any residual bubbles are eliminated again by pressing them toward the membrane edge, and fine adjustments of membrane orientation are made. The very thin residual layer of water entrapped between the lens and the membrane evaporates in a few hours (although the spectacles may be worn immediately), and the result is a firm

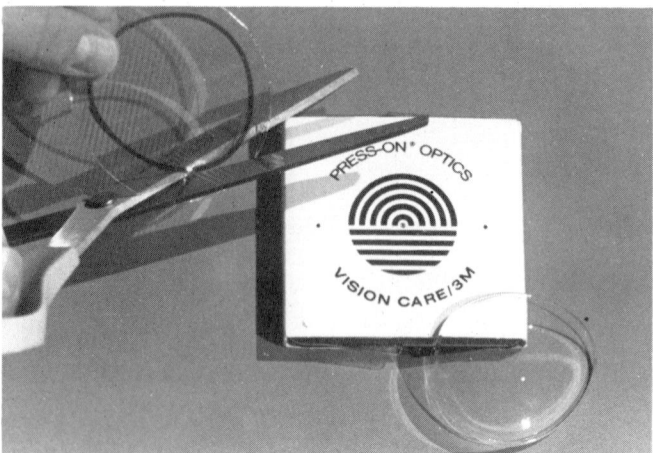

FIGURE 3-3 A Fresnel membrane prism of 20 Δ cut to correspond to the spectacle lens shape.

adherence of the membrane to the spectacle lens. No part of the membrane must overlap the spectacle lens bevel, or the seal will be broken. The lens and membrane are then patted dry with a clean cotton towel.

Provided all air between the spectacle lens and membrane is removed, the membrane will remain firmly adherent to the carrier lens through surface tension for an indefinite period. It can be removed easily, however, because it is not glued to the lens. To remove it requires simply peeling back from the edge. The optics of the spectacle lens are not affected; successive membranes can be applied to the same carrier lens if desired. Used membranes are discarded or recut as necessary and reused without damaging the optical properties of the prism.

The advantages of Fresnel prisms are listed in Table 3-1. The approximately 1 mm thickness (even for prisms of high power) provides for a noticeably thinner edge when moderate to high powers of Fresnel prism are used compared with conventional prisms of the same magnitude (Fig. 3-4). The resulting decrease in weight is substantial and is a major advantage, particularly for infants and older patients with tender noses. The prisms are available in a large range of powers (up to 30 Δ), and consequently the clinician is rarely limited by the magnitude of prism needed since a total of 60 Δ (30 Δ on each spectacle lens) can be applied. This is especially advantageous when a prismatic correction is desired for a patient with a large angle of strabismus. In fact, once an optical prescription requires a total prism amount greater than 20 to 25 Δ, a Fresnel membrane is the only option other than a heavy and unsightly clip-on prism.

Cost is another advantage of Fresnel prisms. They are themselves fairly inexpensive, making them perfect for clinical situations in

TABLE 3-1
Fresnel Membrane Prisms

Advantages	Disadvantages
Available in high powers (to 30 Δ)	Decreases visual acuity
Thin	Decreases contrast sensitivity
Light weight	Visibility of ridges
Large diameter	Reflections and scattered light from prism facets
Easy application	Discolors with time
Localized or sector use on spectacles	Colored fringes
In-office application and modification	Secondary image seen toward base
Fairly inexpensive	

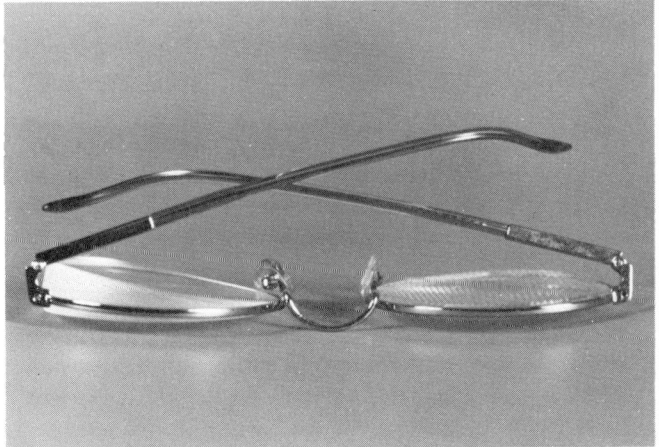

FIGURE 3-4 A base-out prism of 12 Δ in Fresnel membrane form (left lens) and ground-in form (right lens). (Frame and lenses courtesy Family Eyecare Associates, Olympia Fields, Ill.)

which prism is to be worn only temporarily, changes in prism magnitude are anticipated (as in a resolving muscle paresis), or a prism adaptation trial is being performed. For a clinical trial the Fresnel can be easily dispensed in the office and worn for a few hours or days to see if adaptation occurs. Furthermore, Fresnel prisms are ideal when there is initially some uncertainty as to the exact prismatic strength required; they are an inexpensive way to assess the acceptability of proposed prismatic correction, giving the practitioner an opportunity to refine the permanent therapeutic prescription. Once it is certain that the proposed amount of prism is acceptable, new prismatic ophthalmic lenses can be ordered from the laboratory.

Fresnel prisms are perfect for situations in which correction is needed for only one viewing distance or one field of gaze or when different magnitudes of power are needed for different viewing distances or fields of gaze. The membrane is simply cut to the appropriate size and affixed to the desired region of the spectacle lens. This type of prism correction is often referred to as sector Fresnel prism.

Sector Fresnel prisms are often used in the management of strabismic patients. There are many instances when a patient has normal sensorimotor fusion at one distance but not at the others (as when he/she fuses with near viewing but not with far) or when different amounts of prism are required to obtain normal sensory fusion at both distance and near. In these cases Fresnel prisms are easily cut and applied to just one part of the spectacle lens; thus they can be used for one viewing distance only (Fig. 3-5), or two sector Fresnel prisms of different powers can be affixed to the spectacle lenses in the configuration of an executive-style bifocal. Likewise, patients with A or V pattern deviations may require a different amount of prismatic correction for the top half of their spectacle lenses (used for upgaze and primary gaze) as opposed to the bottom half (used for viewing in downgaze, provided they drop their eyes rather than their heads). Patients with noncomitant deviations resulting from a muscle paresis sometimes require prism only in the field of action of the affected muscle. For example, a patient with paresis of the left lateral rectus might require prism correction in left gaze only. The membrane, therefore, would be cut so that it could be applied to the left side of the patient's spectacle lens. Sector Fresnel prism can be used in a similar manner for patients with hemianopic field defects (see Chapter 11). Additionally, a Fresnel membrane prism can correct both a vertical and a horizontal deviation simultaneously when it is applied in an oblique orientation (see Chapters 1 and 8).

Cosmetically the prisms are acceptable, especially when compared with the higher-power ground-in prisms. The conspicuous base that conventional clip-on or ground-in prisms have is absent (Fig. 3-4). The ridges of the Fresnel prism, however, appear as multiple lines across the surface of the lens that are apparent to an observer at close range and may be noticed by the patient (Fig. 3-6). Although they sometimes cause concern, a light tint can be put into the spectacle lenses to mask them.

In addition to the noticeable prism lines, the main disadvantages of Fresnel prisms are a decrease in visual acuity[10,11] and a reduction in contrast sensitivity.[11,12] These negative effects are directly related to the magnitude of prism power.[10-12] Scott[13] noted that prism powers less than or equal to 10 Δ are usually well tolerated and do not result in an acuity reduction greater than one line. Woo et al.,[12] however, have reported that a one line reduction can be expected from a 5 Δ Fresnel prism, three lines from a 15 Δ, four lines from a 20 Δ, and five lines from a 30 Δ. Clinically, this does not always seem to be the case.

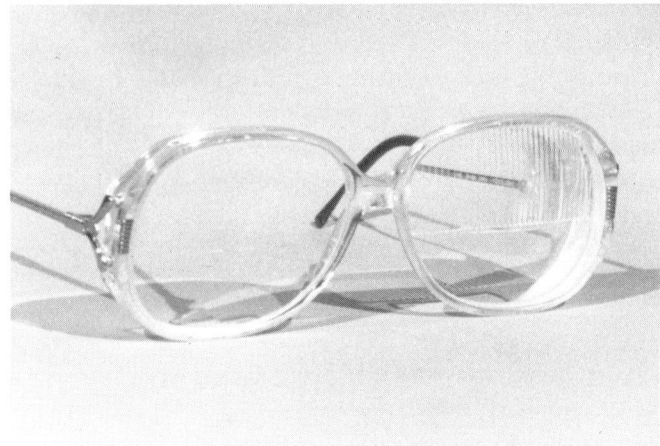

FIGURE 3-5 A sector Fresnel prism. The prescription is OD −4.00 −0.50 × 160, OS −3.00 sph with a +3.00 add OU and 7 Δ BO ground in each eye; a 10 Δ Fresnel membrane prism is placed on the top half of the left lens. (Lenses courtesy Walman Optical, Minneapolis.)

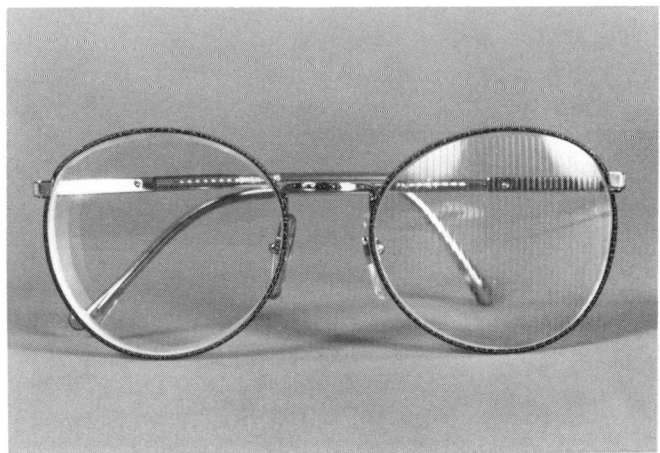

FIGURE 3-6 A base-out prism of 12 Δ in Fresnel membrane form on the left lens and ground-in form on the right. (Frame and lenses courtesy Family Eyecare Associates, Olympia Fields, Ill.)

Contrast sensitivity is reduced at all spatial frequencies, but to a greater degree at the high spatial frequencies.[11,12]

Although the reduction in visual acuity and contrast sensitivity is usually well tolerated by young children, adults seem to be more bothered. When the decreased acuity and contrast are reported to be troublesome, the total magnitude of prescribed prism can be placed over one eye instead of being evenly distributed between the two eyes (see Case Report 1). If only one prism is prescribed, it is usually placed over the poorer-seeing eye, especially in adult patients. A single membrane may be applied over the better-seeing eye, however, if one desires to use the membrane as a form of partial occlusion for amblyopia treatment. If a single membrane is to be oriented to produce a vertical prismatic effect and the vision in both eyes is equal, the prism should be applied over the eye that needs base-down correction (rather than over the eye that needs base-up); the patient will experience less overhead reflection.[14]

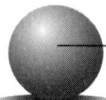

CLINICAL PEARL

If a single Fresnel membrane is to be oriented to produce a vertical prismatic effect and the vision in both eyes is equal, the prism should be applied over the eye that needs base-down correction (rather than over the eye that needs base-up); the patient will experience less overhead reflection.

Other potentially disturbing effects may be reported (Table 3-1). Reflections from the prism facets induce a second image that can be especially annoying when a brightly lit object is being viewed.[10] Colored fringes resulting from chromatic aberration tend to be more pronounced with Fresnel membrane prisms than with ground-in prisms, especially for powers greater than 15 Δ.[10] In addition, the membranes may discolor (turn yellow) with time, especially when exposed to a smoky environment. Perlin and Dziadul[15] suggest that reflections, glare, and contrast reduction can be lessened by incorporating a tint into the carrier lenses or into the Fresnel membrane itself.

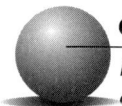

CLINICAL PEARL

Reflections, glare, and contrast reduction may be lessened in a Fresnel prism correction by incorporating a tint into the carrier lenses or into the Fresnel membrane itself.

Prismatic distortions inherent in Fresnel membrane prisms have been compared with those of conventional prisms. Adams et al.[6] investigated five basic optical distortions described by Ogle[16,17]—(1) horizontal magnification, (2) vertical magnification, (3) curvature of vertical lines, (4) asymmetrical horizontal magnification, and (5) angular magnification changes in the vertical meridian with lateral angle—and found that horizontal and vertical magnification becomes quite large with increasing base curve when a conventional prism is used. Fresnel membrane prisms, however, had substantially less overall symmetrical (horizontal and vertical) magnification than similarly powered conventional prisms did and were relatively unaffected by a change in base curve of the spectacle lens. The clinical significance of this finding is that a high-power Fresnel membrane prism may be prescribed over only one eye (for example, when a patient cannot tolerate the decreased visual acuity and contrast sensitivity) without fear of inducing a difference in retinal images due to a dissimilarity in monocular magnification. The differences in performance resulting from the last three distortions were reported to be clinically insignificant. They did, however, lessen with increasing spectacle base curves of up to 9 D.

Vertical Prism Options

Vertical prism may be implemented using any of the previously mentioned methods of prismatic correction: clip-on, decentration, ground-in, Fresnel membrane. In addition, vertical correction can be obtained by prescribing slab-off prism or ordering base-down prism in a contact lens.

Slab-off Prism

Slab-off prisms should be considered for patients who demonstrate a vertical deviation at near point only or one of unequal magnitude at distance and near. Historically, slab-off has been used to correct for the vertical prismatic imbalance induced when anisometropic patients view through their bifocal segments. For many years slab-off lenses were manufactured in glass only and were considered a custom-made job performed only by a surfacing laboratory.

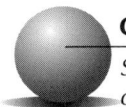

CLINICAL PEARL

Slab-off prisms should be considered for patients who demonstrate a vertical deviation at near point only or one of unequal magnitude at distance and near.

The fabrication of conventional slab-off lenses requires a special grinding process that creates base-up prism in the reading area of the prescription lens by removing a section of glass from the lower portion of the fused multifocal lens (Fig. 3-7, *A*). The slabbed-off prism is taken from the lower half of the front of the weaker plus or stronger minus lens surface, with the top line of the base-up prism zone coinciding with the top of a flat-top bifocal segment. The end result is base-up prism in the lower part of the slab-off lens.

Conventional slab-off lenses are currently available from surfacing laboratories in both glass and CR-39. In addition, there is a premolded CR-39 series of slab-off lenses available in semifinished form that has base-down (rather than base-up) prism applied to the lens with lower minus or higher plus power (Fig. 3-7, B). Because the prism effect is base down, these lenses are called "reverse slab-off." For a given prismatic prescription, reverse slab-off would be provided in the eye opposite the one in which conventional slab-off was prescribed; hence the resultant prism effect would remain the same. It should be noted, however, that when conventional slab-off for one eye and reverse slab-off for the other are prescribed the total amount of prism can be maximized.

Generally, slab-off is not prescribed for amounts less than 1.5 to 2 Δ. Conventional slab-off (base-up) is usually considered a specialty order from the laboratory. Because the grinding process is time consuming and requires a certain level of expertise, the lenses are somewhat costly. However, it is now possible to order semifinished glass lenses with the slab-off correction already ground in on the front surface.[18] Reverse slab-off can also be ordered in semifinished form. Slab-off and

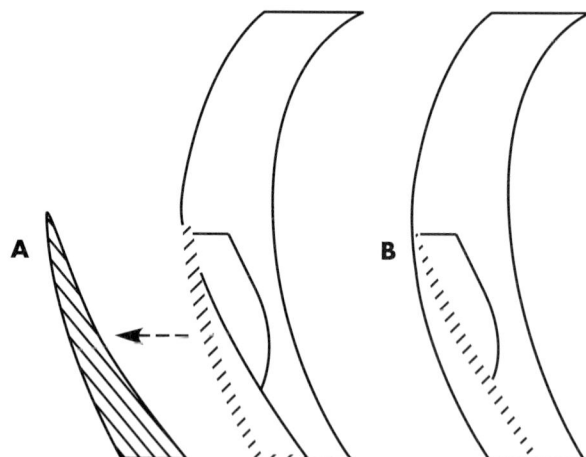

FIGURE 3-7   Slab-off prisms. **A,** Conventional, obtained by a special grinding process that removes a section of glass from the lower part of the lens (fused multifocal in this case). A base-up prismatic effect is created in the lower reading section of the lens. **B,** Reverse, cast-molded on the front surface of the lens. A base-down effect is created in the lower reading section.

reverse slab-off corrections are fabricated for prism powers up to approximately 7 Δ.

Although primarily prescribed for low to moderate vertical imbalances induced when presbyopic patients lower their eyes below the optical centers of anisometropic lenses to read, slab-off also is ideal for patients with vertical deviations that vary in magnitude with distance and near viewing. Ground-in prism can be prescribed to compensate for the distance deviation, and the difference between the distance and near deviations can be compensated by using slab-off prism. For example, assume that the optimum prism prescription is 13 Δ BDOD at distance and 18 Δ BDOD in the reading position at near point. Two separate pairs of glasses could be ordered or, alternatively, the following could be prescribed: OD, 6 Δ BDOD; OS, 7 Δ BUOS (ground in) with 5 Δ slab-off. Because of the considerable laboratory cost, slab-off is usually given only after the practitioner is fairly certain that the proposed amount of vertical prism is acceptable.

Vertical Prism in Contact Lenses

Although base-down vertical prism in contact lenses is routinely employed as a "ballast" for bifocal positioning and stabilizing meridional orientation of toric lenses, its use in the management of vertical deviations is much less common. This is likely due to the misconception that a contact lens containing prism, when placed on the eye, retains only about a fourth of the prismatic power present in air[19,20]—which hypothesis assumes that part of the prismatic effect is neutralized by the tear film, thereby resulting in less refraction of light passing from a contact lens to tears than from a contact lens to air. Reputed clinical support for this hypothesis comes from Filderman,[19] who measured the distance vertical phoria (by von Graefe's method) with the subject wearing a rigid contact lens of a known prismatic power (greater than the habitual vertical phoria). Because the induced vertical phoria created by the contact lens was significantly less than would be predicted by the sum of each subject's habitual phoria (when wearing his/her own nonprismatic contact lens) and the known power of the prismatic contact lens, Filderman concluded that the prismatic power of a contact lens was reduced when worn on the eye.

Bailey[21] and Mandell,[22] however, have shown that placing a prismatic contact lens on the eye does not change the effectivity of the prism. They demonstrated (optically) that the path of a ray through a prism correction is identical regardless of whether a contact lens is placed on the eye. In a recent clinical investigation Con et al.[23] found that the difference between the contact lens prism power in air and the magnitude of the induced vertical phoria measured with the prism on the eye was insignificant, provided there was no binocular fusion. When fusion was not prevented and the subjects were allowed to adapt binocularly for 5 minutes, the phoria was significantly reduced (making it appear that the effectivity of the prism was less when placed on the eye). Therefore the clinical evaluation that Filderman[19] used to support his hypothesis, that the effectivity of a prism contact lens is less when placed on the eye, may in fact have been in error. It appears that his subjects were allowed to view binocularly for unspecified periods after the insertion of a prismatic contact lens and before the von Graefe phorias were measured. Consequently, there was no control for prism adaptation (see Chapter 4), which could well have occurred.

CLINICAL PEARL

Placing a prismatic contact lens on the eye does not change the effectivity of the prism.

The fact that there is no difference in prismatic effectivity between a given amount of prism in a contact lens and the same amount in a spectacle lens applies only for distance viewing.[21] When near targets are being viewed, the prismatic effect of prism in a contact lens is greater than it would be in a spectacle lens. This occurs because, for near viewing conditions, the deviating effect of prism increases as the prism is moved closer to the eye's center of rotation.[2,24] Note, however, that the difference in power often is not clinically significant for low prism powers.

The refractive power of a contact lens also can alter the total prismatic power when the lens rides low. As Mandell[25] points out, a prismatic contact lens can be considered to consist of two parts, a refractive portion and a prismatic base-down (due to gravity) portion. In instances in which the lens rides low or drops down, the line of sight passes not through the optical center of the refractive part but rather above it. Therefore the refractive portion of the lens produces a prismatic effect (just as spectacles do) that can be calculated by Prentice's rule.[2] The total prismatic power of the contact lens is then the sum of the prismatic components resulting from viewing away from the optical center and the actual prism in the lens. Because a low-riding plus lens would induce base-down prism and a minus lens base-up prism (see Case Report 2), the total base-down prismatic power would increase with a low-riding plus lens and decrease with a minus lens. The effect of the refractive portion is obviously dependent on the refractive power of the lens, becoming more significant as the power increases, with plus lenses having the greatest potential for creating base-down prismatic effect. One should keep in mind that if both the patient's lenses ride low and are of similar refractive power there will actually be no net change in the total amount of vertical prism correction.

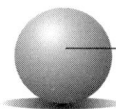

CLINICAL PEARL

The total base-down prismatic power increases with a low-riding plus contact lens and decreases with a low-riding minus lens; however, if both lenses ride low and are of similar refractive power, there will be no net change in the total amount of vertical prism correction.

Unfortunately, large amounts of prism cannot be incorporated into contact lenses without markedly reducing their wearability because of physical discomfort or inadequate lens positioning. The maximum limit before wearability appears to diminish is approximately 3 Δ[26,27] to 4 Δ* for rigid lenses, although there is a report[28] of successful rigid lens fits with up to 5 Δ of incorporated prism. For soft lenses the maximum power than can be incorporated into the lens is approximately 4 Δ†.

Because base-down prism is the only orientation that can be prescribed in contact lenses, it is naturally given to the eye demonstrating the hyperdeviation. The recommendation[29] has been made that when a prism correction is small (1 to 2 Δ) it can be prescribed for both eyes, using a minimum of 1 Δ on the eye that does not require the base-down correction. (An additional prism diopter then would be needed for the hyperdeviated eye to compensate for the 1 Δ BD over the eye not requiring the base-down prism.) This method would be most appropriate in situations in which a spherical lens on one eye and a prismatic lens on the other were not tolerated because of differences in comfort.

It has been suggested[29] that fusional ability and stereoacuity may actually be improved for the patient viewing through a prismatic contact lens correction compared with previously worn prismatic spectacle lenses. Because most lens aberrations and distortions of spectacle lenses are significantly less in contact lenses, higher-quality retinal images result, thereby potentially enhancing sensorimotor fusion.

• Case Reports

I. Combination of Ground-in Prism and a Sector Fresnel Prism

A 76-year-old woman presented with the chief complaint of horizontal double vision present at all distances beyond 3 feet that had begun approximately 5 years previously. It was not associated with any

---

*Personal communication, Art Optical Contact Lens Inc, Grand Rapids, Mich.
†Personal communication, Coast Vision Inc, Huntington Beach, Calif.

trauma or changes in health status, nor were there any other accompanying signs or symptoms. She had been forced to discontinue driving because of the diplopia and had recently begun to sit closer to her television to eliminate the double images.

The patient was currently under ophthalmological care for chronic open-angle glaucoma. The ophthalmologist had prescribed two different pairs of spectacles containing prism. Neither pair, however, eliminated the double vision. She was told that the diplopia was due to a muscle problem, that nothing else could be done, and that she would have to learn to live with it. She had accepted this point of view for several years but then decided to obtain a second opinion. There had been no previous treatment with vision therapy or extraocular muscle surgery, nor was any recommended.

Ocular history revealed myopia, first corrected at age 14, and chronic open-angle glaucoma of 3 years' duration. General health history revealed hypertension, asthma, carotid insufficiency, and a slight potassium deficiency. Current medications included betaxolol (Betoptic) bid, methazolamide (Neptazane) tid, reserpine (Serpasil) qd, dipyridamole (Persantine) tid, theophylline (Theodur) prn, and aspirin qd. Family eye and health histories were unremarkable.

Current spectacle prescription and distance acuities

OD   −3.75 −0.75 × 159   with 8 Δ BO and +3.00 add (20/30)
OS   −3.25 DS   with 6 Δ BO and +3.25 add (20/30)

Spectacle prescription that patient did not like and therefore did not wear

OD   −2.25 −1.25 × 171   with 7 Δ BO and +2.75 add
OS   −3.00 −0.25 × 114   with 2.5 Δ BI (sic), 2.5 Δ BD and +3.00 add

Subjective refraction and distance acuities

OD   −4.00 −0.50 × 160   (20/30) PHNI*
OS   −3.00 DS   (20/30) PHNI

Cover testing though habitual spectacle prescription (with either eye fixating)

(6 m):   Comitant constant alternating esotropia of 10 Δ
(40 cm): 6 Δ of esophoria

Because these measurements were made over the habitual prescription lenses that already contained 14 Δ BO, the actual deviation measured approximately

(6 m):   24 Δ BO
(40 cm): 20 Δ BO

---

*Pinhole, no improvement.

Comitancy testing (versions and Maddox rod)

Comitant deviation

A diagnosis of divergence insufficiency was made.[30] It was our opinion that a prism correction was the most appropriate management plan. After trial framing various amounts of prism, it was determined that an additional 10 Δ BO was needed for distance viewing and that no additional prism was needed for near viewing. Alternative management strategies were to prescribe two pairs of prism glasses, one for distance and one for near, or to prescribe different amounts of prism in the upper and lower portions of the spectacle lenses. We decided to use Fresnel membrane prism as a trial.

Fresnel membrane prisms were applied to the top half of the patient's preferred spectacle lenses (those containing 14 Δ BO); a 5 Δ BO prism was applied to each lens. She was instructed to wear her spectacles with the prism full-time and to return in 2 weeks. At the 2-week follow-up visit, diplopia was no longer present at distance and her eyes were comfortable; however, she complained that the "lines" of the membrane prisms blurred her distance vision. Distance visual acuity through Fresnel prisms was 20/30−3 (versus the original 20/30) in the right eye and 20/40+ (versus the original 20/30) in the left. Cover testing revealed orthophoria at distance and 4 Δ esophoria at near.

Because the spectacle lenses already had significant edge thickness from the myopic prescription, it was impossible to order the needed 24 Δ BO that was required for the top portion and the 14 Δ BO for the bottom portion in ground-in form. Therefore we ordered new spectacle lenses with the most recent refraction and a total of 14 Δ BO prism ground-in, with the intent of adding the additional 10 Δ BO in Fresnel membrane form:

OD　−4.00 −0.50 × 160 with 7 Δ BO and +3.00 add
OS　−3.00 DS with 7 Δ BO and +3.00 add

The major reason for ordering new spectacle lenses was to change the patient's bifocals from a round segment to a flat-top segment. (An executive was not recommended because of the added edge thickness.) We thought the prism would abut the flat-top segment nicely and, consequently, be more cosmetically pleasing and functional in nature (Fig. 3-5).

The patient was seen 3 weeks later for the dispensing of her new spectacles. Her diplopia had not recurred, but she was still disturbed by her decreased acuity because of "the lines" in the Fresnel prism. Although the acuity reduction was relatively minor, she was still disturbed by it. To solve this problem, we replaced her two 5 Δ BO prisms with one 10 Δ BO prism over the top portion of the nondominant (left) eye's lens. She reported improved clarity with a single Fresnel membrane prism as opposed to two membranes.

A 1-month progress evaluation revealed that the patient continued to have clear and comfortable single vision. She then returned to her ophthalmologist for management of her glaucoma and was lost to follow-up.

II. Prism in a Contact Lens and Temporary Fresnel Membrane Prism

A 65-year-old man was referred by an ophthalmologist for a contact lens refitting. He was currently under this physician's care for open-angle glaucoma. The ocular history included cataract surgery and an intraocular implant OD 11 years previously. Six years after the cataract surgery a corneal transplant OD was performed. At that time the intraocular lens implant was removed because of surgical complications.

The patient was a long-time wearer of gas-permeable contact lenses whose present pair was 2.5 years old and had been fitted by another ophthalmologist. He had a history of heart problems and was taking pilocarpine and dipivefrin (Propine) for his glaucoma along with propranolol (Inderal) for his heart. He was satisfied with the comfort and clarity of vision through his contact lenses but was bothered by the presence of intermittent vertical diplopia.

Subjective refraction and distance acuities

OD   −0.75 DS   (20/40) +3.25 add
OS   −12.00 −0.25 × 180   (20/40) +3.25 add

Von Graefe vertical phorias at 6 m and 40 cm

Variable magnitude; 4 Δ left hyperphoria when the left eye's contact lens settled inferiorly

We thought the intermittent vertical diplopia might be due to a prismatic effect induced when the high-minus gas-permeable contact lens rode low. Diplopia was not present immediately after the blink because the upper lid pulled the lens upward so the patient viewed through its optical center. After the blink, however, the heavy minus lens dropped down and settled such that the patient was viewing above the optical center of the lens. Therefore, a base-up prismatic effect was introduced before the left eye.

Originally, we attempted to change the parameters of the contact lens fit to obtain better centration. Multiple attempts, however, were unsuccessful; the high minus lens continued to ride low, with a resultant vertical diplopia. We therefore tried prescribing vertical prism to offset this effect. After trial framing various amounts of vertical prism, we determined that 3 Δ of BDOS at the spectacle plane would eliminate the vertical diplopia. Because a lesser amount is usually needed in a contact lens, 2 Δ was ordered in a gas-permeable lens. A pair of these lenses (OD −0.75 DS, OS −10.50 DS) were ordered, with 2 Δ BD in the left lens. Spectacle lenses were to be worn over the contact lenses:

OD   Plano −0.25 × 180 (20/30+), +3.25 progressive add
OS   +0.25 −0.25 × 180 (20/40), +3.25 progressive add

The patient wore these lenses successfully for 18 months without vertical diplopia. He then returned with the complaint of a constant horizontal diplopia at distance and near. This had started 1 week previously and remained stable. He was unable to identify any event or circumstance coincident with its onset. Medical history had not changed since the last visit.

Pertinent findings were a constant right esotropia that measured 21 Δ BO at distance and 16 Δ BO at near. Version testing revealed an abduction deficit of the left eye. Alternate cover testing in different fields of gaze suggested a paresis of the left lateral rectus. It was empirically determined that 20 Δ BO alleviated the diplopia; therefore, a 20 Δ BO Fresnel membrane prism was applied to the left lens of the spectacle correction (as a temporary measure). The referring ophthalmologist was consulted by phone, and an appointment with the patient's internist made for the following day. Subsequent medical testing revealed that the patient had suffered a minor stroke. He continued to wear the base-out Fresnel membrane prism, and the paresis resolved about a month later. Consequently, the Fresnel prism was no longer necessary and was removed from the patient's spectacles. He has continued to wear the prismatic contact lens, with no complaints of diplopia for the last 3 years.

III. Custom-Made Fused-Prism Spectacle Lenses

A 76-year-old man presented with the complaint of double vision at distance only that was horizontal in orientation, worse in left gaze, and of several months' duration. He reported that it was especially bothersome when driving and he was currently having to close one eye to drive. A thorough medical work-up had been performed by the patient's internist, who believed the diplopia was related to the patient's blood pressure and prescribed metoprolol (Lopressor) for hypertension.

Subjective refraction and acuities

OD   +3.00 −0.75 × 105 (20/25) +2.50 add
OS   +3.00 DS (20/25) +2.50 add

Cover test

(6 m): Constant right 12 Δ esotropia
(40 cm at reading position): 4 Δ exophoria

Maddox rod

(6 m): 12 Δ BO to alignment
(40 cm): ortho to alignment

Versions

Slight abduction deficit OD

Ocular health

Unremarkable except for mild nuclear sclerosis OU

As a trial in the office, a 12 Δ BO Fresnel membrane prism was placed on the patient's right spectacle lens while he viewed a distant target; this resulted in single vision. A sector Fresnel was then cut to fit the top portion of that lens. Because he was wearing executive bifocals, the membrane was cut to fit the entire top portion of the lens starting at the bifocal line. The Fresnel was dispensed that same day to see if it would eliminate the diplopia.

The patient wore the Fresnel successfully for 5 months and then returned to the office wondering if the prism could be put into his glasses. A custom-made executive bifocal with the distance portion (containing 6 Δ BO in each lens) fused to the reading portion (no prism) was ordered (Fig. 3-8). The prescription lenses were OD +3.00 −0.75 × 105, OS + 3.00 DS with 6 Δ BO in the top portion of each lens and a +2.50 add (executive-style bifocal) with no prism in the bottom portion.

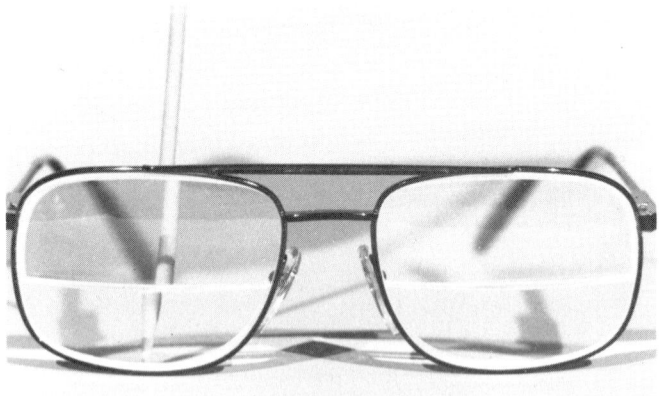

FIGURE 3-8 A custom-made executive bifocal with the distance portion (containing 6 Δ BO in each lens) fused to the reading portion (with no prism). The prescription lenses are OD + 3.00 −0.75 × 105, OS +3.00 DS, with 6 Δ BO in the top portion and a +2.50 executive bifocal with no prism in the bottom portion. (Lenses courtesy Walman Optical, Minneapolis.)

TABLE 3-2
Characteristics of Various Prism Options

	Horizontal prism available	Vertical prism available	Maximum power per lens (Δ)	Available with plano prescription	Localized (sector) use	Appreciable weight increase	Significant edge thickness	"Additional" cost ($) per lens (approx)
Clip-on	Yes	Yes	20	Yes	No	Yes	Yes	13*
Decentration	Yes	Yes	†	No	No	No	†	None
Ground-in	Yes	Yes	≈12	Yes	No§	No <5 Δ / Yes ≥5 Δ	Yes	2 per Δ
Fresnel membrane	Yes	Yes	30	Yes	Yes	No	No	12
Slab-off	No	Yes	≈7 to 8	Yes	Inferior only	Yes	Yes	40
Contact lens	No	BD only	≈4	Yes	No	Yes	Yes	RGP 5 / SCL 25

*Add clip-on frame cost of $12.00.
†Some laboratories will manufacture.
§Depends on lens power, eye size, and interpupillary distance.

Diplopia was completely eliminated and the patient was so pleased that he had a pair made for sunglasses. He wore this prismatic correction successfully for 3 years until he passed away.

SUMMARY

There are several ways to incorporate prism in an optical prescription (Table 3-2). Both horizontal and vertical prismatic corrections can be supplied by clip-on, deliberate decentration, ground-in, or Fresnel membrane prisms. When vertical correction is required, slab-off prism and prismatic contact lenses are additional options. The introduction of Fresnel membrane prisms has considerably increased the practitioner's armamentarium. In most cases the only limitation is one's creativity and willingness to implement different forms of prismatic correction. Attention to practical matters (such as cosmesis, weight, magnitude limitations, and cost of materials) will increase the probability that the patient can successfully accept and adapt to the prismatic correction.

References

1. Jampolsky A, Flom M, Thorson JC: Membrane Fresnel prisms: a new therapeutic device. In Fells P (ed): *First Congress of the International Strabismological Association,* St Louis, 1971, Mosby, pp 183-193.
2. Fannin TE, Grosvenor T: *Clinical optics,* Boston, 1987, Butterworths, pp 93-124, 446.
3. Sheard C: A dozen worth-while points in ocular refraction, *Am J Physiol Opt* 4:443-455, 1923.
4. Morgan MW: Distortions of ophthalmic prisms, *Am J Optom Arch Am Acad Optom* 40:344-350, 1963.
5. Borish IM: *Clinical refraction,* ed 3, Chicago, 1970, Professional Press, p 874.
6. Adams AJ, Kapash RJ, Barkan E: Visual performance and optical properties of Fresnel membrane prisms. I, Distortion, *Am J Optom Arch Am Acad Optom* 48:289-297, 1971.
7. Zamfirescu F, Weiss JB: Prisms in superior oblique palsy. In Moore S, Mein J, Stockbridge L (eds): *Orthoptics past present future,* Miami, 1976, Symposia Specialists, pp 217-221.
8. Miller OE, McLeod JH, Sherwood WT: Thin sheet plastic Fresnel lenses of high aperture, *J Opt Soc Am* 41:807-815, 1951.
9. Flom MC, Adams AJ: Fresnel optics. In Safir A (ed): *Refraction and clinical optics,* Hagerstown, Md, 1980, Harper & Row, pp 293-307.
10. Véronneau-Troutman S: Fresnel prisms and their effects on visual acuity and binocularity, *Trans Am Ophthalmol Soc* 76:610-653, 1978.
11. Lucas BJ, Naito T: Fresnel prisms: their effects on visual acuity and contrast sensitivity. Unpublished paper. Southern California College of Optometry, 1983. (Available from the MB Ketchum Memorial Library, Southern California College of Optometry, Fullerton, Calif)
12. Woo GC, Campbell FW, Ing B: Effect of Fresnel prism dispersion on contrast sensitivity function, *Ophthalmic Physiol Opt* 6:415-418, 1986.

13. Scott WE: Office use of prisms. In *Symposium on Strabismus. Transactions of the New Orleans Academy of Ophthalmology*, St Louis, 1978, Mosby, pp 91-103.
14. Amos JF, Rutstein RP: Vertical deviations. In Amos JF (ed): *Diagnosis and management in vision care*, Boston, 1987, Butterworths, pp 515-583.
15. Perlin RR, Dziadul J: Fresnel prisms for field enhancement of patients with constricted or hemianopic visual fields, *J Am Optom Assoc* 62:58-64, 1991.
16. Ogle KN: Distortion of the image by prisms, *J Opt Soc Am* 41:1023-1028, 1951.
17. Ogle KN: Distortion of the image by ophthalmic prisms, *Arch Ophthalmol* 47:121-131, 1952.
18. Brooks CW: *Understanding lens surfacing*, Boston, 1992, Butterworth-Heinemann, p 286.
19. Filderman IP: The effect of surrounding media on prismatic contact lenses, *Optom Week* 56:19-24, 1965.
20. Soper JW, Girard LJ, Sampson WG: Special designs and fitting techniques. In Girard LJ, Soper JW, Sampson WG (eds): *Corneal contact lenses*, St Louis, 1964, Mosby, pp 290-291.
21. Bailey NJ: Prism in a contact lens, *J Am Optom Assoc* 37:44-45, 1966.
22. Mandell RB: The prism controversy, *J Am Optom Assoc* 38:190, 1967.
23. Con S, Ng J, Carter D, Mandell RB: Solution to the contact lens prism paradox, *Contact Lens Spectrum* 7:52-54, 1992.
24. Obstfeld H: The effect of prismatic spectacle and contact lens corrections on ocular rotation, *Ophthalmic Physiol Opt* 6:233-237, 1986.
25. Mandell RB: Prism power in contact lenses, *Am J Optom Arch Am Acad Optom* 44:573-580, 1967.
26. Bennett AG: *Optics of contact lenses*, ed 4, London, 1974, Association of Dispensing Opticians, p 42.
27. Bailey NJ: Special contact lenses and their applications. III, Prism contact lenses, *Opt J Rev Optom* 97:54-56, 1960.
28. Véronneau-Troutman S: A new optical modality to overcome diplopia, *Trans Am Ophthalmol Soc* 77:181-190, 1979.
29. Ewell DG, Gates H, Remba MJ: Special fitting procedures: the prism ballast contact lens principle. In *Encyclopedia of contact lens practice*, vol 2, South Bend, Ind, 1961, International Optics Publishing, p 45.
30. Scheiman M, Gallaway M, Ciner E: Divergence insufficiency: characteristics, diagnosis, and treatment, *Am J Optom Physiol Opt* 63:425-431, 1986.

Self-Assessment Questions

1. Base-up and base-down prism may be prescribed in all of the following formats except for
   a. ground-in prism
   b. contact lenses
   c. Fresnel membrane prism
   d. slab-off prism

2. With a relatively small eye size and low to moderate refractive error, the maximum amount of prism that can usually be ground into a single spectacle lens is
   a. 2 to 4 Δ
   b. 4 to 6 Δ
   c. 10 to 12 Δ
   d. 18 to 20 Δ

3. You determine that your 28-year-old patient needs 2 Δ BUOD to maintain comfortable and single vision. Her refractive error is +2.00 −2.00 × 180 OU. Which of the following would *not* be an option?
   a. spectacle lenses with prism obtained through decentration
   b. spectacle lenses with ground-in prism split between the two eyes
   c. gas-permeable contact lenses with base-down prism in the left lens
   d. Fresnel membrane prism base-down over the left eye

4. Which of the following would *not* be beneficial in helping to maximize the cosmesis of a pair of spectacles requiring a −3.00 DS refractive correction and 4 Δ of base-out ground-in prism in each eye?
   a. high-index plastic lenses
   b. a small frame size
   c. antireflective coating
   d. an edge treatment (that is, translucent edge coat or roll and polish)
   e. a rimless frame

5. Your patient currently wears a spectacle prescription of OD −1.50 DS with 1 Δ BU, OS −2.00 DS with 1 Δ BD, and informs you that she would like to wear contact lenses. Which of the following statements most accurately reflects what she should be told?
   a. Vertical prism can be prescribed in contact lenses, but it can be incorporated only in soft lenses, not in gas-permeable lenses.

     b. Because the prismatic effect is substantially less in contact lenses than in spectacles, a contract lens correction would not be an effective mode of implementing vertical prism.

     c. A vertical prismatic correction can be ordered using the same prismatic correction as in the spectacle lenses: 1 Δ BU will be incorporated in the right lens, and 1 Δ BD in the left lens.

     d. A vertical prism correction can be ordered with 1 to 2 Δ BD incorporated in the left lens.

Answers: 1. b.   2. c.   3. a.   4. e.   5. d.

4

Prism Adaptation in Heterophoria Patients

Rachel V. North
David B. Henson

Key Terms

prism adaptation	vision therapy	heterophoria
fixation disparity	fusional vergence	anisometropia
orthoptics		

Prism Adaptation

The first report of the phenomenon that we now know as prism adaptation was made by Schubert[1] in 1943. He found that 2 prism diopters (Δ) of induced vertical vergence could be adapted to; in other words, the induced vertical disparity reduced with time. Further evidence of prism adaptation came from researchers[2-5] investigating the phoria position after periods of forced vergence. They found that phoria measurements were affected by measurements of fusional vergence. If positive fusional vergence measurements were made, the subsequent phoria became more esophoric. Similarly, when negative fusional vergence measurements were made the subsequent phoria was more exophoric. This temporary change of the phoria position has been named an aftereffect of or an adaptation to the forced vergence.

The ability of the vergence system to adapt has been investigated further by several researchers,[6-22] who found that the oculomotor system can change the tonic innervation to the extraocular muscles and thereby alter the extent of any phoria. If a prism is placed before an eye to induce either horizontal or vertical disparity, one would expect the measured phoria or fixation disparity to change by an amount equal to the prism power. In actual fact, however, the patient may gradually adapt to the prism; that is, after a short period of binocular viewing, the phoria and fixation disparity return to their baseline values.

Adaptation to Vertical Prism-Induced Phorias

Ogle and Prangen[6] used a fixation disparity technique to measure the rate of adaptation to prism-induced vertical disparities in subjects with normal binocular vision. They found that adaptation to a vertical prism of 2 Δ is usually complete within 3 to 7 minutes and that the adaptive process can be adequately described by a logarithmic curve. If the prism was increased gradually, in 2 Δ steps, the subjects were able to adapt to a total disparity of 6 Δ. If the 6 Δ was worn for an additional hour, then on removal the subjects experienced diplopia for periods of 2 to 16 minutes.

Carter[9] also found that subjects could adapt to vertical prisms. He described an individual with 1 Δ of left hyperphoria, who was prescribed 1 Δ BDOS. After a month of wear this person had returned to the original 1 Δ of left hyperphoria. The prescription was increased to 2 Δ (1 Δ BDOS and 1 Δ BUOD), which again was adapted to after 2 weeks of wear. Finally, the prism was increased to 3 Δ and the person showed adaptation after 2 days. Surprisingly, there were no symptoms before the initial prism prescription and none were reported with subsequent prescriptions.

Henson and North[13] and Sethi and North[15] both found that subjects could adapt to vertical prisms of increasing magnitude. They measured heterophorias using a "flashed" Maddox rod technique in conjunction with a tangent scale. The rod was exposed for 0.25 of a second by means of a photographic shutter placed in front of the left eye and controlled by the subject via a cable release. The shutter was connected electronically to test charts situated at 4 m and 0.4 m in such a way that the chart illumination was extinguished only when the shutter was open. The individual viewed a high-contrast letter chart (with the nonoccluded eye) until the Maddox rod was exposed. This allowed better control of accommodation than is usually obtained with the Maddox rod technique. The muscle light was placed in the center of the test chart. To obtain the baseline phoria measurements, each subject was allowed 15 seconds of binocular viewing followed by 15 seconds of monocular occlusion when the Maddox rod was placed in front of the shutter. At the end of the occlusion period a phoria measurement was made. This procedure was repeated until three identical successive readings were obtained or a total of six measurements were taken, with the mean of the last three used as the baseline phoria. During the next occlusion period a prism was placed in front of the occluded left eye and a phoria measurement was made before any binocular viewing through the prism. This was repeated at least 14 times, with the prism remaining in front of the left eye, and it gave a total period of binocular viewing through the prism of at least 3.5 minutes.

The ability of subjects with normal binocular vision to adapt to 2 Δ of vertical induced disparity was evaluated. Figure 4-1 shows the averaged responses from eight individuals measured from their baseline heterophoria to the insertion of a 2 Δ base-up prism while viewing a chart at 4 m. All the subjects showed rapid adaptation; the phorias were reduced by approximately 1.75 Δ after 3.5 minutes of

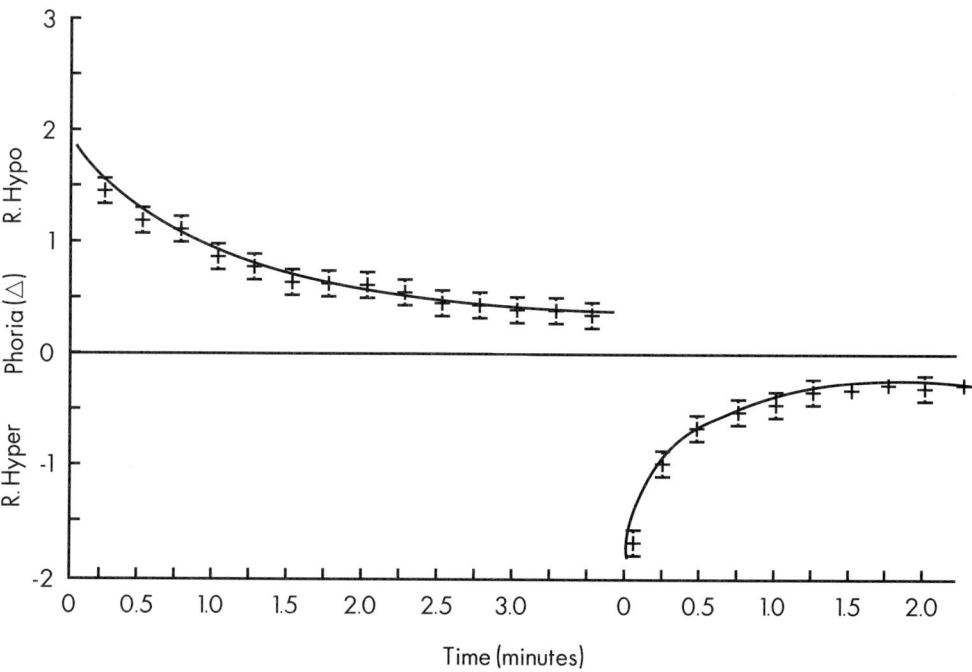

FIGURE 4-1 Change in heterophoria response with the duration of binocular viewing after insertion (above the abscissa) and removal (below the abscissa) of a 2 Δ base-up prism, with fixation at 4 m. Mean of eight subjects who had normal binocular vision. Vertical bars represent ± 1 SE. (From Henson DB, North R: *Am J Optom Physiol Opt* 57:129-137, 1980.)

binocular viewing through the prism. The averaged response after the prism was removed is also shown in Figure 4-1. Note that the initial rate of recovery was slightly faster than the initial rate of adaptation. The adaptation responses were symmetrical for base-up and base-down prisms at both distance and near.

Influence of Vertical Fusion Ability on the Adaptation

If vertical prism disparity is gradually increased in 2 Δ steps, subjects can adapt to a 6 Δ disparity[15]; but if a 6 Δ of disparity is introduced in a single step, the amount of adaptation is markedly reduced. None of the four subjects in Sethi and North's study could achieve fusion when a 6 Δ vertical prism was placed in front of one eye; despite a lack of fusion, however, two did exhibit some adaptation. It appears that the amount of adaptation was related to fusion, because the adaptation increased with an increase in prism magnitude until the prism power fell outside the subjects' fusional amplitudes and then it decreased. Also the larger the prism disparity was, the longer the time taken to achieve fusion (Table 4-1) and the slower the rate of adaptation.

After adaptation the vertical fusional reserves tend to be symmetrical about the newly adapted-to position.[6,9,19] Rutstein and Eskridge,[16] measuring forced vertical vergence fixation disparity curves and the ability of subjects to adapt to a 2 Δ vertical prism worn for 3 hours,

TABLE 4-1

Time (in seconds) When Fusion (if achieved) Occurred during the 3.5 Minutes of Binocular Viewing through the Prism

	JP	BS	VB	RN
Base-up (Δ)				
2	15	15	15	15
4	180	60	Diplopia	75
6	Diplopia	Diplopia	Diplopia	Diplopia
Base-in (Δ)				
6	15	15	10	15
9	Diplopia	Diplopia	15	Diplopia
12	Diplopia	Diplopia	105	Diplopia
Base-out (Δ)				
6	6	3	5	5
12	30	6	10	15
18	40	10	15	30
24	Diplopia	15	20	45

From Sethi B, North RV: *Am J Optom Physiol Opt* 64:263-268, 1987.

found that individuals with the greatest adaptation ability generally had flatter forced-vergence curves.

Adaptation to horizontal prism-induced phorias

Several researchers have investigated adaptation to horizontal prisms in subjects with normal binocular vision. Once again, the oculomotor system demonstrates a remarkable ability to adapt although the adaptation response to horizontal prisms may be very asymmetrical. Ogle et al.[7] reported one subject who took 50 minutes to adapt to a 6 Δ base-in prism and only 10 minutes to a 28 Δ base-out prism. Mitchell and Ellerbrock[8] reported that the adaptation response to base-in and base-out prisms was invariably asymmetrical when the subjects viewed a near target and was in the reverse direction to that found by Ogle et al.[7] at distance. While also investigating adaptation to horizontal prisms, Carter[10] reported that 11 of 13 subjects showed almost total adaptation to the inclusion of their maximum fusible base-out and base-in prisms (up to 10 Δ base-in and 32 Δ base-out) after 15 minutes of wear. He used a distance fixation disparity technique and found that most of the adaptation occurred within the first 5 minutes.

Schor[11] noted that the amount of adaptation was often asymmetrical to horizontal prisms, being greater when the base was in one direction than when it was reversed. He compared the prism-induced fixation disparity with the amount of prism adaptation after 30 seconds of binocular viewing in 14 subjects. Prism values of 1.5 to 6 Δ base-in and base-out were used to force the vergence while the subjects viewed a distant chart. Prism adaptation was defined as the amount of fusional vergence that remained after 40 seconds of monocular occlusion following a 30-second prism adaptation period. Schor[11] found that eight subjects showed greater adaptation to base-out prism than base-in while six had the opposite results. The direction of maximum prism adaptation coincided with the direction in which the prism-induced fixation disparity curve had the lowest values. This agreed with Ogle et al.,[7] who stated that Type II and Type III fixation disparity curves can represent rapid adaptation to base-out and base-in prisms.

Henson and North[13] and North et al.[14] also found asymmetrical adaptation to horizontal prisms when a distant target was viewed. The adaptation to 6 Δ base-out and 6 Δ base-in was measured. All subjects demonstrated an ability to adapt to horizontal prism-induced phorias at both distance and near. The phoria gradually returned toward its baseline value with an increasing duration of binocular viewing. However, the rate of adaptation was asymmetrical to horizontal prisms at distance, being faster to base-out than to base-in prism (Fig. 4-2). At near the responses to horizontal prisms were virtually symmetrical (Fig. 4-3).

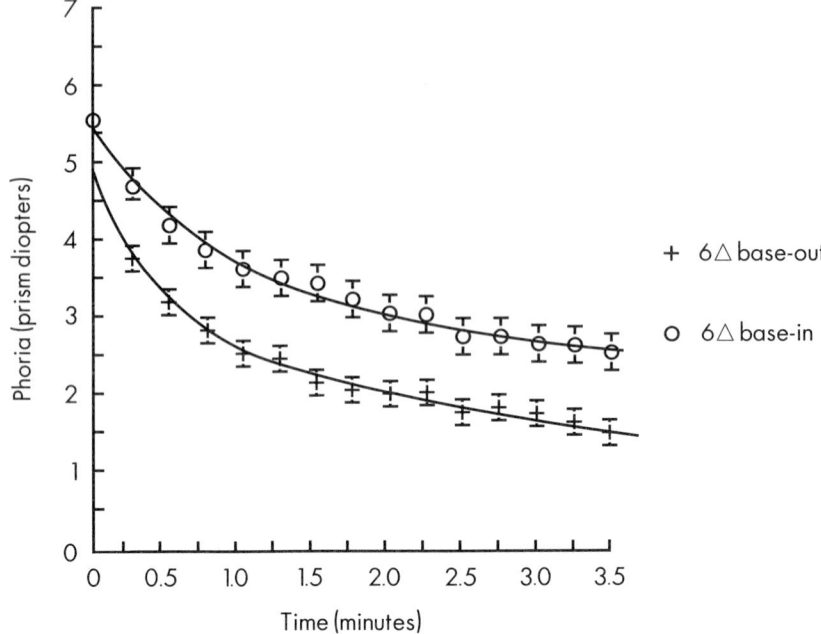

FIGURE 4-2 Change in heterophoria response with the duration of binocular viewing after the insertion of a 6 Δ base-out and a 6 Δ base-in prism, with fixation at 4 m. Mean of 40 subjects. Vertical bars represent ± 1 SE. (From North RV, Sethi B, Owen K: *Ophthalmol Physiol Opt* 10:81-85, 1990.)

Influence of horizontal fusion ability upon adaptation

The amount of adaptation to prisms of increasing magnitude and the relationship to fusional reserves are shown in Figure 4-4. The amount of adaptation increases with increasing prism magnitude until the prism reaches the limit of the subject's fusional reserves; then it levels off or decreases. The rate of adaptation is also inversely related to the time taken for fusion to occur. As the magnitude of the prism increases, the time for fusion increases (Table 4-1) and the rate of adaptation decreases.

Once again, fusional reserves have been found to be symmetrical about the newly adapted position.[9,17]

Spread of Adaptation

The lateral spread of adaptation was investigated by Henson and Dharamshi,[18] who took phoria measurements with the eye in different positions both before and after a subject had adapted to vertical prism. (During adaptation the subject's binocular visual experience was

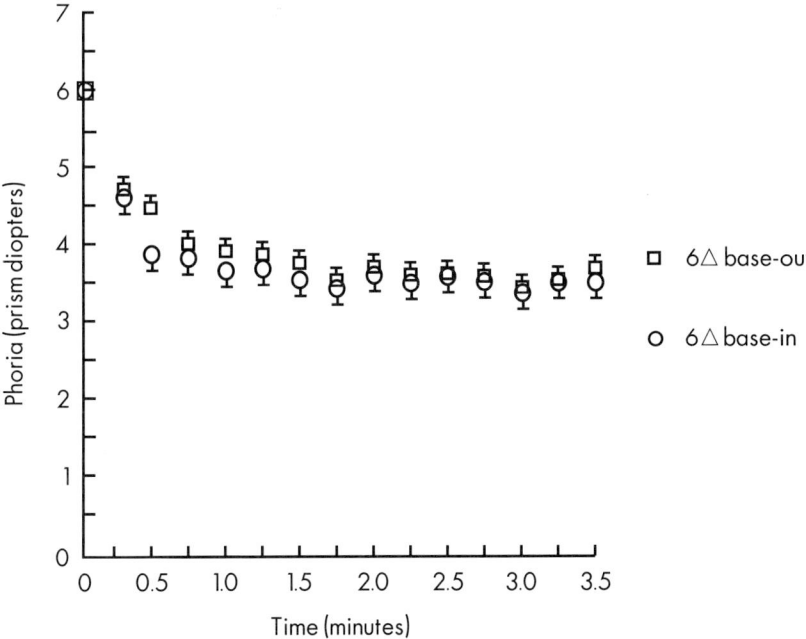

FIGURE 4-3 Change in heterophoria response with the duration of binocular viewing after insertion of a 6 Δ base-out and a 6 Δ base-in prism, with fixation at 40 cm. Mean of 40 subjects. Vertical bars represent ± 1 SE. (From North RV, Sethi B, Owen K: *Ophthalmol Physiol Opt* 10:81-85, 1990.)

confined to the primary position of gaze.) They found that adaptation spread across the retina from the position of binocular visual experience, being maximal at the position where binocular visual experience through the prism was obtained and decreasing with increasing eccentricity from this position. Its spread was found to be greater in the horizontal than in the vertical meridian and to be reduced to only 60% of the maximum 20° from adapted position in the horizontal meridian and 40% in the vertical meridian (Fig. 4-5).

The results of this experiment support the hypothesis that adaptation takes place over limited motor fields, being maximal in the visual direction where binocular visual experience is obtained and then decreasing by an amount dependent upon the angular distance from the direction of binocular visual experience.

Adaptation in Anisometropia

The ability of the oculomotor system to adapt over limited motor fields has been investigated further by using subjects with anisometropia.

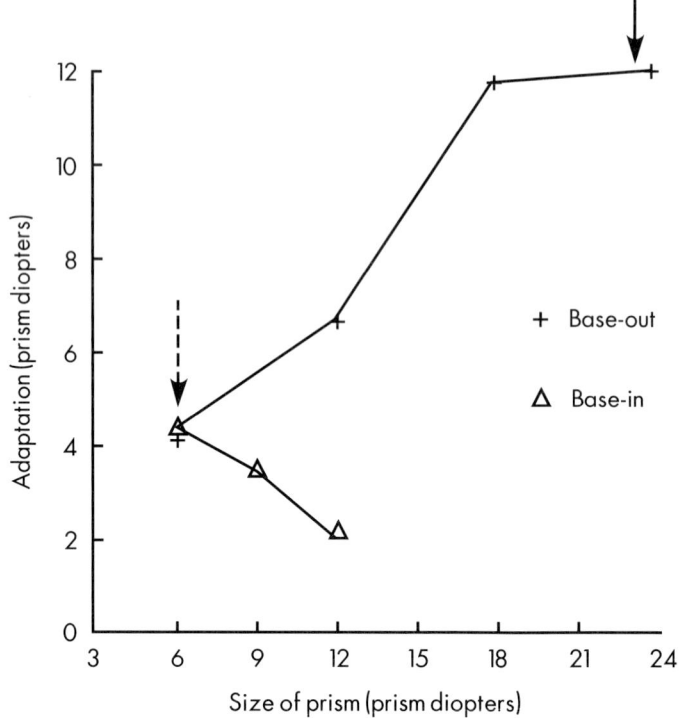

FIGURE 4-4 Amount of adaptation after 3.5 minutes of binocular viewing through horizontal prisms of increasing magnitude. Mean of four subjects. Limit of fusion reserves: convergence (*solid arrow*), divergence (*dashed arrow*). (From Sethi B, North RV: *Am J Optom Physiol Opt* 64:263-268, 1987.)

A spectacle-corrected anisometrope must cope with prismatic disparities that vary with the direction of gaze. Although there may not be any prismatic effect when viewing through the optical centers of the prescription, a vertical prismatic effect is introduced upon elevation or depression of the eyes and a horizontal prismatic effect upon looking to the right or left. The magnitude of this effect is dependent upon eye position. While the amplitude of the induced horizontal effect is usually within the patient's fusion range, this is not always the case for induced vertical prismatic effects.

Several researchers,[7,18-23] however, have reported that the phorias of a spectacle-corrected anisometrope remain approximately the same regardless of the direction of gaze. This finding implies that patients can adapt to prismatic effects which vary across the motor field.

Allen[22] measured the vertical phorias of spectacle-corrected anisometropic subjects with distance and near fixation. To assess the amount of adaptation, he compared the calculated prism at the

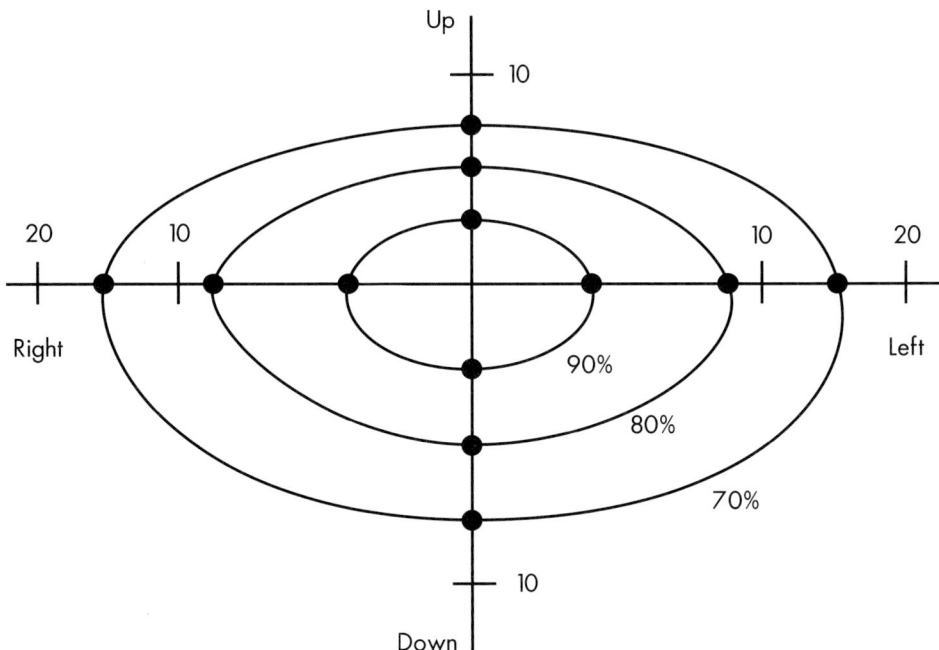

FIGURE 4-5 Spread of adaptation from a single position coinciding with the center of the diagram. (From Henson DB: In Obrecht G, Stark LW [eds]: *Presbyopia research: from molecular biology to visual adaptation*, New York, 1991, Plenum.)

reading position with the actual phoria measured and found that the vertical adaptation was approximately equal to the calculated prismatic effect. However, when the anisometropia was high (over approximately 3 D), he found a lag of adaptation, that is, the prismatic effect was not fully adapted to.

Henson and Dharamshi[18] induced anisometropia by fitting one eye with a soft contact lens and then correcting the induced ametropia with a spectacle lens. The contact/spectacle lens system induced a prismatic effect whose magnitude was dependent upon eye position and the dioptric power of the lens. The subjects' phorias were measured in different directions of gaze. Initially the magnitudes increased as the line of sight moved away from the optical center of the spectacle lenses. Repeat measures taken after a period of adaptation showed the amount of adaptation to be dependent upon eye position.

This was a clear demonstration that the oculomotor system is capable of adapting to induced noncomitant deviations. It is important to note, however, that the rate of adaptation was slower than that experienced with step displacements produced by an ophthalmic prism. The adaptation in the superior field (especially at 22° above the straight-ahead position) was found to be less than that in the inferior field, which was thought to be due to the fact that the subjects were more likely to gain visual experience in the inferior than in the superior motor field. (The subjects performed normal office/laboratory–type tasks during the adaptation period; it would be quite unusual for a subject to spend much time in upward gaze.) This suggestion was confirmed by a modification to the above experiment[23] in which the spectacle lens aperture was reduced with opaque material to allow only an 18° field of view. The rate of adaptation in areas outside the 18° motor field was markedly reduced suggesting that the rate of adaptation is dependent on the amount of binocular visual experience obtained at each position.

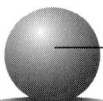

CLINICAL PEARL

The oculomotor system is capable of adapting to induced noncomitant deviations.

If the amount of anisometropia is increased, the fusional vergence demand on the oculomotor system will also be increased. When subjects were fitted with a contact/spectacle lens system that increased the amount of anisometropia, the rate of adaptation was found to be significantly reduced in both the center and the periphery of the motor field. Even at the center, where the fusion demand was small, adaptation was slow. Therefore it did not appear that the slowing of the adaptation rate was due only to an increased demand on the fusion system. This effect can be explained by hypothesizing that the oculomotor system is limited not only by the magnitude of the fusional vergence demand but also by the rate of change of demand with eye position.

There is a marked difference in the rate of adaptation between step and noncomitant displacements. Step displacements appear to be corrected within a period of a few minutes whereas noncomitant ones produced by inducing anisometropia can take several hours. The early results of Henson and Dharamshi[18] demonstrated that adaptation to a step displacement spreads over a fairly large range of directions of gaze. With induced anisometropia this spread could hinder the adaptive process by producing an inappropriate adaptation in adjacent gaze directions. When the eyes move about the motor field in the early stages of adapting, marked adaptation in one direction might occur as a result of spread and be followed by adaptation in the other direction as a result of visual experience. The oculomotor system clearly has the ability to overcome this problem, probably by reducing the width of the adapting channels, but the process places an extra load on the system that tends to reduce the rate of adaptation.

Models of the Adaptation System

Ogle and Prangen[6] suggested that the fusion mechanism responsible for vertical adaptation is mediated by two reflexes—the psycho-optical and the involuntary. The *psycho-optical* reflex operates during adaptation to (1) the vertical vergence demands introduced by fixating points obliquely at near or (2) the varying prismatic effects produced by anisometropic prescriptions. These are likely conditioned and nonstabilizing reflexes initiated to meet the demands of the environment. The *involuntary* reflex is responsible for adaptation to prisms and results directly from optical stimuli, to maintain binocular single vision. It is further divided into a fast system and a slow system. The *fast* system is nonstabilizing and operates when prism vergence measurements are being made; it has vertical limits of $\pm 3 \Delta$. The *slow* system takes between 3 and 6 minutes to operate and results in more stable adaptation to prism; it is therefore stabilizing and can have limits that exceed the fusional vergence reserves.

Schor[12] hypothesized that when a prism is placed before an eye the fast (phasic) fusional vergence system initially responds to the retinal image disparity and its output then acts upon a slow (tonic) fusional vergence system; it is this slow system that stimulates adaptation to the fusional demand. The slow fusional vergence system also reduces, by means of negative feedback, the demand on the fast system. (See Chapter 5.) He also hypothesized that the slow fusional vergence controller must be located before the accommodative convergence and convergence accommodation cross-links since adaptation occurs only with both accommodative and disparity vergences when binocular vision is permitted.

Carter[9] suggested in an earlier paper that the adaptation system operates to reduce the demand or stress placed upon the fusional vergence system.

Adaptation Ability in Subjects with Abnormal Binocular Vision and/or Asthenopia

There are several reports of subjects who lacked or had deficient adaptation systems.[6,7,11] Ogle et al.[7] described seven subjects, most of whom had abnormal binocular vision, who were lacking or who showed partial adaptation ability to horizontal prism. For example, one individual with divergence insufficiency who had suffered from intermittent diplopia at distance for years was prescribed 4Δ base-out over each eye. After 1 month of wear there was no adaptation to the prism and the subject reported relief of symptoms. These findings of Ogle et al.[7] support the suggestion by Carter[9] that an absent or deficient adaptation system causes high distance phorias and patients with high distance phorias and asthenopia should benefit from relieving prisms.

In 1979 Schor[11] investigated three subjects with intermittent esotropias and found that they adapted well to base-in but not to base-out prisms; in addition, their forced-vergence fixation disparity curves had large values in both directions. He suggested[11] that the surprisingly high amounts of fixation disparity in response to base-in prisms could be due to a sensory factor interfering with fusion.

North and Henson[24] examined a total of 15 subjects with binocular vision problems, 14 of whom also had asthenopia. The subjects' abilities to adapt to prisms were examined at the distance at which symptoms occurred (that is, 4 m or 0.4 m). In addition, prism vergences, heterophorias, and associated phorias (using the Mallett unit) were measured. Some subjects also had measurements taken at a distance where they were not symptomatic. A questionnaire that requested details concerning symptoms of blurred vision, diplopia, headaches, and visual fatigue was given and the subjects were then classified into two groups according to their symptoms: (1) "persistent and severe," when one or more of the asthenopic symptoms occurred every time the subject attempted a specific visual task and at a severity that made continuation of the task extremely difficult, and (2) "occasional," when the subject often suffered from one or more of the symptoms while performing a specific visual task.

The responses from three typical subjects are shown in Figure 4-6: SJ, with a normal adaptation response; AJ, with a partial response; and TT, with no response. SJ reported no symptoms, AJ occasional symptoms, and TT persistent and severe symptoms. The amount of adaptation achieved after 105 and 225 seconds was compared with that achieved by the normal group. Adaptation was considered abnormal if it was more than 2 standard deviations from the norm at either of these points (105 and 225 seconds). It was found that most subjects demonstrated abnormal adaptation to base-out and/or base-in prism at both distance and near. Only two subjects adapted normally to horizontal prism at distance; one exhibited an esotropia and was asymptomatic, and the other had an intermittent exotropia that was controlled better at distance than at near. The adaptation to vertical prism was normal in all but two cases. Surprisingly, a poor relationship was found between the amount of adaptation after 225 seconds, the phoria, the prism vergence values, and the presence of fixation disparity. It can be seen in Table 4-2 that subjects may have normal prism vergences but abnormal prism adaptation. (The prism vergences were accepted as normal if within or greater than the normal range.[25,26]) There is also a poor relationship between the amount of adaptation and the direction of the phoria. All the subjects who were exophoric at distance adapted normally to base-out prism, and three who were esophoric adapted normally to base-in prism (Table 4-3).

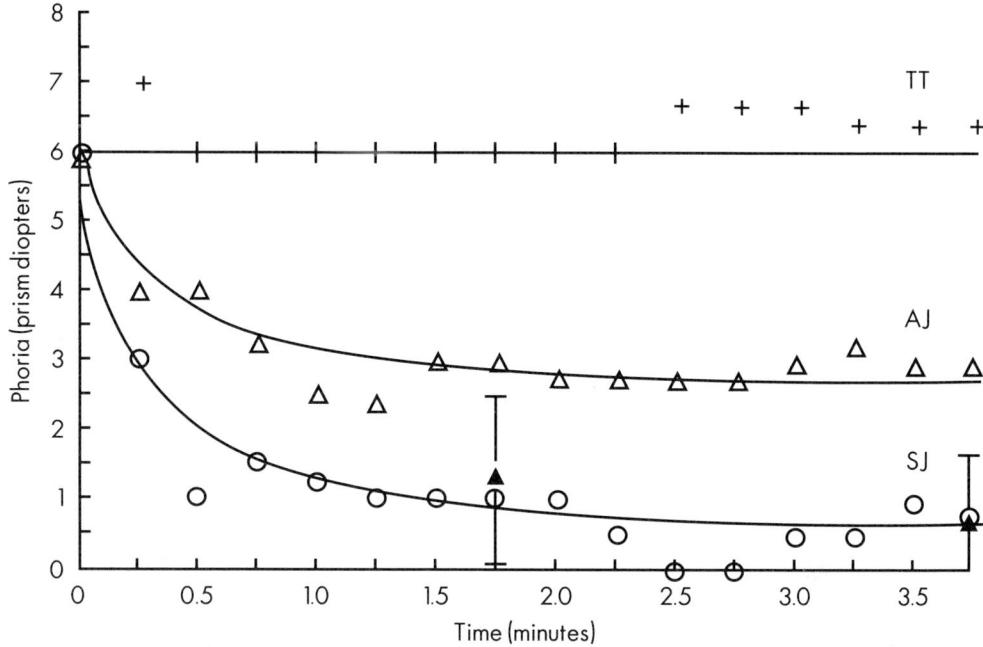

FIGURE 4-6 Adaptation responses of three subjects to 6 Δ of base-out prism, with fixation at 4 m, showing normal (SJ), partial (AJ), and no (TT) adaptation. Vertical bars represent normal values, ± 1 SD. (From North RV, Henson DB: *Am J Optom Physiol Opt* 58:746-752, 1981.)

CLINICAL PEARL

Even if a patient has a normal fast fusional vergence mechanism, (as shown by normal prism vergences), it does not necessarily follow that adaption ability is normal.

Pickwell and Kurtz[27] investigated short-term prism adaptation in subjects with and without symptoms. They also found a low correlation between heterophoria, associated phoria, prism adaptation, and symptoms. They measured the amount of prism adaptation at near after 30 seconds of binocular viewing through 6 Δ base-out and 6 Δ base-in prism, they recorded the phoria directly after a period of binocular viewing; this was therefore a measure of the fast fusional vergence system. Using the same technique they could not differentiate between subjects with and those without symptomatic phorias. Both groups showed adaptation after 30 seconds of binocular viewing through the

TABLE 4-2

Subjects with Abnormal Binocular Vision or Asthenopia Showing Normal Prism Vergences and Adaptation

	Vergence	Adaptation	Both
Distance			
Horizontal	4/5*	2/5	1/5
Vertical	0/4	3/4	0/4
Near			
Horizontal	8/10	1/10	1/10
Vertical	2/5	4/5	1/5

*The denominator is the number of subjects in whom measurements of both prism vergences and adaptation were taken.
From North RV, Henson DB: *Am J Optom Physiol Opt* 58:746-752, 1981.

TABLE 4-3

Subjects with Abnormal Binocular Vision or Asthenopia with Exo- and Esodeviations Showing Normal Adaptation

	Distance (Δ)		Near (Δ)	
	6 base-out	6 base-in	6 base-out	6 base-in
Exodeviation	4/4*	1/4	4/8	4/8
Esodeviation	3/6	2/6	0/3	2/3

*The denominator is the number of subjects in whom both measurements of prism adaptation to base-out and base-in were taken.
From North RV, Henson DB: *Am J Optom Physiol Opt* 58:746-752, 1981.

horizontal prisms, which led them to conclude than an abnormal fast fusional vergence system is not characteristic of a symptomatic phoria.

Effect of Vision Training on the Adaptation System

It has been suggested by Schor[28] that the success of vision training (orthoptic treatment) in relieving symptoms may be due to an improvement in the patient's ability to adapt to prism. Symptomatic stress on the fast fusional vergence system may be relieved by prescribing prism or by giving orthoptic treatment to either increase the rate and magnitude of the adaptation system or increase the velocity of the fast fusional system.

North and Henson[29] examined this topic further by monitoring a population of 15 patients attending the Orthoptic Department of the Bristol Eye Hospital. The patients were divided into two groups. Group 1 consisted of seven patients with convergence insufficiency whose adaptive ability was measured before and after vision training. Group 2 contained eight patients, seven of whom had already received vision therapy for convergence insufficiency and one of whom underwent squint surgery; their adaptive ability was measured after vision training.

An induced disparity of 6 Δ base-out with fixation at 40 cm was used to test adaptive ability in all patients. The distance and near heterophoria, prism vergences at near, and near point of convergence (NPC) were also measured. Vision training normally lasted 8 weeks and consisted of push-ups, physiological diplopia, and fusional reserve exercises.[30] To determine whether there were any learning effects, the same tests were conducted twice on a control group of six subjects with normal binocular vision.

The mean measurements recorded for Group 1 before and after vision training are shown in Table 4-4. Before vision training the mean prism adaptation response fell outside the normal range (mean ±2 SDs). After vision training the responses improved, on average by 2.24 Δ, placing them within but still to one side of the normal range of values (Fig. 4-7). The control group showed a mean increase in adaptation of 0.19 Δ. The NPC also improved in all patients. An improvement of the base-out prism vergences was found in four patients, with a mean increase of 16 Δ. After vision training, all but one of the patients reported either total or partial relief of their symptoms.

The results after vision training from Group 2 are shown in Table 4-5. All the patients had normal base-out prism vergences and NPCs after vision training. Six adapted normally to base-out prism. The two who showed an abnormal adaptation ability reported no relief and only slight relief of their symptoms. Only one patient with an apparently normal prism adaptation response had symptoms, and he suffered from diplopia throughout the test. There was a poor correlation between the amount of prism adaptation and prism vergences and between prism adaptation ability and the NPC.

Discussion

The process of oculomotor adaptation is essential to the visual system, enabling it to compensate for the normal changes in orbital mechanics that occur naturally with age. For example, there is a loss of orbital fat,

TABLE 4-4

Group 1—Mean Measurements Both Before and After Vision Training

	Before	After
Near exophoria (Δ)	4.9	4.4
Near-point convergence (cm)	14.4	7.0
Base-out prism vergences (Δ)	18.5	34.3
Base-out prism adaptation (Δ)	1.63	3.87

From North RV, Henson DB: *Optom Vis Sci* 69:294-299, 1992.

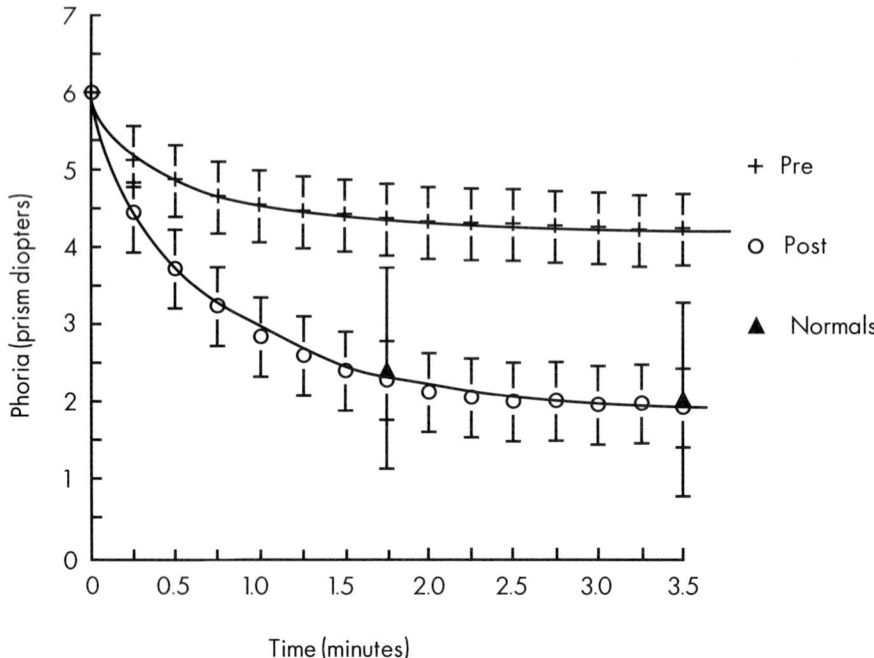

FIGURE 4-7 Change in heterophoria response with duration of binocular viewing after the insertion of 6 Δ base out both before and after visual training. Mean of seven subjects, ± 1 SD. Vertical bars at 105 and 210 seconds represent the 95% confidence limits of normal subjects. (From North RV, Henson DB: *Am J Optom Physiol Opt* 59:983-986, 1982.)

TABLE 4-5

Group 2—Mean Measurements After Vision Training

	Measurement	Subjects within normal range
Base-out prism vergence (Δ)	28.5	7/7
Near-point convergence (cm)	6.6	8/8
Base-out prism adaptation (Δ)	4.22	6/8
Symptoms		2/8

From North RV, Henson DB *Optom Vis Sci,* 69:294-299, 1992.

which results in enophthalmos[31] as well as alterations in muscle structure.[32] These changes require alterations in the patterns of extraocular muscle innervation.

The findings of these studies suggest that normal adaptation to prism-induced heterophorias is associated with comfortable binocular vision. Patients with symptomatic anomalies of binocular vision frequently have an abnormal adaptation system and therefore do not adapt to prism. This inability to adapt appears to be greatest at the distance where symptoms are most severe. In patients who demonstrate no prism adaptation ability a prismatic correction placed in the direction required to correct their symptomatic phoria will usually provide relief of symptoms.[7,10,24,28] Therefore asthenopic subjects with no adaptation ability may find relief of their symptoms by wearing a prism prescription.

CLINICAL PEARL

Normal adaptation to prism-induced heterophorias is associated with comfortable binocular vision. Patients with symptomatic anomalies of binocular vision frequently have an abnormal adaptation system and therefore do not adapt to prism. This inability to adapt appears to be greatest at the distance where symptoms are most severe.

CLINICAL PEARL

In patients who demonstrate no prism adaptation ability a prismatic correction placed in the direction required to correct their symptomatic phoria will usually provide relief of symptoms.

A question frequently posed is "Why do patients who possess normal adaptation ability exhibit a heterophoria and not orthophoria?" North and Henson[24] found that patients could adapt from a prism-induced exophoria back to their baseline esophoria and vice versa. McCormack[33] reported similar responses. Prisms were used to correct the near phoria of 30 patients, of whom 27 adapted from their induced orthophoria back to their habitual phoria. He suggested[33] that the maintenance of an original heterophoria, shown by this response, is a characteristic of normal and comfortable binocular vision; however, it is not essential. Ogle et al.[7] suggested that the adaptation system must be different from or unrelated to those innervational factors responsible for a phoria. It has also been suggested by Crone and Hardjowijoto[34] that maintenance of a heterophoria is due to an abnormal adaptation system that operates around the phoria position instead of around orthophoria. Dowley,[35] investigating the phoria and prism adaptation ability at distance in asymptomatic patients and found different prism adaptation responses to horizontal prisms (6 Δ) in esophorics, exophorics, and orthophorics. Exophores showed a reduced base-out prism response compared to orthophores but a similar base-in prism response. He suggested that exophoria therefore exists due to a partial failure to adapt to base-out prism. Esophores showed a reduced base-in prism response compared to orthophores but a similar base-out response, which implies that esophoria exists due to a partial failure to adapt to base-in prism. He concluded[35] that the presence of heterophoria in normal subjects may be due to partial saturation of prism adaptation.

The success of vision training in relieving symptoms appears to be related to an improvement in adaptation ability. Vision training improves not only the fast fusional vergence mechanism, as shown by the increased prism vergence values, but also the slow fusional vergence system (that is, the adaptation system). Even if a patient has a normal fast fusional vergence mechanism, it does not necessarily follow that adaptation ability is normal. This was shown in studies[24] in which the prism vergences had a poor correlation with adaptation ability; in some patients the prism vergences were found to be normal but the adaptation ability was lacking.

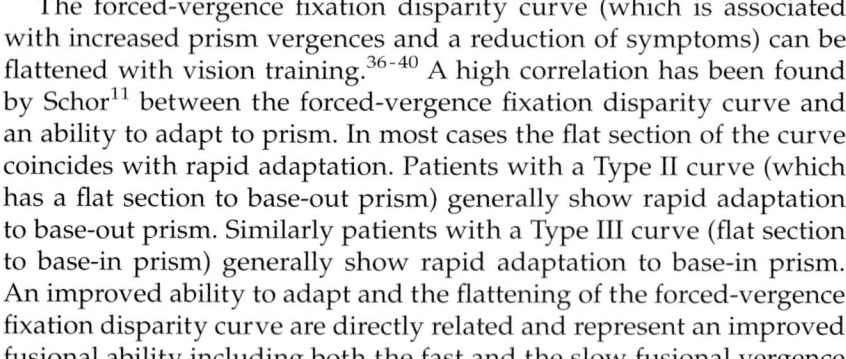

CLINICAL PEARL

The success of vision training in relieving symptoms appears to be related to an improvement in adaptation ability. Vision training improves not only the fast fusional vergence mechanism, as shown by the increased prism vergence values, but also the slow fusional vergence system (that is, the adaptation system).

The forced-vergence fixation disparity curve (which is associated with increased prism vergences and a reduction of symptoms) can be flattened with vision training.[36-40] A high correlation has been found by Schor[11] between the forced-vergence fixation disparity curve and an ability to adapt to prism. In most cases the flat section of the curve coincides with rapid adaptation. Patients with a Type II curve (which has a flat section to base-out prism) generally show rapid adaptation to base-out prism. Similarly patients with a Type III curve (flat section to base-in prism) generally show rapid adaptation to base-in prism. An improved ability to adapt and the flattening of the forced-vergence fixation disparity curve are directly related and represent an improved fusional ability including both the fast and the slow fusional vergence systems.

To summarize, it appears that[41]

1. Adaptation ability in heterophoric patients is associated with comfortable binocular vision.
2. Patients with binocular anomalies producing symptoms invariably have an abnormal adaptation mechanism, with the abnormality greatest at the distance where symptoms are most severe.

3. Adaptation ability may be used as a guide to monitor the effectiveness of vision training. If the patient's adaptation ability improves, it appears likely that his/her symptoms will be relieved. If there is no improvement, it is unlikely that continuing the vision training will provide relief of symptoms and the practitioner should then consider prescribing prism.

CLINICAL PEARL

Adaptation ability may be used as a guide to monitor the effectiveness of vision training. If the patient's adaptation ability improves, it appears likely that his/her symptoms will be relieved. If there is no improvement, it is unlikely that continuing the vision training will provide relief and the practitioner should then consider prescribing prism.

References

1. Schubert G (1943). Cited by Ogle and Prangen, Reference 6.
2. Ellerbrock V, Fry GA: The after-effect induced by vertical divergence, *Am J Optom Arch Am Acad Optom* 18:450-454, 1941.
3. Alpern M: The after effect of lateral duction testing on subsequent phoria measurements, *Am J Optom Arch Am Acad Optom* 23:442-447, 1946.
4. Morgan MW: The direction of visual lines when fusion is broken as in duction tests, *Am J Optom Arch Am Acad Optom* 24:8-12, 1947.
5. Ellerbrock VJ: Tonicity induced by fusional movements, *Am J Optom Arch Am Acad Optom* 27:8-20, 1950.
6. Ogle KN, Prangen A de H: Observations on vertical divergences and hyperphorias, *Arch Ophthalmol* 49:313-334, 1953.
7. Ogle KN, Martens TG, Dyer JA: *Oculomotor imbalance in binocular vision and fixation disparity*, Philadelphia, 1967, Lea and Febiger.
8. Mitchell AM, Ellerbrock VJ: Fixational disparity and the maintenance of fusion in the horizontal meridian, *Am J Optom Arch Am Acad Optom* 32:520-534, 1955.
9. Carter DB: Effects of prolonged wearing of prism, *Am J Optom Arch Am Acad Optom* 40:265-273, 1963.
10. Carter DB: Fixation disparity and heterophoria following prolonged wearing of prisms, *Am J Optom Arch Am Acad Optom* 42:141-152, 1965.
11. Schor CM: The influence of rapid prism adaptation upon fixation disparity, *Vision Res* 19:757-765, 1979.
12. Schor CM: The relationship between fusional vergence eye movements and fixation disparity, *Vision Res* 19:1359-1367, 1979.
13. Henson DB, North R: Adaptation to prism-induced heterophoria, *Am J Optom Physiol Opt* 57:129-137, 1980.
14. North RV, Sethi B, Owen K: Prism adaptation and viewing distance, *Ophthalmic Physiol Opt* 10:81-85, 1990.
15. Sethi B, North RV: Vergence adaptive changes with varying magnitudes of prism-induced disparities and fusional amplitudes, *Am J Optom Physiol Opt* 64:263-268, 1987.
16. Rutstein RP, Eskridge JB: Clinical evaluation of vertical fixation disparity. III, Adaptation to vertical prism, *Am J Optom Physiol Opt* 62:585-590, 1985.

17. Stephens GL, Jones R: Horizontal fusional amplitudes after adaptation to prism, *Ophthalmic Physiol Opt* 10:25-28, 1990.
18. Henson DB, Dharamshi BG: Oculomotor adaptation to induced heterophoria and anisometropia, *Invest Ophthalmol Vis Sci* 22:234-240, 1982.
19. Cusick PL, Hawn HW: Prism compensation in cases of anisometropia, *Arch Ophthalmol* 25:651-654, 1941.
20. Ellerbrock V, Fry GA: Effects induced by anisometropic corrections, *Am J Optom Arch Am Acad Optom* 19:444-459, 1942.
21. Ellerbrock VJ: Further study of effects induced by anisometropic corrections, *Am J Optom Arch Am Acad Optom* 25:430-437, 1948.
22. Allen DC: Vertical prism adaptation in anisometropes, *Am J Optom Physiol Opt* 51:252-259, 1974.
23. Sethi B, Henson DB: Vergence-adaptive change with a prism-induced non-comitant disparity, *Am J Optom Physiol Opt* 62:203-206, 1985.
24. North RV, Henson DB: Adaptation to prism-induced heterophoria in subjects with abnormal binocular vision or asthenopia, *Am J Optom Physiol Opt* 58:746-752, 1981.
25. Morgan MW: The clinical aspects of accommodation and convergence, *Am J Optom Arch Am Acad Optom* 21:301-313, 1944.
26. Borish IM: *Clinical refraction,* ed 3, Chicago, 1970, Professional Press.
27. Pickwell LD, Kurtz BH: Lateral short-term prism adaptation in clinical evaluation, *Ophthalmic Physiol Opt* 6:67-73, 1986.
28. Schor CM: Fixation disparity: a steady state error of disparity-induced vergence, *Am J Optom Physiol Opt* 57:618-631, 1980.
29. North RV, Henson DB: Effect of orthoptics upon the ability of patients to adapt to prism-induced heterophoria, *Am J Optom Physiol Opt* 59:983-986, 1982.
30. Mohindra I, Molinari J: Convergence insufficiency: its diagnosis and management, *Optom Month* 71:222-225, 310-313, 1980.
31. Weale RA: *The aging eye,* London, 1963, HK Lewis.
32. Miller JE: Aging changes in extraocular muscle. In Lennerstrand G, Bach-y-Rita P (eds): Wenner-Gren Center International symposium series. *Basic mechanisms of ocular motility and their clinical implications,* vol 24, Oxford, 1975, Pergamon Press, pp 47-61.
33. McCormack GL: Vergence adaptation maintains heterophoria in normal binocular vision, *Am J Optom Physiol Opt* 62:555-561, 1985.
34. Crone RA, Hardjowijoto S: What is normal binocular vision, *Doc Ophthalmol* 47:163-199, 1979.
35. Dowley D: Heterophoria, *Optom Vis Sci* 67:456-460, 1990.
36. Arner RS, Berger SI, Braverman G, Kaplan M: The clinical significance of the effect of vergence on fixation disparity—a preliminary investigation, *Am J Optom Arch Am Acad Optom* 33:399-409, 1956.
37. Sheedy JE, Saladin JJ: Phoria, vergence, and fixation disparity in oculomotor problems, *Am J Optom Physiol Opt* 54:474-478, 1977.
38. Sheedy JE: Fixation disparity analysis of oculomotor imbalance, *Am J Optom Physiol Opt* 57:632-639, 1980.
39. Cooper J, Selenow A, Ciuffreda KJ, et al: Reduction of asthenopia in patients with convergence insufficiency after fusional vergence training, *Am J Optom Physiol Opt* 60:982-989, 1983.
40. Rutstein RP, Daum KM, Cho M, Eskridge JB: Horizontal and vertical vergence training and its effect on vergences, fixation disparity curves, and prism adaptation. II, Vertical data, *Am J Optom Physiol Opt* 65:8-13, 1988.
41. North RV, Henson DB: The effect of orthoptic treatment upon the vergence adaptation mechanism, *Optom Vis Sci* 69:294-299, 1992.

Self-Assessment Questions

1. After 3.5 minutes of binocular viewing through a 2 Δ vertical prism, how much adaptation will have occurred in a patient with normal binocular vision?
   a. 40%
   b. 50%
   c. 70%
   d. over 80%

2. An asymptomatic patient has a distance oculomotor balance of 6 Δ exophoria with 0.5 Δ of right hyperphoria and near exophoria of 12 Δ and 0.5 Δ of right hyperphoria. Which prescription would you provide?
   a. BUOD
   b. BDOD
   c. BI
   d. none

3. What percentage of adaptation will have spread to a point 20° horizontally from the adapted position?
   a. 60%
   b. 50%
   c. 40%
   d. 10%

4. Which of the following statements is false?
   a. Adaptation occurs to both horizontally and vertically induced-prism disparities.
   b. The rate of adaptation depends on the direction of the prism and the viewing distance.
   c. The adaptation ability cannot be used as a guide to the effectiveness of vision training.
   d. Symptomatic patients with no adaptation ability may benefit from prescriptions that incorporate relieving prisms.

_____

Answers: 1. d.   2. d.   3. a.   4. c.

5

Horizontal Prism Prescription

J. James Saladin

Key Terms

Sheard's criterion	CA/C ratio	control systems
Percival's criterion	heterophoria	analysis
Morgan's norms	disparity vergence	vergence facility
fixation disparity	vision therapy	accommodation
AC/A ratio	vergence adaptation	latent exophoria

In a study of horizontal prism prescription for nonstrabismics, there are several basic questions that need to be answered. Why and when should horizontal prism be prescribed? What are the appropriate directions and amounts? What are the possible extenuating circumstances? A study of methods used in the past for prescribing such prism reveals differences of opinion not only on the methods but also on what constitutes oculomotor imbalance and therefore the reasons for prescribing. The multiplicity of opinions results from a lack of a common conception of the physiology of the oculomotor system. After a review of representative methods used now and in the past, a working model of the oculomotor system will be presented and then a method of prism prescription based on that model will be constructed.

Horizontal oculomotor imbalance exists when the total innervation to the extraocular muscles is inadequate to comfortably obtain and/or maintain ocular alignment. Under the Maddox classification of vergences (Morgan[1]), possible sources of innervation consist of tonic and fusional vergences at distance with accommodative and proximal innervation added at near. Figure 5-1 shows this in diagrammatic form. In both cases (distance and near viewing), fusional vergence is the innervational source designated to make up for the inadequacy of innervation from the other sources. Retinal disparity is the stimulus for fusional vergence, and for that reason the preferred name for fusional vergence has become *disparity* vergence. Henceforth in this chapter, disparity vergence will be the name given to what was once called fusional vergence. At the risk of over-simplification, it is the misuse or overuse of disparity vergence (and the attendant accommodative interaction) that defines oculomotor imbalance in nonstrabis-

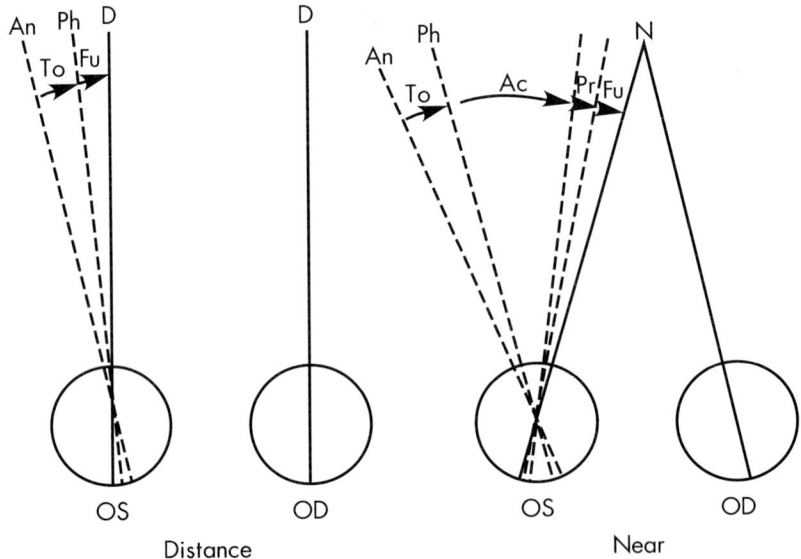

FIGURE 5-1 The vergence system according to Maddox is summarized for both distance and near fixations. For distance fixation, tonic and, if need be, fusional (disparity) vergences are called upon. For near fixation, tonic, accommodative, and proximal vergences are used, with fusional vergence being called on to correct any inaccuracy in the sum of the other three. *D,* Position of the distance target; *N,* position of the near target; *An,* anatomical position of rest; *Ph,* physiological position of rest; *To,* angle overcome through tonic innervation; *Fu,* angle overcome through fusional vergence (may be in either direction); *Pr,* proximal convergence angle; *Ac,* accommodative convergence angle.

mics. Horizontal prism should be prescribed to relieve stress on the disparity vergence mechanism, but only after the more basic problems have been corrected.

In the past, *stress* (here defined as the force exerted from any source) on the disparity vergence system was determined by measuring the horizontal phoria. The ability to withstand that stress was estimated by measuring the disparity vergence ranges. The prism prescription direction was determined by giving esophores base-out and exophores base-in. The amount was determined in different ways. In general, though, methods designed for diagnostics were adapted for prescriptive purposes and could be separated into those based on intrasubject comparisons and those based on intersubject comparisons.[2] Study of Percival's[3] and Sheard's[4] criteria will suffice to acquaint the reader with intrasubject comparisons whereas a knowledge of the use of Morgan's[5] norms will be adequate for understanding intersubject methods.

Percival and Sheard developed criteria that are examples of the use of intrasubject comparison. For both, the data from one test were to be compared with data from another test and in every case to be obtained from the same person.

Percival's criterion states that *a patient's demand point (zero phoria) should be in the middle third (area of comfort) of the relative vergence range.* For example, with vergence blur as the deciding value, the negative range from zero might be 12 prism diopters (Δ) of divergence ability and the positive range 24 Δ of convergence ability, with the total vergence range being 36 Δ. In this case the demand point would fall just inside the middle third of the total range (Fig. 5-2, *A*). The criterion would also be met if divergence ability were 24 Δ and convergence ability 12 Δ. Any combination of convergence and divergence ability would work as long as the vergence demand point fell within the middle third. If the divergence ability were 6 Δ and the convergence ability 30 Δ, the total convergence ability would be 36 Δ; but now the demand point would not be in the *middle third*. To meet Percival's criterion, 6 Δ of base-out prism would be required (Fig. 5-2, *B*). The criterion was intended for use equally in esophores and exophores.

There are two important points to make when Percival's criterion is discussed. One is that neither the magnitude nor the direction of the heterophoria is a consideration. The other is that a practitioner can make any patient who has originally met Percival's criterion not meet it by expanding the vergence ranges through orthoptics. For instance, positive disparity vergence training can easily increase the positive vergence limits, thereby moving the middle third in a convergent (or eso) direction. Most practitioners would agree that this is a theoretical consequence resulting from a strict application of the criterion that leads to an implausible conclusion.

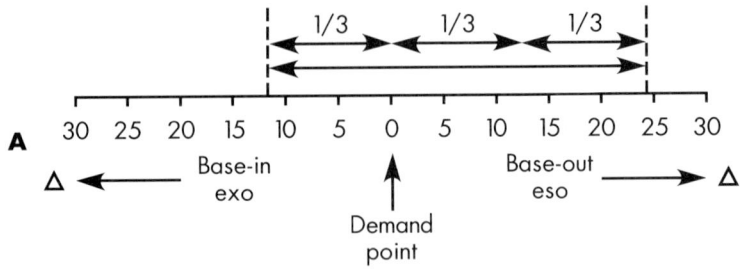

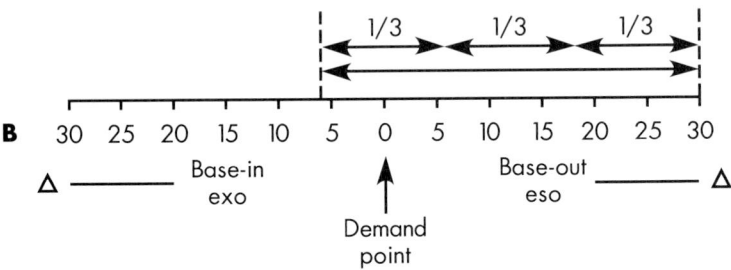

FIGURE 5-2 Percival's criterion states that the vergence demand point should fall within the middle third of the range of relative vergence. In **A** the demand point falls just at the left edge of the middle third of the range between the vergence blur points (12 Δ base-in to 24 Δ base-out); therefore Percival's criterion is just met. In **B** the relative vergence range is from 6 Δ base-in to 30 Δ base-out, for a total vergence range of 36 Δ. The middle third would be from 6 Δ base-out to 18 Δ base-out; the demand does not fall in the middle third. The prescription of 6 Δ of base-out would move the demand to the middle third.

Sheard's criterion[4] compares the heterophoric amount to the opposing vergence. Briefly, it states that *the opposing vergence range (to first sustained blur) should be at least twice the phoric amount.* Sheard did not have any particular statistical evidence for this criterion but believed that any system, whether physical, financial, or physiological, should have a certain amount of reserve strength if it was going to resist the forces put upon it over time. It seemed to work well in the clinic and has become a part of the optometric lore. As an example (Fig. 5-3), consider an 8 Δ exophore with a 10 Δ base-out–to–blur vergence range. This patient would need the base-out–to–blur expanded to 16 Δ (twice the phoric amount of 8 Δ) *or* 2 Δ base-in to be prescribed. Figure 5-3 shows that the prescription of 2 Δ base-in would decrease the phoria to 6 Δ of exophoria *and* increase the base-out–to–blur vergence range by 2 Δ at the same time. As with Percival's criterion, Sheard's was intended to apply equally to esophores and exophores.

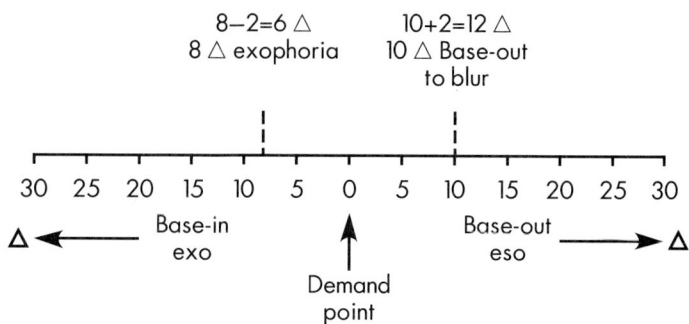

FIGURE 5-3 Sheard's criterion is met if the relative vergence range opposite the phoria is twice the phoric amount. In the example the patient has 8 Δ of exophoria with an inadequate base-out–to–blur vergence value of 10 Δ. Sheard's criterion is not met, because 2 × 8 Δ = 16 Δ not 10 Δ. Two prism diopters of base-in prism would reduce the phoria by 2 Δ and increase the base-out vergence range by 2 Δ; therefore the remaining phoric value would be 6 Δ and the base-out vergence range would be 12 Δ. Sheard's criterion would be met.

Morgan's norms[5] (Table 5-1) were developed from clinical data on some 800 pre-presbyopic patients. The far and near phorias, along with the blur, break, and recovery of vergence ranges, and the gradient AC/A ratio were all assigned normal ranges based on the clinical data. If a patient's data were within the range of normalcy, he/she was not expected to have symptoms based on oculomotor dysfunction, since the average person did not have such symptoms. (That was the way the theory went anyway.) Morgan himself fully understood the assumptions inherent in this approach and was not convinced that they were warranted. The more prominent assumptions were that phoria and vergence readings were adequate to detect oculomotor dysfunction and that data gathered from Morgan's subpopulation could produce ranges that would be appropriate for other subpopulations (for instance, the presbyopic or the pediatric subpopulations). The use of Morgan's complete technique also involved comparing certain groups of test data; but for the purposes of our discussion, we can approach the technique in a simplified manner. If the patient's data did not fall within the normative ranges, then prism or lenses were prescribed to enable them to do so. For instance (Fig. 5-4), if the phoria at near were 3 Δ eso and the normal range at near was ortho to 6 Δ exo, then 3 Δ of base-out prism would be needed to move the phoria point to just inside the range of normalcy. Similar methods could be applied if a vergence point were outside normal ranges. In practice, Morgan insisted that a *pattern* of abnormal data points should exist and that the patient should have symptoms attributable to oculomotor dysfunction before he would prescribe

TABLE 5-1

Morgan's Norms

Test	Mean	(SD)
6 m phoria	1 exo	(2)
Positive vergences (Δ)		
Blur	9	(4)
Break	19	(8)
Recovery	10	(4)
Negative vergences (Δ)		
Break	7	(3)
Recovery	4	(2)
40 cm phoria	3 exo	(5)
Positive vergences (Δ)		
Blur	17	(5)
Break	21	(6)
Recovery	11	(7)
Negative vergences (Δ)		
Blur	13	(4)
Break	21	(4)
Recovery	13	(5)
Dynamic retinoscopy	+1.37 D	(0.37)
Monocular cross cylinder	+1.00 D	(0.50)
Binocular cross cylinder	+0.50 D	(0.50)
Positive relative accommodation	−2.37 D	(1.12)
Negative relative accommodation	+2.00 D	(0.50)
Gradient AC/A	4/1	(2)

From Morgan MW: *Am J Optom Arch Am Acad Optom* 21:301-313, 1944.

prescribe for the dysfunction. He also tended to use the norms specifically for differential diagnoses of oculomotor dysfunction and then to combine this knowledge with Sheard's or Percival's criterion and known physiological principles for the actual determination of a prescription. Speaking of the Sheard, Percival, and normative approaches,[6] he believed, "In general, it is found that all three methods give similar results, and it is only rarely that data will be found which do not lead to the same conclusion regardless of which of the three methods is used."

The use of fixation disparity for the determination of oculomotor imbalance and subsequent lens or prism prescription is considerably different from the methods previously mentioned. Fixation disparity is a condition wherein the images of an object fixated by both eyes do not stimulate exactly corresponding points but do fall within Panum's areas and therefore are seen singly. For the greater part of the past 100 years, *fixation disparity* has been thought of as a small part of the phoria that is left over after motor fusion and sensory fusion have both done their best to achieve alignment. As such, the thinking went, it should be eliminated, which would show that the sum of sensory and motor fusion is adequate to achieve exact alignment. Ogle et al.[7]

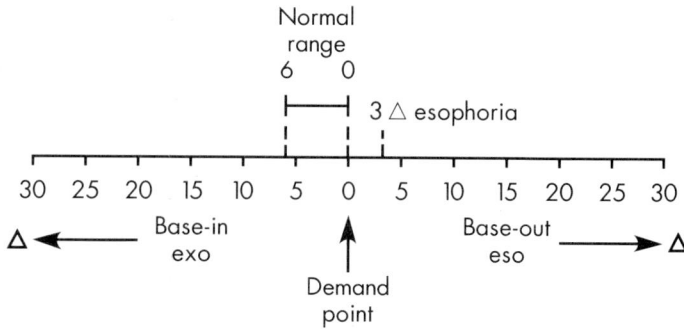

FIGURE 5-4 A normative (Morgan's values) approach. The patient is 3 Δ esophoric at near. The range of normalcy for a near heterophoria is ortho to 6 Δ exo. A prescription of 3 Δ base-out would create functional orthophoria; therefore, if the phoria were again measured through the prescribed prism, orthophoria would be found.

laid much of the theoretical background for fixation disparity, but Mallett[8] is given credit as the first to consistently propound fixation disparity for the management of oculomotor imbalance. His idea was to neutralize it through lenses or prisms. As will be explained later in this chapter, his concept was a step in the right direction but was deserving of further development. The Mallett system (instrument and technique) was used in the late 1960s and early 1970s in the United States. My experience (as well as that of others with whom I worked) was that it held for vertical oculomotor imbalances but was unreliable for horizontal imbalances (see Chapter 6).

All the methods of prescribing prism thus far mentioned are effective to some extent. Most of the time the practitioner ends up prescribing about the same amount and direction of prism (or the commensurate amount of minus or plus lens) no matter which method is used; but there are some unsettling questions about the process. Why sometimes (and more often than is comfortable intellectually) does the patient not accept the prism prescription? Why is there not a direct link between known physiology, the patient's symptoms, and the treatment technique? No unifying concept has been proposed. The rest of this chapter will concentrate on answering these questions, constructing that unifying concept, and bringing into the overall picture some of the newer concepts in oculomotor physiology.

Pathophysiology

For any observation distance other than infinity the eyes must converge because there is a horizontal separation between them. The amount of this convergence is dependent upon the distance between the eyes and the distance from the eyes to the fixated object. The eyes must also accommodate appropriately for the fixation distance. It is this need for proper convergence and accommodation and for agreement between the two that provides the seed for most oculomotor dysfunction. In the present discussion we are interested mainly in (1) the convergence aspect and (2) accommodation only as it relates to convergence.

According to Maddox's classification of vergences, tonic vergence provides the innervation to move the eyes from the anatomical to the physiological position of rest, and it is this physiological position that provides the starting convergence point for optometric measurements. The physiological position of rest is the vergence position that the eyes assume under dissociated (unfused) conditions with accommodation relaxed. In clinical terms, it is the distance phoria position. If it does not provide parallel visual axes, then a distance heterophoria exists and disparity vergence must be called into play to make up for the inappropriateness of tonic vergence (Fig. 5-1).

How does the system know when and how to make up for this inadequacy? Except for the extreme periphery, each point on one retina is paired with a point on the other retina. Both points report their stimulation to the same group of cells in the occipital cortex and therefore signal a visual event in the same position with respect to the fixated object. Such pairs of points on the retinas are called *corresponding points*. If a fixated object is not projected onto corresponding retinal points, the visual system can compute how much it misses and whether convergence or divergence is needed to make it fall on those points. Until the image of an object falls on corresponding retinal points, it will be retinally disparate (that is, retinal disparity exists for that object).

Under simultaneous stimulation of both eyes, an "area of forgiveness" exists about each corresponding point. If an object is imaged on the retinas not exactly on corresponding points but within the areas of forgiveness (Panum's areas) about those points, the perceptual system simply says, "Close enough! There must be only one visual event in the 'out there' called visual space." Even though the person is perceiving one visual event or object, the visual system also knows that corresponding points are not being stimulated and can process the information as to both amount and direction. Figure 5-5 illustrates a distant fixation point that is not being imaged exactly on corresponding points but is within Panum's area of one eye and is perceptually associated with the stimulated point in the other eye. This lack of exactness is, of course, retinal disparity, but since the fixation point and Panum's areas are concerned, it is called fixation disparity. The system uses retinal disparity as the stimulus for a disparity vergence movement. The system knows *when* a deficiency in tonic vergence exists for distant fixation because a disparity exists. It also knows whether to *diverge* or

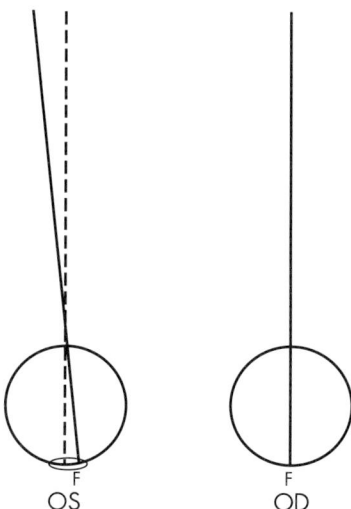

FIGURE 5-5 When a patient fixates a distant object, the visual axes should be parallel. Note that the left axis is slightly divergent. The small circle about the fovea (*F*) represents Panum's area in the left eye, which under binocular conditions corresponds to the fovea of the right eye. Here the patient will see the fixation object as single even though the images do not fall on exactly corresponding points. An exo fixation disparity then occurs. If an eso disparity had occurred, the left eye would have been slightly converged. In actual practice, fixation disparity angles can be split between the eyes and can have both motor and sensory components, a complication of much theoretical but not much clinical interest.

converge because of the direction of the disparity; and, in addition, it knows *how much* to move because of the amount of the disparity.

Now stereopsis enters into the picture. Figure 5-6 shows that if lines are drawn from each pair of corresponding points through the center of the exit pupil the intersection of each pair of lines will itself form a curved line in space, the horopter. This represents the zero depth position. Objects in space are judged either farther or nearer than one another with respect to the horopter. If only the horopter that forms from using the retinal points along the horizontal meridian is considered, Figure 5-6 will serve as an example. *X* is the fixation point and is imaged directly onto the absolute centers of the two foveas. *Q* represents any point formed by the intersection of the lines from any pair of corresponding points. Hence "all the *Q*s" are perceptually judged to be the same distance from the observer as the fixation point. Now look at *Y*. It does not fall on corresponding points. If the disparity is large enough, it will even be seen double. Furthermore, *Y* is imaged on temporal retinas of both eyes and thus the left eye sees the right image and the right eye the left image. The diplopia

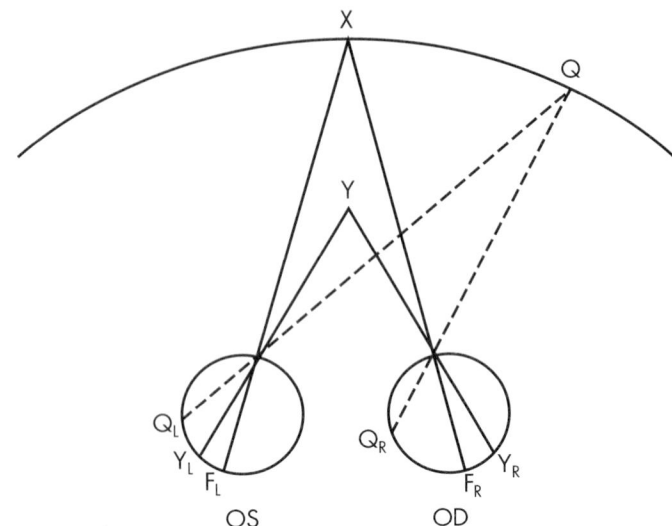

FIGURE 5-6 The patient is fixating point X, which is imaged on the two foveas (F_R and F_L). Q represents any point on the horopter, here shown by the *curved line*. Point Y is not on the horopter and therefore will not be imaged on corresponding points. Here it is seen to be imaged on Y_R and Y_L, which are both on the temporal retina. Note that corresponding points are always on nasal-temporal sides of the retina and cannot be on temporal-temporal or nasal-nasal sides. In this example crossed disparity (or diplopia) would signal that a convergence movement was needed and/or Y was closer than X.

is crossed. If Y were on the far side of X, it would be imaged on nasal retinas, and the diplopia would be uncrossed. Therefore the disparity has a sign depending upon whether the disparity is crossed or uncrossed. It is obvious, from looking at the diagram, that the farther Y is from X along the midline the greater will be the disparity; therefore disparity has an amount. The direction and amount of the disparity are reported to a stereoscopic perceptual center and the person reports a very distinct and singular perception of depth called stereopsis.

Disparity-driven vergence becomes involved when the person is no longer satisfied looking at point X in Figure 5-6 but wants to look at point Y. This fusion reflex is psycho-optical in nature, because first the person must *want* to change fixation and then the optically driven portion can perform the actual change in fixation. If the process is broken up into steps, the movement is more understandable. Once the command is given to look at point Y, the disparity is read for direction and amount. This is accomplished through disparity detectors, which are actual physiological entities in the cortex.[9] In Figure 5-7, either the

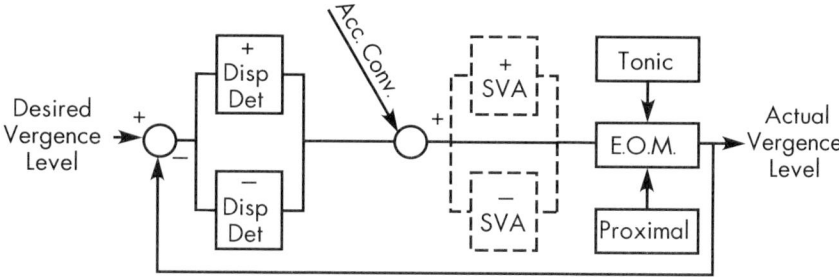

FIGURE 5-7 The left side of the diagram represents the desired vergence level, and the right side the actual vergence level. The task is to make the actual vergence level match the desired. The *line* running below the drawing from the right side returning back to the left represents the feedback of the output result into the input. The difference between the output and the input is computed at the *little circle* on the left and is fed as a disparity into the disparity detectors (*Disp det*). These exist as either crossed (+) or uncrossed (−). Here the signal is read for amount and direction and is then sent to the extraocular muscles (*E.O.M.*), which are also receiving signals from tonic and proximal innervation sources. The innervation for accommodative convergence (*Acc. Conv.*) enters into the system between the disparity detectors and the slow vergence adaptation (*SVA*) mechanisms. See the text for a discussion of the action of slow vergence adaptation mechanisms.

uncrossed (−) or the crossed (+) disparity detectors read the disparity for amount. The movement begins and is continuously tracked by comparing the actual vergence level with the desired vergence level. Think of it as subtracting the actual from the desired vergence level. In the example the amount of disparity should grow less as movement continues. The line going under the bottom of the drawing shows how the actual vergence position is fed back and subtracted from the desired vergence position. Since a subtraction is occurring, the process is called negative feedback. Obviously, when the difference between the actual and desired positions is zero the disparity is zero and the movement is complete.

In actual practice two other sources of innervation can be called upon to help move fixation from point *X* to point *Y*: accommodative convergence and proximal convergence inputs are indicated in Figure 5-7. The person has clinical orthophoria at this time if the sum total of the tonic, accommodative, and proximal innervation is exactly correct. No additional innervation is needed from the disparity vergence system for the person to have steady bifixation on point *Y*. If fusion is broken, the eyes will not move. But what if the sum total of tonic, accommodative, and proximal innervations is not exactly correct for the creation of orthophoria? The movement will then cease, with disparity remaining. The disparity detectors will read the disparity for direction and amount, and since the patient desires fixation a reflex disparity vergence movement will occur. If the disparity is brought to zero through the movement, first thought would suggest that the movement is complete and all is well. The problem is revealed as one realizes that the fixation disparity detectors must be emitting a steady amount of innervation to hold the eyes in that vergence position. The system provides for this small steady-state amount of innervation by leaving a little bit of disparity—called fixation disparity, as it is commonly thought of in a clinical setting. Thus we come to a pivotal concept: *Fixation disparity exists to provide a steady input of innervation that will hold fixation against the stress for misalignment*. Note that under steady-state (unchanging) conditions the input to the disparity detectors in Figure 5-7 is fixation disparity. Fixation disparity detectors require quite a bit of disparity input to provide a given amount of innervational output, and they also fatigue quickly. Therefore if the phoric amount is large, they must provide a large amount of innervation and are prone to fatigue.

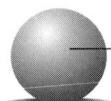

CLINICAL PEARL

Fixation disparity exists to provide a steady input of innervation that will hold fixation against the stress for misalignment.

Another mechanism is available to provide innervation to the extraocular muscles. Called the slow vergence adaptation mechanism, it is situated in a position to receive the innervation from disparity detectors and to multiply that innervation (Fig. 5-7). Normally it has a high output to input ratio and, compared to the disparity detectors, is resistant to fatigue. Actual cells have been found in the midbrain above the third nerve nucleus with characteristics that would lead one to suspect they are responsible for this mechanism.[10] Compared to the disparity detectors, however, the slow vergence adaptation mechanism is, as its name implies, slow (on the order of a few seconds) to respond.

When the disparity vergence movement as a whole is considered, it can be seen to consist of three integrated segments—first, the person becomes dissatisfied with his/her current vergence level; then, a psycho-optical response is invoked that causes retinal disparity to be read for amount and direction; and then, the resulting eye movement is tracked by negative feedback mechanisms until the total tonic, proximal, and accommodative innervations join the innervation produced by the disparity detectors to align the image within Panum's areas. If there is a large phoria, considerable fixation disparity must remain to provoke sufficient response from the disparity detectors. If this continues for more than a couple of seconds, the appropriate slow vergence adaptation mechanism begins to multiply its input from the disparity detectors and cause additional innervation to be created. The negative feedback mechanism then adjusts the input into the disparity detectors. As the innervation becomes increasingly furnished by the slow vergence adaptation mechanism, the fixation disparity can be reduced. Ultimately, a steady-state balance is worked out to provide the needed innervation with appropriate input from tonic, proximal, accommodative, disparity detector, and slow vergence mechanisms. Remember, however, that fixation disparity can be reduced to very little but it cannot be reduced to nothing if the slow vergence adaptation mechanism is going to receive a regulated input. And this is the reason why the concept of "neutralizing fixation disparity" is misleading. We should set as our goal in prescribing prism (or appropriate lenses, or appropriate vision therapy) for horizontal heterophorias the reduction and stabilization of fixation disparity, not its elimination. As a simplistic example, the first disparity-driven vergence movement of the day, as soon as a person awakens, should leave a large fixation disparity for a brief second or two while the slow vergence adaptation mechanism comes up to adequate output, and the disparity detectors power down to a small stable output and stay at that level all day. If this were exactly true, the near and far phorias would have to be the same. In reality the slow vergence adaptation mechanism does not easily lose its output with time even though its input ceases through monocular or even binocular (sleep) occlusion.[11]

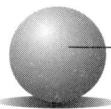

CLINICAL PEARL

Our goal in prescribing prism (or appropriate lenses, or appropriate vision therapy) for horizontal heterophorias is the reduction and stabilization of fixation disparity, not its elimination.

A similar but more simple process occurs with the accommodative mechanism (Fig. 5-8). Here the blur detectors detect a blur. Most probably the system is started in the proper direction by volition (blur has no directional sign) and the reduction in blur is monitored by a negative feedback mechanism. The process continues until input to the blur detectors (that is, blur) exactly provides the needed innervation to the ciliary muscle. (There is good reason to believe that a slow accommodative adaptation mechanism operates in a parallel fashion

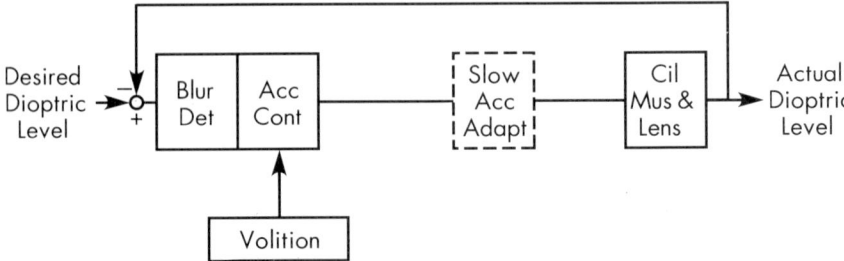

FIGURE 5-8 The left side represents the desired dioptric level, and the right side the actual dioptric level, of the accommodative mechanism. The difference is computed at the *little circle* on the left and is fed as a blur into the blur detectors (*Blur Det*), which report directly to the accommodative controller (*Acc Cont*). The controller also receives innervation from volition. The innervational output from the controller is sent to the ciliary muscle and lens (*Cil Mus & Lens*) and accommodative change is effected. The output is then monitored via the feedback line running from the *Actual* to the *Desired* sides of the diagram. The slow accommodative adaptation (*Slow Acc Adapt*), which is explained in the text, is represented by *dashed lines* because its effect is not yet understood.

to the slow vergence adaptation mechanism[12]; but since the characteristics of this mechanism are still under investigation, I will only mention it here.) The steady-state input to the blur detectors is provided by accommodative lag. Therefore, the reduction and stabilization of this lag, but not its elimination, should be a therapeutic goal. The concept of an accommodative mechanism is mentioned because both accommodation and disparity vergence must coordinate their actions in the final vergence movement.

Figure 5-9 is a clinically applicable working model of the whole system. Note that the two subsystems are related through the accommodative-convergence and convergence-accommodation linkages. Just as any accommodation change will cause a change in vergence state, so any disparity vergence change will cause a change in the state of accommodation. Further explanation is given later in this chapter.

Thus far, my comments have been confined mainly to static aspects. Dynamic (time-dependent) aspects must also be considered. A visual system may have a very powerful slow vergence adaptation mechanism; but if it takes minutes to build up to full power, it is of little practical use. A person may meet all the oculomotor diagnostic criteria thus far discussed but not be able to perform the visual tasks encountered in daily living. These people have difficulty with vergence facility; that is, they cannot quickly overcome a vergence change. Not Sheard's or Percival's or Morgan's diagnostics is equipped to detect dynamic vergence (that is, *facility*) problems.

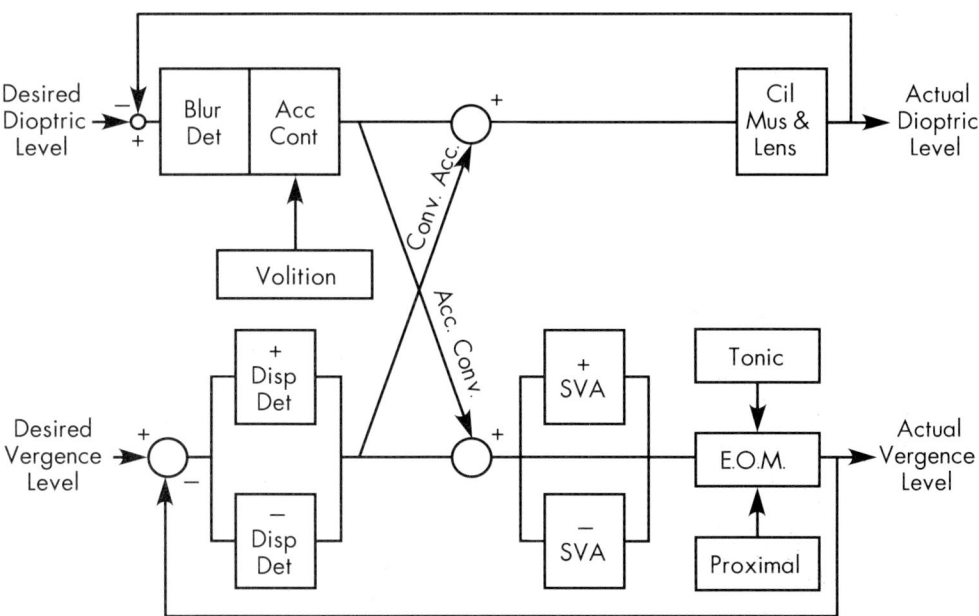

FIGURE 5-9 Figures 5-7 and 5-8 are combined. The connecting links are accommodative convergence and convergence accommodation. The resulting diagram can be thought of as a physiological model, because its implications constitute known actions of the actual physiological system. Although a physiological model does not have to have an exact anatomical correlate to be useful, this one does have sufficient correlation to be appealing to the practical mind of a clinician.

Vergence facility testing can be done[13] and will provide a measure of the dynamic aspects.

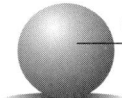

CLINICAL PEARL

Not Sheard's or Percival's or Morgan's diagnostics is equipped to detect vergence facility problems.

Forced-vergence fixation disparity curves (see the appendix at the end of this chapter) can also be used. Because of the time constraint in operation during measurement of a fixation disparity curve, a facility problem will show up as a steepening of the curve, often accompanied by a large amount of fixation disparity. The rule to remember is that in taking the data for a fixation disparity curve, be sure to determine the fixation disparity within 15 seconds of prism insertion or else remove the prism for 15 seconds before refining the measurement.

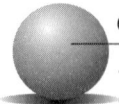

CLINICAL PEARL

In taking the data for a fixation disparity curve, be sure to determine the fixation disparity within 15 seconds of prism insertion or else remove the prism for 15 seconds before refining the measurement.

To understand the pathophysiology of the system, you should ask, what might go wrong? Study of Figure 5-9 will help answer the question. If the disparity detectors are not processing the disparity information properly, automatic regulation of the disparity vergence mechanism will not occur. Certainly suppression (and therefore anything that stimulates suppression) will be a problem. If the slow vergence adaptation mechanism is not operating properly with respect to either static or dynamic aspects, undue demands are made on the disparity detectors and fixation disparity increases. If it increases too much, the process becomes self-defeating because of the size of the central Panum areas.[14] On the accommodative side, nonrecognition of the blur signal will reduce accommodative convergence, and therefore the need for disparity vergence innervation will change, very probably putting additional demands on the disparity detectors. Any lack of stability in the slow accommodative adaptation mechanism will also cause a change in the innervation pattern of the disparity vergence mechanism.

General Concepts of Prism Prescription

Before the clinician even thinks of prescribing prism or vision therapy, a careful refraction should be performed. Quite often, just clearing up and balancing the retinal images will strengthen the oculomotor system sufficiently for it to overcome the stresses put upon it. As the saying goes, "Hang glass first!" The problem is that the system often takes time to adjust to the improved sensory input, and a quick phoria test or vergence measurement performed immediately after determining and providing the refractive correction may be misleading. What will the system be like after wearing the appropriate refractive correction for 2 or 3 weeks? A common example often occurs in preteen children who have gained a diopter or two of myopia since their last glasses were prescribed. At near, their habitual prescription has been seriously under-minused, which has created a near exophoria (because of the loss of accommodative convergence) and necessitated the use of considerable positive disparity vergence. The patient develops the habit of "turning on" a certain amount of positive disparity vergence when a near task is to be performed. Because of this habit, merely removing the need for a disparity vergence does not itself remove the vergence. The near phoria measurement becomes less exo (or more eso) than it will be 2 or 3 weeks later after the habit has had time to wear off. Vergence ranges also shift toward divergence as the habit disappears. Similar scenarios can occur when latent hyperopia is corrected; in this case the initial oculomotor testing will show less eso than will be apparent later. These changes of habit are, of course, largely due to readjustment of the adaptation mechanisms in the accommodative and in the disparity vergence systems.

CLINICAL PEARL

Before prescribing prism or vision therapy, perform a careful refraction. Quite often, just clearing up and balancing the retinal images will strengthen the oculomotor system sufficiently for it to overcome the stresses put upon it.

In 1977 Sheedy and Saladin[15] published a paper in which they measured the phorias, vergences, and fixation disparity curves of 28 optometry students without symptoms and 32 orthoptic clinic patients who had symptoms. They used stepwise discriminant analysis to determine which clinical measures were the best discriminators between symptomatic and asymptomatic esophores and exophores. Sheard's criterion, followed by the angular amount of fixation disparity, was most valuable in dealing with exophores; and in dealing with esophores the absolute value of the phoria, followed by the slope of the fixation disparity curve, was most instructive.

This type of statistical question makes sense from a clinical point of view, because if the clinician is going to perform two tests he/she will want to perform tests that offer different information. For instance, *Sheard's criterion* by itself did an excellent job of separating the symptomatic from the asymptomatic in exophores; but when it was misleading or indecisive, the *angular amount of fixation disparity* did a good job separating out the remaining cases. This suggests that the fixation disparity amount was measuring some aspect of horizontal oculomotor balance that was not ascertained by a phoria-vergence comparison. In contrast, for esophores, the *absolute amount of the phoria* was most discriminative (that is, the greater the esophoria, the greater the probability that the patient would be symptomatic); but when it was misleading or indecisive, the *slope of the fixation disparity curve* was the test most likely to offer new information. Once again, fixation disparity had within it some measure of oculomotor dysfunction above and beyond that indicated by the phoria, although the phoria itself had an input into the fixation disparity measurement. Practically speaking, the clinician could apply this knowledge by using Sheard's

criterion on exophores and taking a simple phoria measure on esophores. If a patient is symptomatic, the failure to meet Sheard's
criterion in an exophore or the possession of significant deviation in
an esophore will essentially answer the diagnostic question. If an
exophoric patient were symptomatic but met Sheard's criterion, or an
esophoric patient had much stronger symptoms than seemed justified
by the phoric amount (a clinical judgment), then a fixation disparity
curve would be the next test to perform. And it might very likely
show an abnormality.

A third clinical measure, the *vergence recovery value*, was also found
to be highly significant in esophores. The third variable in exophores,
however, was the *prism neutralization of fixation disparity* (but its
significance was not high). A study of the relevant diagnostic variables for exophores and esophores gives scientific credence to what
clinicians have known empirically for years—esophoria cannot be
thought of as the mirror image of exophoria for diagnostic purposes.
This lack of symmetry also holds for the management of esophoria
and exophoria. The Sheedy-Saladin study gave some statistical credence to the classic 2/1 base-out vergence range–to–exophoria ratio
given by the Sheard criterion. The ratio based on the data in this study
was 2.1/1. Since Sheard[4] purportedly used only a clinical estimate to
set that ratio, he was proven to be remarkably prescient.

CLINICAL PEARL

*If a patient is symptomatic, the failure to meet Sheard's criterion for an
exophore or the possession of significant deviation for an esophore will
essentially answer the diagnostic question.*

Because the method of case selection may have biased the symptomatic group in their 1977 paper, Sheedy and Saladin[16] redid that
study with a new group of subjects and reported these results in a
1978 paper. In the new paper the subjects were all taken from one
population, a group of optometry students, but because this was a
nonclinical population, the strength of symptoms (and therefore of the
clinical signs) was undoubtedly less. Of the 103 subjects, 33 had
definite symptoms, 44 no symptoms, and 26 marginal symptoms. In
an attempt to sharpen the statistical difference, this marginal group
was removed from the study. Once again, Sheard's criterion was the
overall best test for discrimination and was much better for exophores
than for esophores. In this study Percival's criterion was good for
esophores but it was a Percival's based on break or recovery, not the
conventional Percival's using the blur vergence findings. The fixation
disparity variables were good second-line choices for tests. Again,

however, they appeared to be testing something a bit different from whatever the phorias and vergences were testing. The fixation disparity variables of most use were the curve type, slope, and angular amount of fixation disparity.

With all these data, one would think that if a patient presents with common symptoms (headache, difficulty focusing, rubbing eyes, sleepiness, etc.), is exophoric, and does not meet Sheard's criterion, it would be necessary only to prescribe prism to meet Sheard's criterion to produce a successful case. Worrell, Hirsch, and Morgan[17] put this idea to the test and found that such an application of Sheard's criterion was anything but universally successful. In fact, only the subjects who were presbyopic exophores wearing bifocals at near gave any preference for the prism. In contrast, esophores preferred base-out prism, and the greater the esophoria the greater was their preference. Why the seeming inconsistency? Worrell et al.[17] prescribed the prism to 1/3 Δ, which meant that they were probably dealing with small amounts of prism. Prescribing to 1/3 Δ implies that there are some steep cutoffs between the symptomatic and asymptomatic patients as far as oculomotor imbalance is concerned. The data of Worrell et al. would seem to imply that the cutoff is much more steep for esophores than for exophores. A clinician should not expect 1 or 2 Δ of base-in prism (prescribed to meet Sheard's criterion) to create a happy patient out of a symptomatic exophore. Although a small amount of prism may be significant for an esophore, it is the presence of the prism that helps not whether it was prescribed by Sheard's criterion, Percival's criterion, or any other prescription scheme. Sheard's and Percival's criteria, along with comparison to Morgan's norms, are better diagnostic than therapeutic standards. They tell the practitioner when the symptoms match the signs sufficiently for there to be reasonable expectation of some cause-and-effect relationship. If a person gets sleepy after reading for 15 minutes, and has 8 Δ of exophoria at near with only 6 Δ of base-out vergence–to–blur, then oculomotor dysfunction is a very real possibility as a cause for the sleepiness. If Sheard's criterion can be met with 3.5 Δ of base-in prism, would 3 Δ be inadequate and 3.5 translate the patient to oculomotor Nirvana? Of course not! If prism were going to help, 2 Δ would help a little bit and 4 Δ would help even more. The patient's response to the prism will depend on his/her asthenopia threshold and on other aspects of the oculomotor balance that are not described in phoria-opposing vergence comparisons.

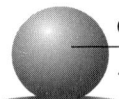

CLINICAL PEARL

Sheard's and Percivals's criteria, along with comparison to Morgan's norms, are better diagnostic than therapeutic standards.

What are the aspects of oculomotor balance that are (and are not) reflected in phoria-opposing vergence comparisons? The heterophoric amount describes the load (stress) put on the disparity vergence system. The opposing vergence is a measure of the system's fusional reserve ability, as Sheard suggested, but that merely names the phenomenon; it does not explain it. A complete understanding of the vergence system is beyond the scope of this chapter and is not really needed here. What the clinician needs is a way to estimate *how* the disparity vergence system is coping with the stress put on the system by the phoria (and any other sources of stress). Earlier in this chapter I explained that the disparity vergence system is self-regulating, that the accommodative system is self-regulating, and that the two act together in mutual self-regulation through the accommodative-convergence and convergence-accommodation linkages (Fig. 5-9). The fixation disparity necessary to support a disparity vergence system can be looked upon as a gauge showing how well the system is operating. If very little fixation disparity is being required, the system is not being strained. If a large amount of fixation disparity is present, the system is being strained. One person's oculomotor system may be able to support 8 Δ of exophoria with little fixation disparity while another's may need considerable fixation disparity to support it.

Figure 5-10 is a function based on data from Ogle[18] (and reinforced by my clinical experience) showing the average amounts of fixation disparity needed to support a given esophoria and exophoria. Note that it is linear, with a steep slope on the esophoria side, but is decidedly less steep and less linear on the exophoria side. As a rule, under the fixation disparity testing conditions (largely dependent on the 1.5° diameter fusion locks) used by Ogle[18] and by Sheedy and Saladin,[15] it takes about 1 minute of arc or slightly more of fixation disparity to support 1 Δ of esophoria but much less to support 1 Δ of exophoria. Now one can understand why Sheedy and Saladin[15] found that the phoric amount was a good indicator of stress on the system for esophores—stress increases fairly linearly with the amount of the esophoria. It also presents a good idea (though not a complete idea) of how to prescribe prism for esophores: any amount of base-out prism up to the phoric amount will help. Certainly one would want to reduce the fixation disparity to within the limits of central Panum's areas, which have working radius of 3 to 4 minutes of arc.

Why is the exo side of the function in Figure 5-10 different from the eso side? It would seem that, as a rule, it takes much less exo fixation disparity to support 1 Δ of exophoria than is the case for eso fixation disparity and esophoria. The difference lies in the slow vergence adaptation mechanisms. The positive (exo disparity) system is inherently more powerful than the negative system. This should come as no surprise to optometrists—it is common knowledge that the average base-in vergence finding is much less than the base-out finding

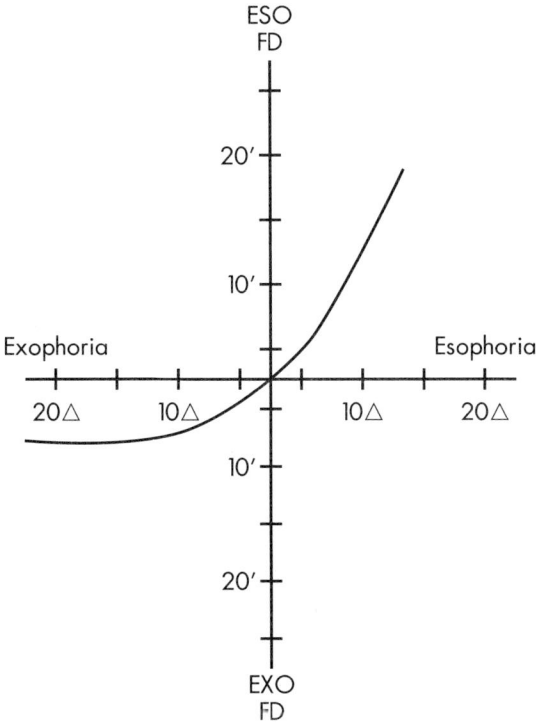

FIGURE 5-10 The amount and direction of dissociated phoria with the accompanying fixation disparity angle. Note the linear relationship between fixation disparity *(FD)* and the phoric amount on the esophoric *(right)* side of the graph. Each prism diopter of esophoria is associated with slightly more than 1 minute of arc of eso fixation disparity. On the exophoric *(left)* side a small amount of exo fixation disparity is associated with a broad range of exophoric amounts. (Modified from Ogle KN: *Binocular vision,* New York, 1964, Hafner, p 75.)

and the base-out side is more easily expandable with orthoptics than the base-in side. The output/input ratio for the positive slow vergence adaptation mechanism seems inherently better than that for the negative slow vergence adaptation mechanism. So, the innervation to extraocular muscles must come much more from the disparity detectors, in the case of esophoria, and much less from those detectors in the case of exophoria. How can one test for the strength of negative or uncrossed disparity detectors in esophores when one does not have a device to measure fixation disparity? The answer is, "Look at the vergence recovery findings." I use the 1:1 rule: a 1 Δ esophore should be able to fuse 1 Δ of base-in, a 2 Δ esophore, 2 Δ of base-in, etc., when the prism is inserted. I prefer to use individual prisms with rapid insertion rather than Risley prisms with a more gradual ramp-type insertion. Quite often, in uncomplicated cases, I prescribe sufficient prism to meet this 1:1 rule, offering as statistical support the fact that the vergence recovery finding was very high on the list of important parameters in both Sheedy-Saladin papers.[15,16] At any rate, any amount of base-out prism, up to the phoric amount, will help. And this brings up the question as to why a variant of Percival's criterion worked and Sheard's did not for esophores. Percival's criterion induces some (moderate) amount of base-in vergence ability on the system; it cannot be met without at least some base-in vergence ability, since the greater the esophoria usually the greater will be the *base-out* vergence ability and the greater then must be the *base-in* vergence ability to meet that criterion. Sheard's criterion is inadequate for esophores because it is based on the blur finding and can be met with little or no base-in recovery.

Sheard's criterion is determined by comparing the phoric amount (determined usually by the von Graefe or Maddox rod method) to the base-out–to–blur finding determined with Risley prisms. Thus the situation is set up for a ramp vergence stimulus that is almost perfect for testing the slow vergence adaptation system. If the slow vergence adaptation system is functioning properly, fixation disparity need not change or at most need change only very little. This explains the exo side of Figure 5-10. I have already established that the positive side of the disparity vergence system relies mainly on the slow vergence adaptation system. Sheard's criterion is largely a function of this system and therefore is ideal for testing the patency of the positive disparity vergence system.

A forced-vergence fixation disparity curve shows how the system will function as the vergence load on the disparity vergence system varies. Unless the amount of phoria is constant at all distances, the load on the vergence system must vary with the fixation distance. The slope of the fixation disparity curve is an indicator of how the system can manage changes in phoria or (synonymously here) load. It is my contention that a major source of asthenopia is overuse or misuse of the disparity detectors. If the slope of the curve is steep, then fixation disparity is changing to provide varied innervation to the extraocular muscles. The slow vergence adaptation mechanism is not reacting at all, or is not reacting quickly enough, to provide adequate relief. If sufficient prism is prescribed to lessen the fixation disparity to a comfortable level but the curve is steep, the prism prescription should be of some help although it will not relieve all the symptoms. Later in the chapter the difference in management of basic exo and convergence insufficiency cases will provide an example.

The next aspect of a fixation disparity curve that has diagnostic significance is the curve type (Fig. 5-11). *Type I* is the expected; it shows the functioning of both eso and exo disparity detectors[19] by the presence of an upsweep on the left side and a downsweep on the right

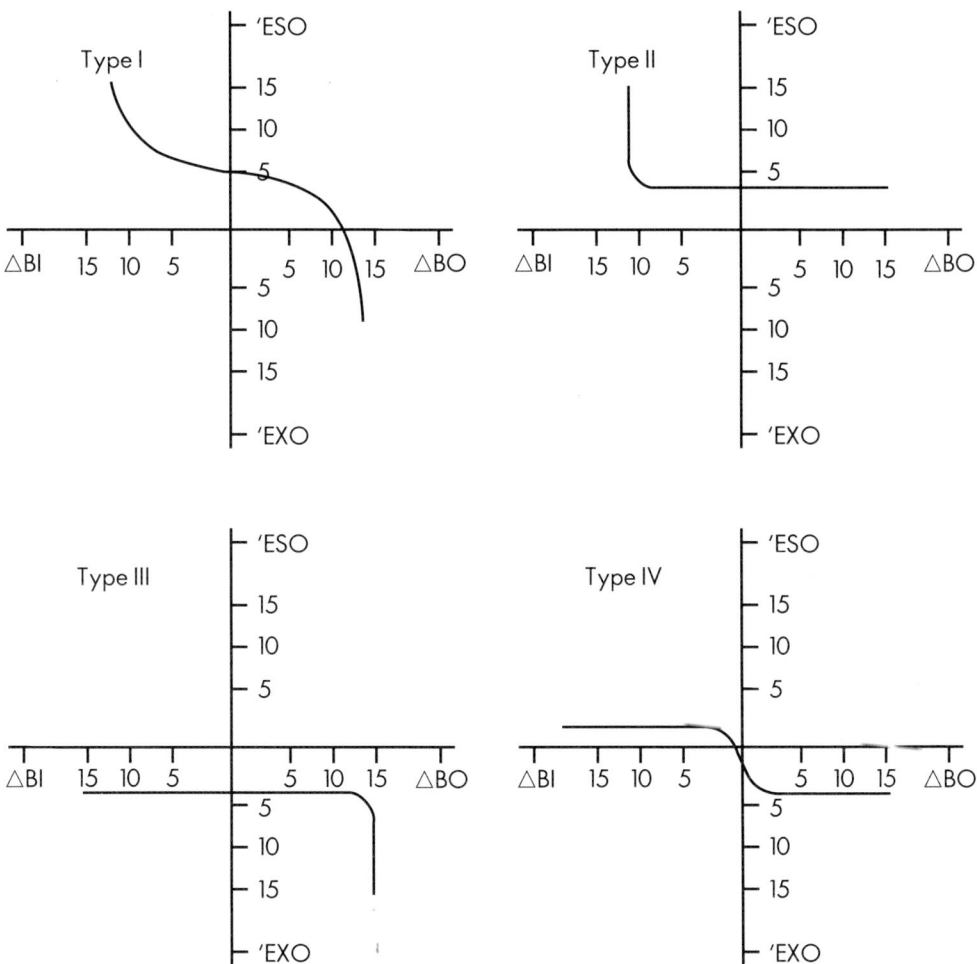

FIGURE 5-11 The forced-vergence fixation disparity curve types as described by Ogle.[18]

side of the curve. Any functioning of the slow vergence adaptation mechanisms will be shown by the presence of a middle, flatter portion of the curve between the upsweep and the downsweep. *Type II* curves are associated with esophorias and indicate a lack of exo disparity detector function. The disparity vergence system in these patients operates by varying the amount of eso fixation disparity. There is no intercept on the horizontal axis. For Type II curve cases the goal of prism prescription is to reduce fixation disparity to acceptable limits (as little eso fixation disparity as possible) and then provide some base-in and base-out slow vergence adaptation. This is another way of saying "Prescribe to a flat spot on the curve." It has been my clinical experience that such patients are never completely satisfied—residual symptoms remain. Because of the natural limitations on the negative disparity system, that system never seems as good as the positive. Type II curves indicate that the prognosis for vision therapy management is not good. In another paper,[20] my co-workers and I explain how the best stereopsis scores occur with a slight bit of exophoria. Any esophoria compromises the stereoscopic threshold.[21] Because of the close association between disparity vergence systems and stereopsis, I offer the idea that what holds for stereopsis will also be relevant for the disparity vergence system.

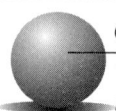

CLINICAL PEARL

Type II fixation disparity curves indicate that the prognosis for vision therapy management is not good. In contrast, a prism prescription is not particularly desirable for Type III and Type IV cases because vision therapy has such a good record of success.

Type III systems are almost always associated with exophorias and suggest a lack of eso disparity detector function. For these cases, prism prescription is not particularly desirable because vision therapy has such a good record of success. A comparatively modest investment in vision therapy will almost always convert a Type III to a Type I, and the patient's symptoms will abate. Prism prescribed to a flatter (and necessarily lesser exo fixation disparity) can be prescribed, but it is supportive, not curative. The question remains unanswered in my mind as to why Type III curves can so easily be converted into Type I curves but Type II curves cannot.

A *Type IV* curve indicates that the reflex nature of the fusional vergence system has been sorely compromised. I believe that the person is using volition to align the eyes and thus to replace the automatic reflex-driven accommodative and disparity vergence systems. These patients will tell you that they consciously aim their eyes. Vision therapy to restore the reflex nature of the oculomotor system (both disparity *and* accommodative vergence) will create an asymptomatic patient with a normal Type I curve. Once again, prism prescription is not indicated because it does not address the problem.

Neutralization of fixation disparity by the appropriate choice of lenses or prism can sometimes work; but it works because fixation disparity is reduced and stabilized, not because fixation disparity has been neutralized. Obviously, when the fixation disparity has been neutralized it has been reduced to a minimum, but there is a theoretical gulf between the two approaches. Note that the Sheedy-Saladin studies[15,16] both showed that it was the angular amount of fixation disparity in minutes of arc that was the better discriminator, not the amount of prism required for neutralization of the fixation disparity. As stated before, the goal is to reduce and stabilize fixation disparity to a reasonable amount, not eliminate it. The aspects that are missing when one tries to simply minimize or neutralize fixation disparity are the fixation disparity curve slope and type. To the extent that curve slope and type are relevant in a particular case, prism prescription by either fixation disparity reduction or neutralization has problems.

Study of the fixation disparity curves of exophores[22] has revealed the reason why Sheard's criterion often fails for small-angle exophores but seems to be much more reliable for large angle exophores. It is because the small base-out vergence amount required to meet this criterion for small amounts (<4 Δ) of exophoria can be composed almost entirely of voluntary accommodative convergence. No real disparity-driven vergence need be involved. In these small-angle cases, 2 or 3 Δ of base-out vergence stimulus would cause an immediate and precipitous drop-off toward exo fixation disparity. Now that this principle is understood, a clinician need not necessarily measure a fixation disparity curve on a small-angle exophore with symptoms but can simply realize that the patient does have an oculomotor imbalance, even though Sheard's criterion is met, and then act accordingly. As will be seen in the next section, the patient can be treated for having poor positive disparity vergence ability.

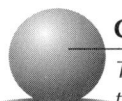

CLINICAL PEARL

The reason why Sheard's criterion often fails for small-angle exophores is that the base-out vergence amount required to meet this criterion can be composed almost entirely of voluntary accommodative convergence.

Duane-White Syndrome Interpretation

Horizontal oculomotor imbalance will respond to prism prescription depending on the type of imbalance. Although the Duane-White classification system for horizontal imbalance has some conceptual flaws as originally proposed, the modern interpretation is workable and is commonly used as a method to classify *static* horizontal oculomotor imbalances. Dynamic (time-dependent) factors are not commonly considered in making a Duane-White diagnosis. Syndromes that require exophoria at distance are convergence insufficiency, basic exo, and divergence excess—depending upon whether the AC/A ratio is low ($<4/1$), normal ($4/1$ to $6/1$), or high ($>6/1$). Syndromes that require esophoria at distance are divergence insufficiency, basic esophoria, and convergence excess—again depending on whether the AC/A ratio is low, normal, or high. (See Wick[23] for a modern optometric interpretation of these syndromes.)

The most common Duane-White syndrome is convergence insufficiency. These patients do not respond consistently to prism prescription for the relief of their symptoms. Roy and Saladin (unpublished observations) subjected six patients with convergence insufficiency to a 30-minute reading task. A fixation disparity curve was performed on all six before and after the task. The fixation disparity curves showed an increased fixation disparity on the base-out side, as would be predicted from fatigue effects. At another time the patients wore 4 Δ of base-in prism and the entire sequence was repeated. After accounting for 2 Δ of latent exophoria, the averaged fixation disparity curve showed improvement when the before and after curves were compared to those curves done without the base-in prism. Subjectively, the patients reported no improvement with the base-in prism. Although the Worrell, Hirsch, and Morgan[17] study was not specific to convergence insufficiency, it did agree with the Roy and Saladin study. The mark of a convergent insufficient fixation disparity curve[19] is a sharp drop-off on the base-out side (Fig. 5-12). Quite often there is an accompanying large exo fixation disparity. If the prism can reduce this to normal amounts (< 6 minutes of exo fixation disparity with a 1.5° fusion lock), an improvement may be experienced by the patient. If, however, the slow vergence adaptation mechanism is slow in reacting, or the patient has learned to habitually substitute voluntary accommodative convergence for positive disparity vergence, the prism will not be corrective. At any rate, the prescription of base-in prism for convergence insufficiency is not the desired approach. The condition is readily treated with vision therapy, which may be corrective, while a prism prescription is merely supportive.

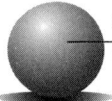

CLINICAL PEARL

The prescription of base-in prism for convergence insufficiency is not the desired approach. The condition is readily treated with vision therapy, which may be corrective, while a prism prescription is merely supportive.

Uncomplicated basic exophoria can be treated with prisms. Often there is considerable positive slow-vergence ability available. If prism is prescribed according to Sheard's criterion, the origin of the fixation disparity curve will be moved to the left by the amount of the prism and the whole curve will move upward because less fixation disparity is needed. The complications begin when a latent exophoria exists.[22] An indication of latent exophoria can be detected by observing a large flat spot in the curve on the *base-in* side past the amount of the

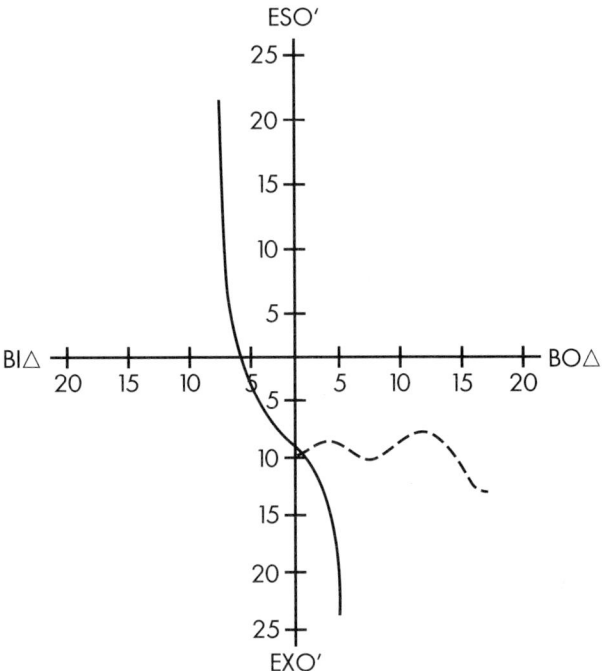

FIGURE 5-12 The forced-vergence fixation disparity curve of a convergent-insufficient patient. Note the steep slope and the large fixation disparity at the vertical axis intercept, along with the drop-off on the base-out side. The drop-off means that there is very little positive slow vergence adaptation occurring under the testing conditions. The *dashed line* shows what usually happens to the curve if the patient uses volition to support convergence as a base-out prism is applied.

manifest exophoria (Fig. 5-13). Why should a large base-in vergence ability develop in an exophore? There certainly is no teleological need for it. The explanation is that the apparent flat spot in the curve on the base-in side is not active stimulation of the *negative* slow vergence adaptation mechanism but rather is relaxation of the *positive* slow-vergence adaptation mechanism; hence the latent exophoria. If a latent exophoria exists, any clinically reasonable amount of long-term prism (6 Δ at most) will probably be insufficient to satisfy the patient's needs. As in patients with convergence insufficiency, it is better then to use vision therapy than base-in prism. Vision therapy will also be needed if the patient has learned to substitute voluntary accommodative convergence for real positive disparity vergence. Here the reflex operation of both the disparity vergence mechanism and the blur-driven accommodative mechanism have to be restored.[19]

The forced-vergence cover test is a way to test for latent exophoria when a fixation disparity curve method or occlusion is not a viable

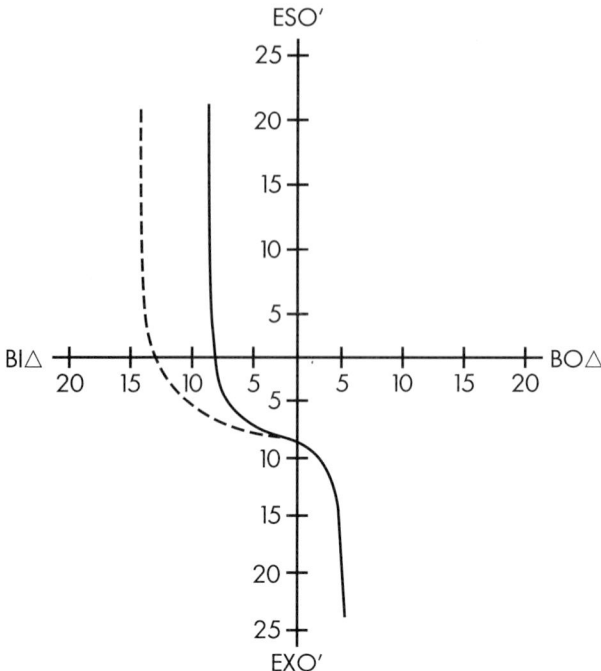

FIGURE 5-13 The *continuous line* represents the fixation disparity curve of a typical 6 or 7 Δ exophore. Note that there is a base-in width to the curve of about the amount of the exophoria; in other words, the fixation disparity neutralizes (horizontal axis intercept) at about the same amount as the exophoria. There remains very little base-out width to the curve; thus the curve drops off quite rapidly as base-out prism is applied. This patient should be symptomatic. The *dashed line* changes the curve to one suggesting that a latent exophoria exists. Now the prism neutralization point is considerably larger than the exophoric amount.

alternative. It is a variant of the alternate cover test at distance: neutralize the exo movement with base-in prism and let the patient look about the room through the prism for at least 20 seconds; then redo the alternate cover test, and if movement of the eyes is still neutralized or an exo movement is seen add 2 Δ of base-in. It is very important not to let the patient see without having to fuse through the prism. Have the patient look about the room through the increased amount of base-in prism for at least 20 seconds and then perform the alternate cover test again. If no movement or exo movement is seen, increase the prism by another 2 Δ, have the patient fuse for 20 seconds, and repeat the cover test. This process should be continued until eso movement is seen on the cover test, and then the previous amount of base-in prism is inserted. The beginning amount of exophoria and another 4 Δ is subtracted; the *remaining* base-in prism will be a measure of the amount of latent exo. Clinical experience has shown that a normal person has about 4 Δ of adaptation on this test, which is why the additional 4 Δ are subtracted. Recently Sethi and North[24] found that the most any of four normal subjects would adapt to base-in prism was 4 Δ (with 15 seconds of adaptation time); this lent some published evidence to the use of 4 Δ of expected normal base-in adaptation. I consider any latency of more than the normal 4 Δ to be diagnostically significant and also that, if prism is to be prescribed, it will have to be prescribed in an amount that is probably impractical. Therefore latent exophoria is an indicator for vision therapy rather than a prism correction.

CLINICAL PEARL

The presence of a latent exophoria in a patient with a basic exophoria is an indicator for vision therapy rather than a prism correction. If a latent exophoria is absent, prescribe sufficient prism to meet Sheard's criterion.

Divergence excess patients present a special challenge in that they actually have two problems. The first is the large excess exo posture at distance, and the second is the high AC/A ratio. High AC/A ratios severely stress the oculomotor system because they change the load on the disparity vergence system as fixation distance is changed; thus the disparity detectors are constantly having to adjust their output and are therefore subject to fatigue. High AC/A ratios also magnify the effect of accommodative system noise on the disparity vergence system through the accommodative convergence link. This must be tracked and countered by the fixation disparity detectors, thereby putting even more fatigue pressure on those detectors. High AC/A patients require more plus power for near tasks to reduce the change in their accommodative convergence as fixation distance is changed. This puts the state of accommodation closer to the dark focus, where noise in the accommodative system is apt to be less. Bifocals are a better choice than reading glasses because the add is always available. An add sufficient to make the near and far phorias approximately equal is almost mandatory, and then the patient can be treated as a basic exo. Base-in prism to meet Sheard's criterion should be acceptable, provided a latent exophoria does not exist and the patient continues to rely on a reflex blur drive rather than on volition for the accommodative mechanism. If the amount of prism needed is too large to be practical for long-term wear, vision therapy may be used to augment the prism prescription approach. Over-minusing the distance prescription may help temporarily to build sensory fusion but should not be thought of as a long-term solution.

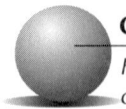

CLINICAL PEARL

High AC/A patients require relative convex power for near tasks to reduce the change in their accommodative convergence as fixation distance is changed. The convex power also puts the state of accommodation closer to the dark focus, where noise in the accommodative system is apt to be less. Bifocals are a better choice than reading glasses, because the add is always available.

Convergence excess (eso at distance with a high AC/A ratio) must be managed with a bifocal or at least a special near prescription that will reduce the esophoria at near. Here again, the high AC/A ratio must be dealt with. Prism prescription at near to reduce the esophoria will not produce the same physiological situation that a near add will, even though the amount of remaining esophoria may be the same. The only reason to prescribe prism in a convergence excess case is to relieve a basic esophoric posture at distance. Then, once the near add is in place, the patient can be treated as a basic eso.

I readily prescribe base-out prism for basic eso patients, particularly if they are already wearing glasses. A moderate amount of base-out prism can dramatically reduce symptoms. As a rule, the more base-out prescribed, up to the phoric amount, the better the patient will like it, provided other considerations (like distortion, weight, and cosmesis) do not become a problem. This is in keeping with the results of Sheedy and Saladin's studies.[15,16]

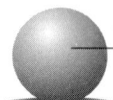

CLINICAL PEARL

A moderate amount of base-out prism for basic eso patients can dramatically reduce symptoms.

Since one usually does not want to prescribe more prism than is necessary, how much is necessary? The 1:1 rule is good to follow: prescribe sufficient prism that the patient has 1 Δ of base-in recovery for each prism diopter of esophoria. For instance (Fig. 5-14), suppose a patient has 6 Δ of esophoria with only 2 Δ of base-in recovery; 2 Δ of base-out prism would reduce the phoria by 2 and increase the base-in recovery by 2, leaving 4 Δ of esophoria and 4 Δ of base-in recovery through the prism. Thus 2 Δ of base-out prism would be the minimum but more would be better, up to a maximum of 6 Δ. As additional information, the optometrist can overprescribe base-out prism, within reason, for an esophore and keep a satisfied patient; but if base-in is overprescribed for an exophore, a decidedly unhappy patient will likely result.

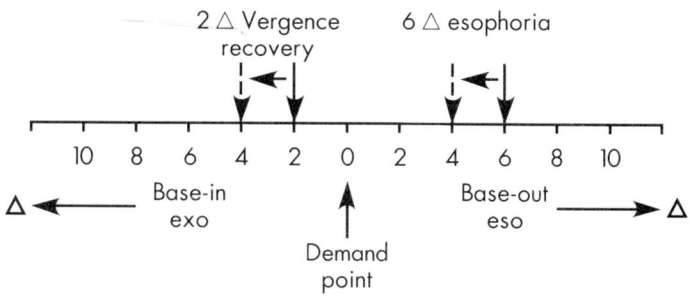

FIGURE 5-14 The 1:1 esophoria to base-in recovery rule. In this example the patient has a 6 Δ esophoria with 2 Δ of base-in recovery. Two prism diopters of base-out prism in the prescription should reduce the phoria by 2 Δ and increase the recovery by 2 Δ.

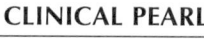

CLINICAL PEARL

The optometrist can overprescribe base-out prism, within reason, for an esophore and keep a satisfied patient; but if base-in is overprescribed for an exophore, a decidedly unhappy patient will likely result.

In the case of divergence insufficiency (eso at distance with a low AC/A ratio), the patient's complaint is often about distance vision. Prescribe sufficient prism to meet the 1:1 criterion at distance. It has been my experience that patients seem to have little trouble with near vision if the amount of base-out prism that must be prescribed to solve the distance problem creates a slight exophoria at near.

At times, a vertical phoria complicates what would otherwise be a simple Duane-White case. I prefer to give the vertical phoria a higher priority for prism prescription than the horizontal; in other words, make sure the vertical problem is taken care of before horizontal prism or horizontal vision therapy is prescribed.

CLINICAL PEARL

Give the vertical phoria a higher priority for prism prescription than the horizontal; in other words, make sure the vertical problem is taken care of before horizontal prism or horizontal vision therapy is prescribed.

If vertical prism cannot be prescribed in the amount needed (see Chapter 6), for whatever reason, the wisest course is to attend to any refractive error and treat the horizontal problem vigorously.[25] Be aware that exophorias greater than 12 to 15 Δ are almost always accompanied by a *false* (that is, secondary) vertical phoria, which is false because it is not there when the eyes are in the fused condition, but is there when the nonfixating eye assumes the exophoric position during a von Graefe or Maddox rod phoria measurement. Check for this type of phoria by measuring the vertical fixation disparity. If the phoria is false, there will be no vertical disparity; if it is *true* (that is, primary) a vertical disparity will be present.

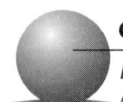

CLINICAL PEARL

Exophorias greater than 12 to 15 Δ are almost always accompanied by a false (that is, secondary) vertical phoria. Check for this by measuring the vertical fixation disparity. If the phoria is false, there will be no vertical disparity; if it is true (that is, primary), a vertical disparity will be present.

Additional Considerations

Thus far, dynamic problems have been mentioned only in the pathophysiology section of this chapter. Remember: dynamic problems are concerned with facility—both vergence facility and accommodative facility. In other words, the response is adequate in amplitude but slow or subject to fatigue. It would seem obvious that such problems are, by their very nature, not particularly amenable to prism (or lens) therapy. If a patient has a facility problem alone, not in conjunction with a static problem, the preferred treatment is vision therapy. An exception would occur when a facility problem is secondary to a static problem. For instance, a basic exo deviation could be the root condition, with a facility problem part of the sequelae.

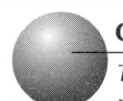

CLINICAL PEARL

The difference between static and dynamic problems is that static problems are more likely treatable with prism, dynamic problems with vision therapy.

The possibility of an anisophoria is always present but frequently forgotten. The patient usually reads in slight downgaze, and we tend to test from the primary position of gaze. A disagreement can therefore result between the patient's symptoms and the signs gathered by the optometric tests. Patients suspected of having oculomotor dysfunction should always be checked for anisophoria. If it is found, prism can be prescribed for the condition at the preferred gaze angle, and perhaps in a task-specific spectacle form, but a general skills vision therapy program will likely be more appropriate.

Inexperienced clinicians are often bothered by the observation that introducing convex power for the compensation of presbyopia brings with it greater exophoria at near. Often Sheard's criterion is not met and the data lie outside standard norms. In 1864, Donders[26] noted that corrected presbyopes seldom made complaints about their near vision that could be blamed on binocular difficulties. Morgan and Peters[27] stated that only rarely does a presbyope complain of asthenopia. Sheedy and Saladin[28] showed that there was indeed a difference in the muscle balance at near between presbyopes and nonpresbyopes if the muscle balance was ascertained in the usual phoria-vergence manner; but, curiously, there was no difference as to asthenopic symptoms. The clue to the difference lay in a comparison of the fixation disparity curves. When the curves for both groups were taken through +2.50 D lenses, they were definitely flatter. By a system of elimination, the authors concluded that presbyopes were using accommodative convergence innervation to overcome the exophoria while nonpresbyopes were being forced to rely on disparity vergence. Therefore the presbyopes were "playing the game of binocularity" differently from the way nonpresbyopes did because they could use accommodative convergence without having to concern themselves with a change in accommodation. They had learned the "trick" of using accommodative convergence in lieu of disparity vergence. It has been my clinical experience that beginning presbyopes (up to a +1.50 add) may have asthenopia or even diplopia when they first wear bifocals. They may have to be taught to use voluntary convergence to overcome the exophoria. This small amount of vision therapy is preferrable to the time and expense of trying to obtain prism in the bifocal segment. Prism is not a good idea here unless the patient has significant exophoria at distance.

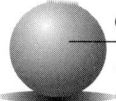

CLINICAL PEARL

For beginning presbyopes whose exophoria at near causes asthenopia or diplopia with bifocal correction, prism is not a good idea; vision therapy is the preferred treatment.

If the conventional tests for near-point balance are inappropriate for presbyopes, what can be used? The clinical question is "Will the patient experience diplopia through the intended near-point prescription?" I check by doing a slow alternate cover test through the intended near-point prescription with the patient reading. As the cover paddle is moved from eye to eye several times, the amount of exo movement often builds. When it seems to reach a steady amount, I remove the cover paddle and look for recovery of fusion. If a fusion movement is seen, then the patient has used either disparity vergence or voluntary vergence to furnish the innervation. Either way is acceptable. If the patient reports diplopia and I see no movement, vision therapy is a consideration, as stated in the previous paragraph. However, if the patient has no diplopia and has not complained of it through the habitual prescription, I explain that suppression is probably occurring and, if reading has been comfortable in the past, I recommend no further treatment.

When a prism prescription is considered for patients younger than 13 years, particularly those with high AC/A ratios, the clinician should be aware of the effects of convergence-accommodation. A complete discussion is beyond the scope of this chapter, but a few comments are in order. Just as accommodation brings with it convergence in accordance with the AC/A ratio, so disparity convergence causes a certain amount of accommodation in accordance with the CA/C ratio. Whereas the AC/A ratio is relatively stable over the working range of accommodation and the pre-presbyopic years, the CA/C ratio is inclined to change. When the AC/A and CA/C ratios are reciprocally equal (a condition that may occur in young persons with high AC/A ratios), the powers of accommodation-convergence and convergence-accommodation to influence the overall system are approximately equal.[29] This sets up a potentially unstable situation. A simple application of one of the rules for prism prescription will not yield the predictable result. An esophoria measured under dissociated conditions fails to predict the esophoric stress encountered under associated conditions. Therefore a relatively small amount of prism can relieve quite a large amount of stress on the binocular system. A slightly different but similarly beneficial sequence of events occurs that permits a relatively small plus add to have a larger effect on binocular stress than would be predicted from a simple computation based on the AC/A ratio. Therefore the effect works out to the good no matter whether the practitioner uses prisms or lenses to reduce the stress, *on esophores*. For exophores, similar statements can be made, but the buffering action of the positive slow vergence adaptation mechanism weakens the effect. Because of its complexity, the interaction of the AC/A and CA/C ratios in the binocular systems of younger patients is not well understood; but the application of control systems analysis offers the promise of further understanding.

Summary

Successful prescription of horizontal prism depends on a successful attempt at differential diagnosis. Exophores are sufficiently different from esophores to require different diagnostic and therapeutic concepts. In addition, exophores differ among themselves in their responses to prism. The same can be said of esophores. Once again, differential diagnosis is the key.

Given a successful differential diagnosis, it is possible in most cases to reduce the content of this chapter to a manageable number of concepts as far as the clinical prescription of horizontal prism is concerned:

1. If an exophoric patient has symptoms attributable to oculomotor imbalance, Sheard's criterion should verify the diagnosis. A fixation disparity curve and/or vergence facility test should be performed if Sheard's criterion is met but the patient is symptomatic. Be aware of the possibility of latent exophoria, of the consequences of using volition to support positive disparity vergence, and of a false vertical imbalance.

2. If the patient is an esophore, the 1:1 rule for comparing the amount of esophoria to the amount of base-in recovery should confirm the diagnosis. Keep in mind, however, that a large amount of esophoria is itself diagnostic. If the diagnosis remains in doubt, a fixation disparity curve and/or vergence facility test can be performed.

3. Basic esophorias may be helped by prescribing sufficient prism to meet the 1:1 criterion. Prism can be prescribed to put the operating point (origin of the fixation disparity curve) on a flat spot in the curve; but, if the patient has a Type II fixation disparity curve, expect residual symptoms.

4. For basic exophorias, prescribe sufficient prism to meet Sheard's criterion. The presence of a latent exophoria is a complication that may militate against prism prescription.

5. For convergence excess and divergence excess, plus lenses at near should be used to create the basic pattern and then a prism prescribed accordingly. Vision therapy may be needed if the amount of prism required is not practical for long-term use.

6. For the patient with convergence insufficiency, make every effort to treat with vision therapy. Prescribe prism to meet Sheard's criterion only as a last resort. Be aware that Sheard's criterion is not applicable for small amounts of exophoria.

7. In the case of a patient with divergence insufficiency, prescribe enough base-out prism to meet the 1:1 rule at distance. The patient will probably be adequately served at near with this prescription.

8. Keep in mind the difference between static and dynamic problems: static problems are more likely treatable with prism, dynamic problems with vision therapy.

Appendix

Generation of a Horizontal Forced-Vergence Fixation Disparity Curve with a Disparometer[30]

1. The patient should view the Disparometer (Fig. 5-15) through the near prescription and in a comfortable reading position.
2. Direct the patient's attention to the letters at the side of the aperture with *vertical* lines in it.
3. *Before* putting polarizing spectacles on the patient, perform a trial run to make sure the patient understands the task—which is to clear the print at the side of the aperture, look at the vertical lines in the aperture, and report when the lines are directly one over the other. The horizontal spacing between the lines can be varied by
   a. Having the patient turn the knob on the back of the Disparometer, until the lines appear one over the other or
   b. Turning the knob yourself and having the patient report when the top line is directly over the bottom one
   If the patient performs the task correctly, the Disparometer should read 0 minutes of arc and the lines should appear aligned.
4. When you are satisfied that the patient can accomplish the task, put polarizing spectacles on the patient (over a near prescription, if necessary) and note that the right eye sees the top line and the left eye the bottom line in the Disparometer aperture.
5. The first datum point is determined with no prism in front of the patient. Have the patient look at and clear the letters to the side of the aperture and then look at the vertical lines and report when they are aligned. There is no time limit on this judgment.
6. The second datum point is determined by placing 2 to 4 Δ of base-in prism in front of one eye. There is a *15-second* time limit on this judgment. If the task is not completed in 15 seconds, remove the prism for at least 15 seconds of rest before reinserting the prism and having the patient complete the task.
7. The third datum point is determined with 2 to 4 Δ of base-out prism in front of one eye. Again, allow only 15 seconds for the task to be accomplished.
8. Choose a base-in prism amount that will stress the fusional limits, place it in front of one eye, and determine the fixation disparity. You may have to choose more than one point to complete the shape of the negative side of the curve.
9. Choose a base-out prism amount that will stress the fusional limits and have the patient repeat the task. More than one trial may have to be run, at increasing base-out prism powers, before the shape of the positive side of the curve is determined.

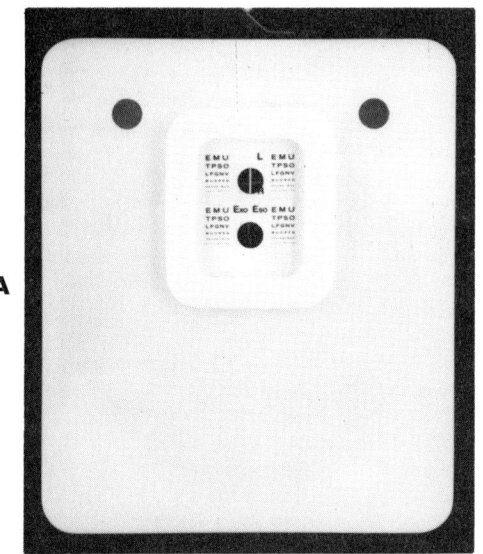
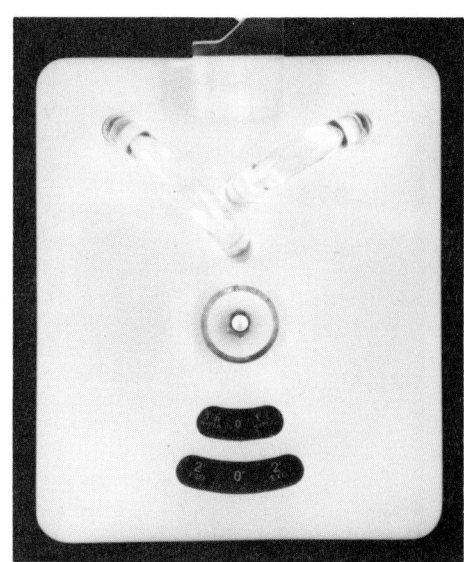

FIGURE 5-15 A, Front or patient side of the Disparometer. **B,** Back side.

References

1. Morgan MW: The Maddox analysis of vergence. In Schor CM, Ciuffreda KJ (eds): *Vergence eye movements: basic and clinical aspects,* Boston, 1983, Butterworths, pp 15-21.
2. Sheedy JE, Saladin JJ: Validity of diagnostic criteria and case analysis in binocular vision disorders. In Schor CM, Ciuffreda KJ (eds): *Vergence eye movements: basic and clinical aspects,* Boston, 1983, Butterworths, pp 517-540.
3. Percival AS: The relation of convergence to accommodation and its practical bearing, *Ophthalmic Rev* 11:313-328, 1892.
4. Sheard C: Zones of ocular comfort, *Am J Optom Arch Am Acad Optom* 7:9-25, 1930.
5. Morgan MW: The clinical aspects of accommodation and convergence, *Am J Optom Arch Am Acad Optom* 21:301-313, 1944.
6. Morgan MW: Anomalies of the visual neuromuscular system of the aging patient and their correction. In Hirsch MJ, Wick RE (eds): *Vision of the aging patient,* Philadelphia, 1960, Chilton, pp 113-145.
7. Ogle KN, Martens TG, Dyer JA: *Oculomotor imbalance in binocular vision and fixation disparity,* Philadelphia, 1967, Lea & Febiger.
8. Mallett RFJ: The investigation of heterophoria at near and a new fixation disparity technique, *Optician* 148:547-551, 1964.
9. Barlow HB, Blakemore C, Pettigrew JD: The neural mechanism of binocular depth discrimination, *J Physiol [Lond]* 193:327-342, 1967.
10. Mays LE, Porter JD, Gamlin PDR, Tello CA: Neural control of vergence eye movements: neurons encoding vergence velocity, *J Neurophysiol* 56:1007-1021, 1986.

11. Marlow FW: Prolonged monocular occlusion as a test for muscle balance, *Am J Ophthalmol* 4:238-250, 1921.
12. Schor CM, Kotulak JC, Tsuetaki T: Adaptation of tonic accommodation reduces accommodative lag and is masked in darkness, *Invest Ophthalmol Vis Sci* 27:820-827, 1986.
13. Griffin JR: *Binocular anomalies procedures for vision therapy,* Chicago, 1982, Professional Press, pp 398-402.
14. Saladin JJ, Carr LW: Fusion lock diameter and the forced vergence fixation disparity curve, *Am J Optom Physiol Opt* 60:933-943, 1983.
15. Sheedy JE, Saladin JJ: Phoria, vergence, and fixation disparity in oculomotor problems, *Am J Optom Physiol Opt* 54:474-478, 1977.
16. Sheedy JE, Saladin JJ: Association of symptoms with measures of oculomotor deficiencies, *Am J Optom Physiol Opt* 55:670-676, 1978.
17. Worrell BE, Hirsch MJ, Morgan MW: An evaluation of prism prescribed by Sheard's criterion, *Am J Optom Arch Am Acad Optom* 48:373-376, 1971.
18. Ogle KN: *Researches in binocular vision,* New York, 1964, Hafner, p 75.
19. Saladin JJ: Convergence insufficiency, fixation disparity, and control systems analysis, *Am J Optom Physiol Opt* 63:645-653, 1986.
20. Saladin JJ, Alspaugh DH, Penrod LR: Effect of vision therapy on stereophotogrammetric profiling: a controlled clinical trial, *Am J Optom Physiol Opt* 65:325-330, 1988.
21. Moore RH, Bryan WE: The practical application of research on visual factors in stereoplotting, *Photogrammetric Engin* 30:991-999, 1020, 1964.
22. Saladin JJ: Interpretation of divergent oculomotor imbalance through control system analysis, *Am J Optom Physiol Opt* 65:439-447, 1988.
23. Wick BC: Horizontal deviations. In Amos JF (ed): *Diagnosis and management in vision care,* Boston, 1987, Butterworths, pp 461-510.
24. Sethi B, North RV: Vergence adaptive changes with varying magnitudes of prism-induced disparities and fusional amplitudes, *Am J Optom Physiol Opt* 64:263-268, 1987.
25. Cooper J: Orthoptic treatment of vertical deviations, *J Am Optom Assoc* 59:463-468, 1988.
26. Donders FC: *On the anomalies of accommodation and refraction of the eye,* London, 1864, New Sydenham Society Press, p 215.
27. Morgan MW, Peters HB: Accommodative-convergence in presbyopia, *Am J Optom Arch Am Acad Optom* 28:3-10, 1951.
28. Sheedy JE, Saladin JJ: Exophoria at near in presbyopia, *Am J Optom Physiol Opt* 52:474-481, 1975.
29. Schor CM: Analysis of tonic and accommodative vergence disorders of binocular vision, *Am J Optom Physiol Opt* 60:1-14, 1983.
30. Sheedy JE: Actual measurement of fixation disparity and its use in diagnosis and treatment, *J Am Optom Assoc* 51:1079-1084, 1980.

Self-Assessment Questions

1. For general purposes, the first choice in prescribing a prism for exophores is one
   a. that meets Sheard's criterion
   b. that meets Percival's criterion
   c. that fits a flat spot on the fixation disparity curve
   d. that neutralizes the fixation disparity
   e. in which the base-out recovery is at least equal to the amount of exophoria

2. Which of the following Duane-White classifications of esophoria is most amenable to *simple* base-out prism prescription?
   a. convergence excess
   b. divergence insufficiency
   c. basic eso
   d. mixed eso

3. For general purposes, the first choice in prescribing prism for esophores is one
   a. that meets Sheard's criterion
   b. that meets Percival's criterion
   c. that fits a flat spot on the fixation disparity curve
   d. that neutralizes the fixation disparity
   e. in which the esophoric amount is equal to the base-in recovery

4. The best principle for using fixation disparity in the treatment of oculomotor dysfunction is to seek to
   a. neutralize it with prism or lenses
   b. minimize and stabilize it
   c. maximize it with vision therapy to the point where the patient will know when it occurs and voluntarily control it
   d. create a Type I fixation disparity curve pattern with vision therapy

Answers: 1. a.   2. c.   3. e.   4. b.

6

Prescribing Prism for Patients With Vertical Heterophoria

Bruce Wick

Key Terms

flip-prism test	Disparometer	prolonged occlusion test
fixation disparity	associated phoria	
vertical vergence	latent hyperphoria	prism adaptation

Clinicians are typically concerned that a vertical prism prescription might be required when a patient has a vertical heterophoria and symptoms such as frequent loss of place while reading or occasional vertical diplopia. Several techniques have been described that can be used to determine the amount of prism to prescribe when a symptomatic patient has a vertical heterophoria. For example, recommendations have been to make vertical prism prescription decisions based on one or more of the following factors: the magnitude of the vertical heterophoria, the vertical vergence ranges, flip-prism tests, or vertical fixation disparity measurements. However, in spite of (or perhaps because of) these numerous recommendations, the precise methods for prescribing vertical prism have not been well defined. As a result, the prescription of vertical prism is often deferred in clinical practice because of uncertainty on the part of the clinician as to the best course of action. In this chapter I discuss the most popular prism-prescribing techniques and make recommendations for clinical determination of vertical prism prescriptions.

Methods of Determining Vertical Prism Correction

Magnitude of the Heterophoria

The magnitude of a vertical heterophoria is often used to determine the vertical prism prescription. The dissociating techniques for measuring such magnitudes include the alternate cover test,[1] Maddox rod,[2] and von Graefe test.[3] The primary advantage of these tests is that they are simple modifications of the standard dissociating techniques used to measure horizontal heterophorias and as such they are generally familiar to most clinicians. Table 6-1 lists some advantages and disadvantages of these measures.

Numerous suggestions have been made by clinical researchers as to how the magnitude of a vertical heterophoria might influence decisions concerning the amount of vertical prism to prescribe. Unfortunately, the clinician can easily become confused because of the considerable variation in prism amount that may be prescribed using the various recommendations. For example, Hansell and Reber[4] recommended prescribing prism power that corrects one third of the hyperphoria. Emsley[5] and Maddox[6] suggested prescribing vertical prism equal to two thirds of the vertical heterophoria, and Giles[7] advised correcting three fourths of the vertical heterophoria. Duke-Elder[8] and Peter[9] believed that a nearly complete correction (or perhaps 0.5 Δ less) should be given for hyperphorias greater than 1 Δ, and Hugonnier et al.[10] recommended complete prismatic correction when the vertical deviation is small.

The varying opinions of these authorities have forced many clinicians to rely on rough guidelines or rules of thumb when prescribing vertical prism. For example, Krimsky[11] did not even suggest a specific

TABLE 6-1
Tests of Dissociated Vertical Heterophoria

Test	Advantages	Disadvantages
Alternate cover	Rapid, objective	Difficult to see small deviations, requires accurate fixation
Maddox rod	Rapid, accurate	Suppression invalidates, subjective
von Graefe	Rapid, accurate	Suppression invalidates, subjective

amount but stated that each case should be considered individually and the weakest prism that will relieve symptoms and restore binocularity should be used. However, the method that should be used to determine the "weakest" prism is not clear, and an anecdotal method has been presented that involves placing a prism with its base in the appropriate direction in the trial frame along with the refractive correction and evaluating the patient's visual acuity or comfort. The lack of standardization, along with the variety of guidelines for using dissociated vertical heterophoria measurements to prescribe vertical prism, implies that a more definitive management regimen than prescribing based on the vertical heterophoria measurement should be sought.

Vertical Vergence Ranges

Methods of determining the amount of prism to prescribe based on vertical vergence ranges vary from that of Tait[12] (who recommended prescribing the amount of vertical prism that requires the patient to use one fifth of the vertical fusional amplitude to oppose the deviation) to that described below (balancing the vertical vergences). Another method involves prescribing prism to balance the recovery values when they closely agree with the direction of the heterophoria; Borish[13] suggested that balancing the recovery values may yield a prism correction that is more readily accepted subjectively.

Balancing the vertical vergence measurements has probably been the method of choice for determining a vertical prism correction for most clinicians. When prescribing based on vertical vergence ranges, one measures the vertical vergence reserves, typically using the rotary prisms of the phoropter. With the patient viewing a horizontal line of letters, vertical prism power is slowly increased using base-down prism over one eye (supravergence, Fig. 6-1) until fusion is interrupted (that is, the patient reports diplopia) and then the prism is reduced until fusion is recovered. In the typical clinical procedure, the measurement is then repeated using base-up prism over the same eye (infravergence). Patients without a vertical heterophoria will generally have supravergence and infravergence ranges that are basically equal for each eye.[14] For example, the left infravergence value will equal the right supravergence value. Thus vertical vergences generally need to be measured over only one eye. Prism that balances the break values may be determined by the formula:

Correcting prism = (Base-down to break − Base-up to break)/2

If the resultant is plus, prism is prescribed base-down; if minus, it is prescribed base-up. For example, if there is 3 Δ of right hyperphoria with 6 Δ/3 Δ of right supravergence and 4 Δ/2 Δ of right infravergence, then 1 Δ BDOD would equalize the break values (6 − 4 Δ)/2 = 2 Δ/2 = 1 Δ. The prescribed prism would thus balance the vertical vergence break values, its amount being usually one half to two thirds the actual vertical heterophoria.

Due to the variability of vertical vergence measurements, a potential problem arises when prescribing vertical prism based on vertical vergence ranges. It has been reported[15,16] that vertical heterophorias and fusional vergence amplitudes can be affected by residual tonicity with the result that vertical vergence magnitudes are affected by the

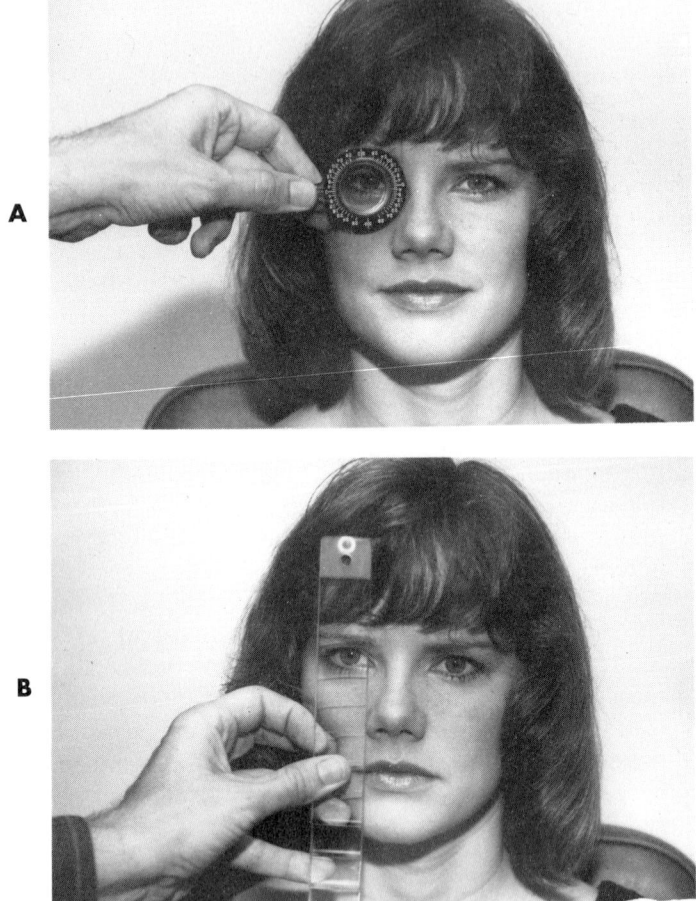

FIGURE 6-1 Vertical vergence testing can be performed with rotary prisms, **A,** a prism bar, **B,** or the phoropter, **C.** As the patient views a horizontal line of letters, vertical prism power is slowly increased by means of base-down prism over one eye (causing supravergence) until diplopia occurs and the prism is then reduced until recovery of fusion occurs. Changes in prism power should be at a slow and steady rate.

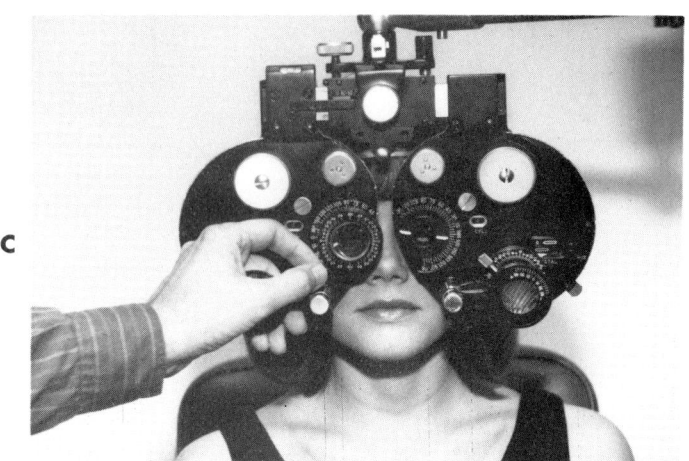

C

FIGURE 6-1, Cont'd.

muscles initially stimulated. For example, if left supravergence is measured first, the left infravergence value is reduced by the amount that tonicity is altered by the first vergence stimulation. Clinically, the problem of altering tonicity during vertical vergence measurements is easily circumvented by first assessing the compensating fusional vergence range and then measuring the opposing fusional vergence range on the fellow eye. Thus, if a right hyperphoria is present, the right infravergence should be measured first and compared to the left infravergence (that is, right supravergence). This avoids the effect of residual tonicity on the fusional vergence reserves. Alternatively, to allow residual tonic innervation to subside, assessment of the opposing vergence can be postponed to the end of the examination.

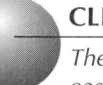

CLINICAL PEARL

The problem of altering tonicity during vertical vergence measurements is easily circumvented by first assessing the compensating fusional vergence range and then measuring the opposing fusional vergence range on the fellow eye. Alternatively, to allow residual tonic innervation to subside, assessment of the opposing vergence can be postponed to the end of the examination.

Vertical vergence measures may also be influenced by factors such as the speed with which the prism disparity is introduced,[17] the distance at which the measurement is taken,[18] and the actual vertical deviation.[13a] The large dependance of the vertical vergence ranges on the measurement technique used, along with the possibility that residual tonicity may affect the measurement results, suggests that vertical prism prescription decisions based upon the vertical vergence range measurement may not always yield the appropriate prism.

Flip Prism

Eskridge[19] suggested that a 3 Δ hand-held prism could be used for determining the amount of vertical prism to prescribe when the patient has a hyperphoria (Fig. 6-2). As the patient views a horizontal row of 0.75 m print, the prism is flipped from base-down to base-up

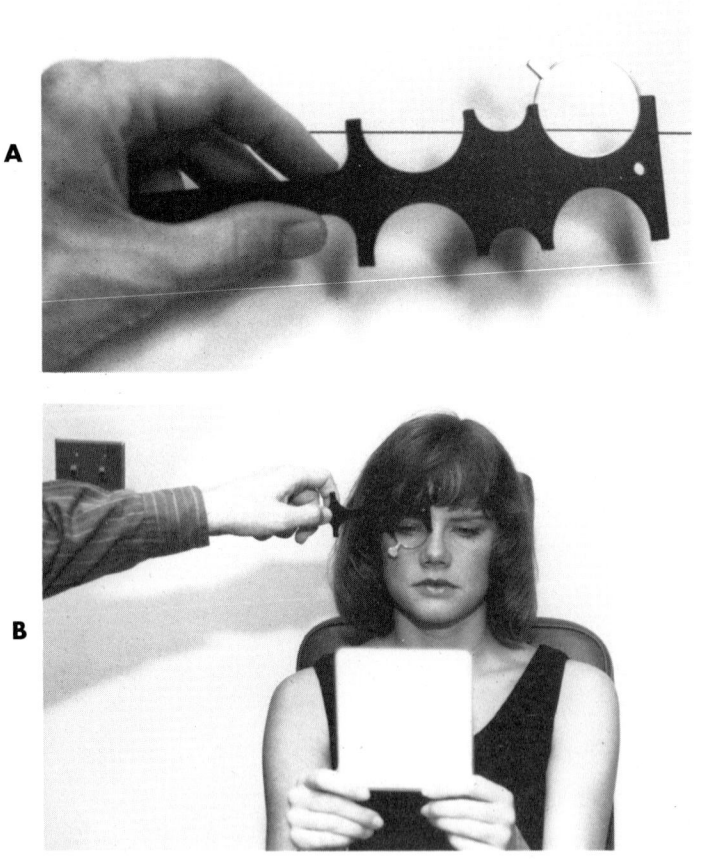

A

B

FIGURE 6-2 A 3 Δ prism in a hand-held rotatable mount, **A,** can be used to test for vertical hyperphoria and to determine the amount of correction that should be prescribed. As the patient views a horizontal row of 0.75 m print, the prism is flipped from base-down to base-up and the vertical separation of images in each presentation is reported, **B.**

and the vertical separation of images in each presentation is reported. The direction of the prism base when the images are seen closer together should correspond to the direction of the vertical heterophoria seen on dissociated testing. For example, a right hyperphoria is indicated if the images are closer when the flip prism is base-up before the left eye. The prism power to be prescribed is determined by placing a diagnostic prism base-down in front of the right eye and increasing the amount until the image separation is equidistant for successive presentations of the flip prism. The flip-prism test is very sensitive, since bisection tasks are performed easily by most patients and the testing procedure approximately doubles small existing vertical heterophorias. However, the test measures the deviation while the patient is diplopic (rather than fused), which is a potential problem since fusion leads to changes in the binocular alignment of the eyes because of vergence adaptation.[20] As a result, assessment using the diplopic images seen during the flip-prism test may provide an overestimation of the prism required by some patients.

Fixation Disparity

The principle of fixation disparity testing is to measure the direction and magnitude of a vertical deviation under conditions when fusion is present. Since the deviation is measured while the patient is fusing, fixation disparity tests probably correlate best with symptoms of vertical heterophorias, just as they do for horizontal deviations.[21,22] In addition to assessment of the vertical associated phoria, the effects of small amounts of horizontal prism on the vertical associated phoria should be determined.

Forced-vergence fixation disparity curves

Vertical forced-vergence fixation disparity curves can be generated by measuring the fixation disparity through various amounts of vertical prism. The results, plotted graphically, compose the forced-vergence curve. Forced-vergence curves are useful primarily when contemplating and monitoring a vertical vergence therapy program. If there is a vertical heterophoria, the graphical presentation of the data constructed from these measures are typically not curved but rather are linear.[23] As a result, the associated phoria measure (described below) is the clinically used assessment for most patients.

The Disparometer* is the most commonly used instrument for clinical measurement of fixation disparity curves. Other instruments include the Woolf† and Wesson‡ cards (Fig. 6-3). The most affordable and readily available of all these instruments is the Wesson card.

---

*Vision Analysis, Walnut Creek, Calif. 94596.
†Bruce Wick, University of Houston, Houston, Texas 77204.
‡Michael Wesson, University of Alabama, Birmingham 35294.

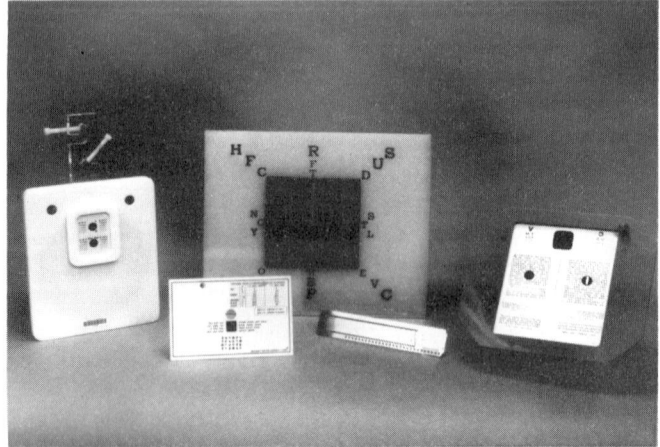

FIGURE 6-3 Instruments (left to right) for clinical measurement of fixation disparity curve parameters include the Disparometer, the Wesson card, the Wolf test, the AO vectographic slide, the Mallett near unit, and the Turville test (not pictured). During each of these tests most of the visual field is visible to both eyes and thus can be fused. However, a portion of the central field is visible only to one or the other eye, because of either polarized filters or a septum (as in the Turville test).

Phoropter setup for measurement of vertical fixation disparity

Regardless of the instrument used, the basic technique for setup is similar. Place the test instrument on the near-point rod with the target plane at 40 cm and the overhead light aimed at the test card. Set the patient's interpupillary distance and desired lens correction. Insert polarizing filters in the phoropter or have the patient wear polarizers. Position the patient behind the phoropter with the Risley prisms set at zero in front of each eye. When using the Disparometer, set the disparity reading to zero with the knob on the back of the instrument. Fixation disparity tests can be performed at distance (with a distance Disparometer) or near. To measure the vertical fixation disparity curve, use the phoropter setup described above and place the Risley prisms in the vertical prism position zeroed in front of each eye.

The Disparometer consists of two 1.5° circular targets, each containing two oppositely polarized lines. The upper circle is used for vertical fixation disparity measurement (Fig. 6-4). The left horizontal line is seen by the left eye, and the right horizontal line by the right eye.

Disappearance of an entire line indicates suppression. The letters surrounding the circles help stabilize accommodation. Modification of the instrument by using thin strips of black tape on the plastic protector over sections of the nonius lines (Fig. 6-4) aids in keeping accommodation at the plane of regard. The circle provides the fusion lock. When using the Disparometer to measure fixation disparity parameters, turn the knob at the rear of the Disparometer and offset the horizontally oriented nonius lines to approximately 5 seconds of left hyperdisparity. Have the patient report the relative placement of the left line; if it appears higher, reduce the hyperdisparity in 1-second steps until alignment is reported. Note the disparity in the window on the back of the instrument and continue to reduce the hyper (or increase the hypo) until misalignment is observed in the opposite direction. The midpoint of the range between alignment in one direction and alignment in the other is the actual fixation disparity measurement. When using the Woolf or Wesson cards, follow the same procedure except have the patient report the amount and direction of disparity directly from observations of the card.

Begin with Risley prisms, measuring the binocular response at other vergence demands. Create vergence demand in 0.5 Δ steps, with a 0.5 Δ base-up presentation before the dominant eye and subsequently alternating base-down with base-up presentations. The patient's eyes should be closed for approximately 15 seconds between subsequent measurements. If vergence demands are always in the same direction or the eyes are not closed between measurements, the curve shape may be artificially altered due to prism adaptation.[24]

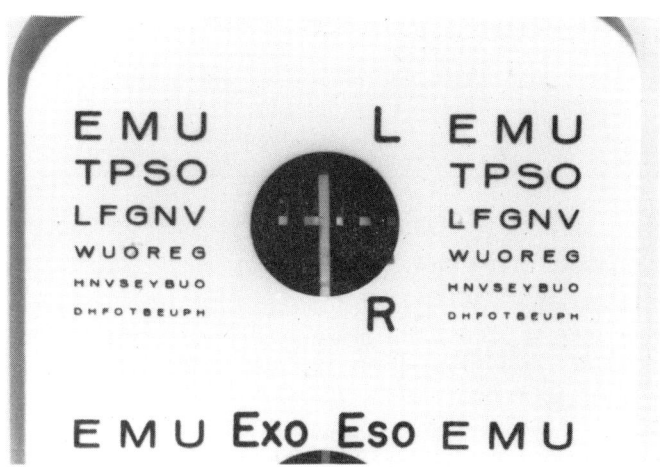

FIGURE 6-4 The letters around the *circle* of the Disparometer help stabilize accommodation. Modification of the instrument by means of black tape on the plastic protector over sections of the nonius lines aids in keeping accommodation at the plane of regard. The circle provides the fusion lock.

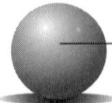

CLINICAL PEARL

Base-up and base-down presentations should be alternated, and the patients' eyes should be closed for approximately 15 seconds between vertical fixation disparity measurements.

Diplopia or suppression marks the end point of the curve. When the patient reports difficulty with the observations because of instability of the nonius lines, it helps to cover one nonious line and present it briefly ("flash" it) a number of times at each setting until the patient reports alignment. Ocassionally there will be diplopia for base-up vergence when the patient can still fuse base-down vergence demands (or vice versa). If diplopia occurs prematurely, vergence demands are alternated between the appropriate base-up and a base-down demand that the patient can just fuse. The base-up demands are graphed, and the last base-down demand to be graphed is the one before fusion was lost. This measurement technique is used so that alternating vergence demands can be presented to maintain the curve shape. After all measurements are complete, the results are graphed.

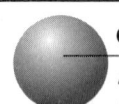

CLINICAL PEARL

If the patient reports difficulty with fixation disparity observations because of instability of the nonius lines, cover one eye (thereby eliminating its nonius line) and then present the line briefly ("flash" it) a number of times at each setting until the patient reports alignment.

Graphing findings

When forced-vergence fixation disparity findings are being graphed, hyper is above the horizontal axis, hypo below, base-down to the right, and base-up to the left (Fig. 6-5). Using the graph paper designed for fixation disparity curves, mark the midpoint of the interval where the patient reported alignment on the Y axis with an *x* and the interval ranges with *horizontal dashes* (Fig. 6-5). Make sure to note the interval ranges, because they may change with vision training. Record the Y intercept, X intercept, and slope on the top of the record. The Y intercept indicates the fixation disparity, and the X intercept the associated phoria measurement (prism required to reduce fixation disparity to zero). The slope is most frequently mea-

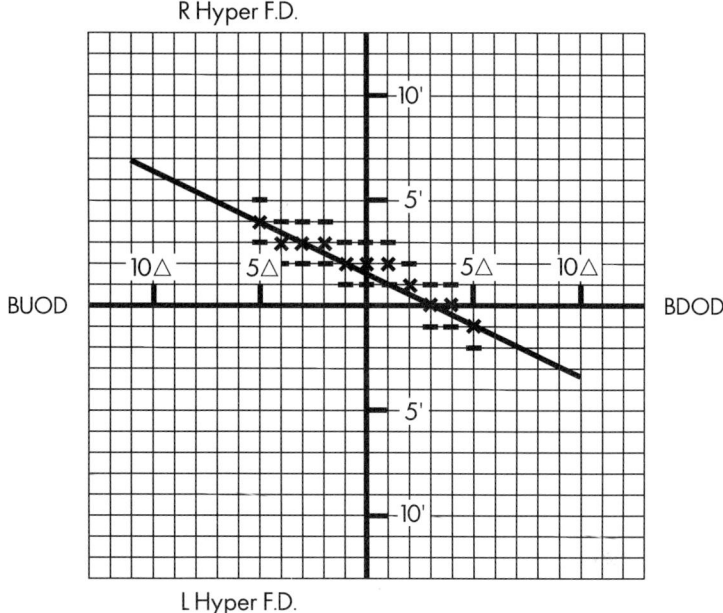

FIGURE 6-5 The vertical fixation disparity graph is typically linear for about 85% of patients tested. Although it is nonlinear for 15% of patients, only 5 to 10% have a clinically significant nonlinearity. As a result, the prism indicated by the associated phoria measure (that is, the amount needed to reduce fixation disparity to zero, *arrow*) can be prescribed in virtually all cases.

sured about the Y intercept (between 1.5 Δ base-down and 1.5 Δ base-up) since that is considered to reflect the vergence eye position where the patient habitually functions. Measure and record the slope as the change in minutes of arc/3 Δ (1.5 Δ BU to 1.5 Δ BD).

Vertical fixation disparity curve types

Although there are four types of horizontal fixation disparity curves, vertical graphs are frequently linear. This linear response pattern was originally reported by Ogle.[17] Rutstein and Eskridge[25] later suggested that all vertical fixation disparities are linear for patients with normal binocular vision. Petito and Wick[26] confirmed that most vertical fixation disparity curves are linear but suggested that about 5 to 10% of subjects have a clinically significant nonlinearity. Generally, vertical fixation disparity graphs are linear enough that vertical prism can be prescribed in an amount that reduces the fixation disparity to zero (associated phoria).

Prism Prescription Decisions

Forced-Vergence Curves

In the case of vertical deviations, the reduction to zero of the vertical misalignment of targets under binocular viewing conditions (that is, associated phoria; see next section) is the most accurate and readily accepted method of precise prism prescribing. It also results in the prescription of the least amount of prism that will relieve symptoms. The primary clinical value of the vertical forced-vergence fixation disparity curve is to develop and monitor vertical vergence therapy programs.

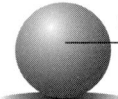

CLINICAL PEARL

In the case of vertical deviations, the reduction to zero of the vertical misalignment of targets under binocular viewing conditions (that is, associated phoria) is the most accurate and readily accepted method of precise prism prescribing. It also results in the prescription of the least amount of prism that will relieve symptoms.

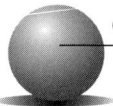

CLINICAL PEARL

The primary clinical value of the vertical forced-vergence fixation disparity curve is to develop and monitor vertical vergence therapy programs.

Vertical associated phoria

The most useful component of fixation disparity testing in diagnosis of vertical deviations is measurement of the vertical associated phoria (prism to reduce the fixation disparity to zero). In addition to the previously described Disparometer and Woolf and Wesson cards, associated phoria measures can be made using the AO vectographic slide, Turville test, and Mallett near unit. During each of these tests most of the visual field is visible to both eyes and thus can be fused. However, a portion of the central field is visible to only one eye or the other because of either a septum (Turville test) or polarized filters (Disparometer, Woolf and Wesson cards, AO vectograph, Mallett).

To evaluate the vertical associated phoria, have the patient view the horizontal lines on the test being used (for instance, the upper circle on the Disparometer). Be sure that each horizontally oriented line is seen simultaneously. If there is no suppression, ask whether the lines appear to be straight across from one another. If one line appears lower, base-down prism is placed before that eye until the patient reports alignment. The reverse is true if a line appears higher (that is, base-up prism is placed before the eye that sees the higher line). Measurement of the vertical associated phoria is complete when there is stable alignment of the nonius lines through the vertical prism. The amount and direction of the prism should be recorded. When a test that has a central fusion lock is used (such as the AO vectographic slide or the Mallett near unit) (Fig. 6-6), the recording should also include information concerning whether one eye or the other tends to deviate (that is, right or left hyper) and whether more prism is required before one eye than the other to reduce the fixation disparity to zero (associated phoria).

A valuable addition to vertical-associated phoria evaluation can be used to ensure that the end point has been reached. The principle is to align the eyes vertically so that no alteration in ocular alignment occurs when the patient blinks. This stable end point can be achieved by interposing vertical prism until the nonius lines seem to be stable through the prism. Then the patient closes both eyes for 1 or 2 seconds. The task is to notice, when the eyes are first opened, whether the nonius lines are exactly aligned or whether one or the other moves up or down to align. The open-close eyes procedure is repeated, and the prism prescription modified in 0.5 Δ steps until the lines appear stable upon opening the eyes and subsequently remain aligned. Frequently a small increase in vertical prism is required from that found during the standard eyes-open associated phoria measure to reach the stable end point of continuous alignment of the lines after opening the eyes.

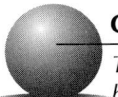

CLINICAL PEARL

To ensure that the end point in the vertical associated phoria evaluation has been reached, have the patient close both eyes for 1 or 2 seconds and then report, when the eyes are first opened, whether the nonius lines are exactly aligned or whether one or the other moves up or down to align. If the nonius lines do not align exactly upon opening, modify the prism prescription in 0.5 Δ steps until the nonius lines appear stable and remain aligned.

For over 30 years assessment of the vertical associated phoria has been known as a method of prescribing prism in vertical heterophorias. In general, when the lines remain aligned immediately after the eyes have been opened again, the amount of prism that reduces the fixation disparity to zero can be prescribed with confidence as the amount that will dramatically relieve the patient's symptoms. For example, Morgan[27] measured the associated phoria by assessing patients' ability to detect alignment differences observed in a row of

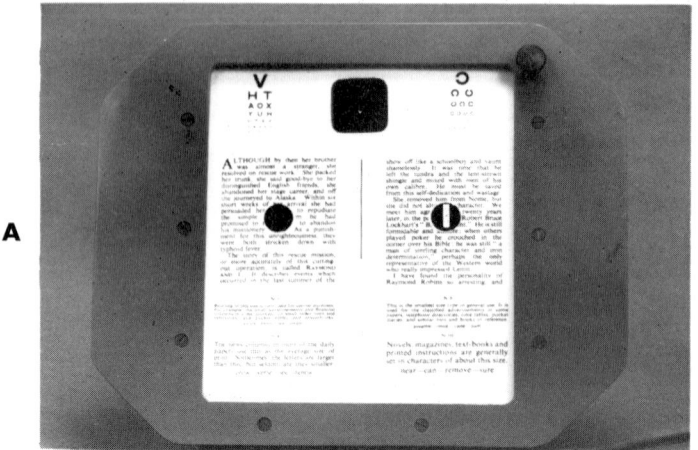

or more accurately of this cutting-out operation, is called RAYMOND AND I. It describes events which occurred in the last summer of the show off like a school show of like a schoolboy and vaunt shamelessly. It ... e that he left the tundra and th ... wn shingle and mixed with m ... wn calibre. He must be saved ... self-dedication and wastage. She removed him from Nome, but she did not alter his character. We meet hime again twenty years later, in the patronage of Robert Bruce Lockhart. Heis still formidable and austere; when others pl

FIGURE 6-6 The Mallett near unit consists of two circular targets containing two oppositely polarized lines. The *right circle* is used for vertical fixation disparity measurement, **A.** The *left horizontal line* is seen by the left eye, and the *right horizontal line* by the right eye. When there is a fixation disparity and only one eye deviates, the patient will report that the target seen by that eye is misaligned while the other target remains aligned with the central fixation lock, **B.**

20/30 letters interrupted by a septum. Of the 215 patients, 98.6% noticed the difference created by a 0.5 Δ vertical prism. Based on the perceived vertical misalignment, prism was prescribed for 15% of the patients whom Morgan tested and over 90% of them successfully wore the prism. The results of Morgan's work concerning prescription of vertical prism were supported by Elvin[28] and Tubis.[29] Based on these workers' results, it is advisable to prescribe prism that is equal in magnitude to the vertical associated phoria. Prescription of as little as 0.5 Δ vertical prism can be expected to have beneficial effects on fusion and patient comfort. Since these measures are easily made and because they successfully reduce symptoms, determination of the vertical associated phoria has become the test of choice in determining the prism to prescribe for vertical heterophoria.

Case Study 1   *Prescribing Vertical Prism Based on Associated Phoria*

A 19-year-old woman complained of blur at near, slow reading, loss of place while reading, reading the same line when going back to the beginning of a line, and headaches (eyelid/brow area) after approximately 30 minutes of reading. She stated that blinking cleared the near blur. The current spectacle prescription was essentially the same as her refractive findings.

OD −0.75 DS   (20/15)
OS −1.25 DS   (20/15)

All further testing was performed through the habitual spectacle lenses. Cover test and Maddox rod testing revealed 3.5 Δ of left hyperphoria In all fields of gaze at distance and near. Vertical vergence ranges were

Left supra 7 Δ/5 Δ
Left infra 1.5 Δ/1 Δ

Associated phoria testing revealed 1.75 Δ left hyper-associated phoria at distance (AO vectographic adult slide) and near (Mallett near unit). Accommodative and horizontal vergence findings were normal.

   Based on these examination findings, the habitual spectacle correction was judged to be adequate, as were accommodative and horizontal fusional abilities. Prescribing with measures of the dissociated heterophoria forces a decision to prescribe somewhere between 1 and 3.5 Δ depending upon the philosophy followed. Prescribing by balancing the vertical vergence ranges would suggest a need for 2.75 Δ BDOS. Associated phoria testing indicated a need to prescribe 1.75 Δ BDOS.

   The myopic correction alone, and then with the addition of 1.75 Δ BDOS, was placed in a trial frame and the patient was allowed to read for 10 to 15 minutes under both conditions. She expressed a feeling of markedly reduced eyestrain and more accurate eye movements (easier returning to the next line of letters) with the prism, which was then prescribed. With the new prescription, the patient no longer lost her place while reading, had no more headaches, and enjoyed substantially increased reading speed.

Horizontal prism corrections

Small amounts of horizontal prism have been shown[30] to reduce the vertical associated phoria to zero in some patients. The number of patients who respond in this manner is unknown, however, since most practitioners prescribe only vertical prism for these patients and do not even investigate the effect of horizontal prism. When small amounts of horizontal prism (less than 2.5 Δ) are successful in eliminating a vertical associated phoria, the patient is usually better managed by a brief vision therapy program emphasizing horizontal vergence and antisuppression therapy. Such programs are almost invariably effective, eliminating the need for any type of prism.

CLINICAL PEARL

When small amounts of horizontal prism (less than 2.5 Δ) are successful in eliminating a vertical associated phoria, the patient is usually better managed by a brief vision therapy program emphasizing horizontal vergence and antisuppression therapy.

Other Considerations in Prescription of Vertical Prism

Regardless of the examination technique used, decisions concerning the prescription of prism for a patient with vertical heterophoria are often complicated by the differing combinations of symptoms and heterophorias that exist. As illustrated in Table 6-2, when a hyperphoric patient is truly asymptomatic, management is frequently deferred (Table 6-2, row 2). On the other hand, it is possible that the patient has remained asymptomatic by avoiding symptom-causing tasks rather than by being truly asymptomatic; in these instances treatment may be indicated.

Diagnostic Occlusion and Prism Prescriptions for Latent Hyperphoria

Some of the most difficult management decisions in clinical practice arise when the patient has symptoms suggesting a vertical deviation but no vertical heterophoria is evident on routine clinical testing (Table 6-2, row 5). Small latent vertical heterophorias can cause patients to be symptomatic. And, just as with some deviations of larger amounts, these vertical deviations may become manifest only with prolonged occlusion.[31] In these instances occlusion is used in the differential diagnosis of vertical heterophoria, just as it often is in a patient suspected of having aniseikonia.[32] When occlusion relieves the symptoms, the cause is usually found to be some handicap to binocular vision.[33]

TABLE 6-2

Clinical Management of Vertical Heterophoria

Vertical deviation	Symptoms	Diagnostic occlusion	Treatment	Percent of patients
1. None present	None	No	None	80
2. Phoria or fixation disparity	None	No	Usually none; consider if avoiding tasks	3
3. Phoria and fixation disparity	Yes	No	Prescribe prism based on vertical associated phoria	12
4. Fixation disparity only	Yes	No	Prescribe prism based on vertical associated phoria	3
5. None on routine testing	Yes	Yes (1 day over eye that tends to have hyper)	Prescribe prism based on vertical associated phoria seen after diagnostic occlusion	2

Prism corrections for latent vertical deviations are based on the associated phoria, severity of symptoms, and monocular occlusion. The patient with latent hyperphoria can be managed successfully following the procedures listed in Table 6-2, row 5. Typically, the hyperphoric eye should be occluded and the patient tested after 24 hours of total occlusion. The occasionally difficult decision concerning which eye is the hyperphoric one is based on alternate cover testing (including patient observations of the phi phenomenon), vertical fixation disparity curves, and reports of vertical instability of the horizontal nonius lines on fixation disparity testing. Monocular occlusion is used to unmask the vertical deviation by first determining, from the fixation disparity curves and dissociated phoria measurements, which eye has a tendency to be hyperphoric and then occluding that eye for 24 hours. When the patient returns the next day (still occluded), dissociated phoria measurements are taken at distance and near immediately after removal of the patch (while not allowing fusion to occur.) With the amount determined during dissociated phoria testing as the starting prism, vertical fixation disparity measurements are taken in the manner described previously. Vertical prism that neutralizes the vertical fixation disparity (associated phoria) can be prescribed; vertical vergence therapy may also be considered.

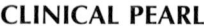

CLINICAL PEARL

Diagnostic occlusion is used when a latent vertical heterophoria is suspected. Typically, the hyperphoric eye should be occluded and the patient tested after 24 hours of total occlusion.

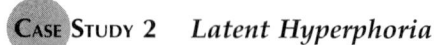

CASE STUDY 2   *Latent Hyperphoria*

An 11-year-old boy had difficulty reading rapidly because of frequent loss of place while reading. He often read the same line when going back to the beginning of a line and had frequent frontal headaches after reading. The current spectacle prescription was essentially the same as the refractive findings:

OD −2.50 DS   (20/15)
OS −2.25 DS   (20/15)

Cover test and Maddox rod testing revealed 1 Δ of exophoria in all fields of gaze at distance and near. The vertical associated phoria findings were orthophoria at distance and an unstable 0.75 Δ left hyper associated phoria at near that increased with time. Accommodative and horizontal vergence findings were normal. Vertical vergence ranges were symmetrical at distance and near.

Although the habitual spectacle correction as well as accommodative and horizontal fusional abilities seemed adequate, the instability and variability of the vertical associated phoria measurement suggested a latent left hyperphoria. Diagnostic occlusion was used for further assessment. The patient was instructed to patch the left eye constantly 24 hours before the follow-up examination. During that examination the patch was removed and fusion was prevented until associated phoria measurements were taken. Associated phoria testing at distance revealed 2.75 Δ left hyperphoria. Cover testing at distance revealed 2 Δ left hyperphoria.

The patient was allowed to read for 10 to 15 minutes with the myopic correction alone and then with the addition of 2.75 Δ BDOS. He expressed a feeling of less eyestrain and more comfortable reading (easier returning to the next line of letters) with the additional 2.75 Δ BDOS, which was then prescribed. With the new prescription the patient initially experienced mild discomfort that subsided in less than 30 minutes. At a 2-year follow-up he reported no recurrence of losing his place while reading.

Out-of-Phoropter Testing

Regardless of which prescribing philosophy will be used for determination of a vertical prism prescription, the clinician should consider the characteristic head postures that patients with hyperphorias often assume. Frequently patients with a significant vertical heterophoria in the primary position tend to tilt or turn their head to a position that allows more comfortable binocular vision. For many of these patients, testing through the phoropter is not appropriate and trial frame evaluation using the best correction will often give a better evaluation of the habitual binocular status.

Testing out of the phoropter is especially valuable when a patient has significant anisometropia and may benefit from the prescription of slab-off prism. Assessing the vertical associated phoria in downgaze gives a much better determination of the amount of slab-off prism to prescribe than calculating the amount that might be needed from the anisometropia. Invariably, when the deviation is measured in downgaze (for example, by assessing the associated phoria), the amount of prism required is less than might be expected based on calculation.

CASE STUDY 3   *Prescribing Slab-Off Prism*

A 60-year-old man complained of transient vertical diplopia when reading following bilateral corneal transplants (hydrops resulting as a sequela of keratoconus) and cataract extraction with intraocular lens implants. The refractive findings were

OD −1.00−5.00 × 060 (20/25)   +2.75 add
OS + 4.00−3.50 × 085 (20/30+) +2.75 add

Cover test and Maddox rod testing through the habitual spectacle lenses revealed 1 Δ of right hyperphoria in all horizontal fields of gaze at distance. Vertical vergence ranges were

Right supra 3 Δ/2 Δ
Right infra 1 Δ/0

Associated phoria testing showed 1 Δ of right hyper-associated phoria at distance. There were no changes in associated phoria response as the patient shifted into lateral gaze. He required a near addition of +2.75 D. His bifocal forced him to look 10 cm below the distance optical centers; in this position of downgaze and looking through the distance correction, the 1 Δ BDOD prism found at distance, and the near addition, there was a 1.25 Δ right hyper associated phoria at near.

Prescribing distance prism could be done using measures of the dissociated heterophoria, balancing the vertical vergence ranges, or testing for an associated phoria. All these indicated a need to prescribe about

1 Δ BDOD. Associated phoria testing at near suggested the need for an additional 1.25 Δ slab-off from the right lens even though calculating the slab-off prism suggested a need for up to 5 Δ (5 D of anisometropia × 1 cm downgaze = 5 Δ).

The refractive correction with 1 Δ BDOD, and then with the addition of 1.25 Δ BDOD for near, was placed in a trial frame. After reading for 10 to 15 minutes under both conditions, he noticed no diplopia and more comfortable reading with the additional near prism in downgaze. This was prescribed in slab-off form. With the new prescription, the patient reported clear single binocular vision while reading.

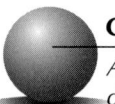

CLINICAL PEARL
Assessing the vertical associated phoria in downgaze gives a much better determination of the amount of slab-off prism to prescribe than calculating the amount that might be needed from the anisometropia.

Split the Prism?

When the amount of prism to prescribe has been determined, the clinician must decide how much to place in each lens. The typical procedure is to split the prism equally between eyes if there is more than 1.25 Δ and to prescribe all the prism before one eye if there is 1 Δ or less. Although splitting the prism between eyes generally works well, there are times when more prism should be placed in front of one eye. Unequal prisms are generally indicated when the patient reports that one eye consistently tends to go higher (or lower) on associated phoria testing with tests that have a *central fusion lock* (AO Vectographic slide, Mallett near unit). In these instances placing all or more of the prism before the eye that deviates tends to yield a more comfortable prism prescription. Such determination can be made reliably only when the associated phoria is tested using measures that have a central fusion lock.

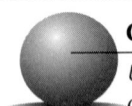

CLINICAL PEARL
Unequal prisms are generally indicated when the patient reports that one eye consistently tends to go higher (or lower) on associated phoria testing with tests that have a central fusion lock. In these instances placing all or more of the prism before the eye that deviates tends to yield a more comfortable prism prescription.

CASE STUDY 4 *Prescribing Unequal Prism Before Each Eye*

A 47-year-old woman complained of transient vertical diplopia of many years' duration. The refractive findings were

OD −5.00 −1.00 × 160 (20/15)
OS −4.75 −1.25 × 005 (20/20+)

Cover test and Maddox rod testing through the refractive findings revealed 7 Δ of right hyperphoria in all fields of gaze at distance and near. Vertical vergence ranges were

Right supra   10 Δ/8 Δ
Right infra   1 Δ/0

On associated phoria testing the patient consistently reported that the right nonius line was higher than the left. There was a 6 Δ right hyper-associated phoria at distance, and the most stable alignment of the nonius lines on the AO vectographic adult slide was achieved with 4.5 Δ BDOD and 1.5 Δ BUOS. There were no changes in associated phoria response as the patient shifted vision into lateral gaze. She required a near addition of +1.50 D. In downgaze through the near addition there was no change in the right hyper-associated phoria.

The refractive correction with 6 Δ split between the two eyes and then with 4.5 Δ BDOD and 1.5 Δ BUOS was placed into a trial frame and the patient was allowed to read and gaze around the room under both conditions. She noticed no diplopia and was more comfortable reading with the unequal prism prescription.

Form of the Prism Correction*

Spectacle lenses

Approximately 10 Δ of vertical prism can be prescribed per spectacle lens (20 Δ total). When prism is prescribed in spectacle lenses, the front curve should be steepened about 2.0 D more than what would be used in a stock lens for the patient's refractive correction. For example, if the stock front curve is 6.50 D, consider using an 8.50 front curve. Steepening the front curve (with an upper limit of about 9.00 D) helps reduce the annoying reflections that sometimes occur with prism prescriptions. Antireflective coatings, frame-matching edge coats, and polished lens edges also help make the final prescription more acceptable. Antireflective coatings are especially important when there are small refractive corrections because a small refractive correction combined with vertical prism often has the most severe internal reflections.

---

*See Chapter 3 for a more complete treatment of this issue.

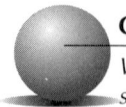

CLINICAL PEARL

When prism is prescribed in spectacle lenses, the front curve should be steepened about 2.0 D more than what would be used in a stock lens for the patient's refractive correction (with an upper limit of about 9.00 D); this will help reduce the annoying reflections that sometimes occur with prism prescriptions.

Contact lenses

Approximately 4 Δ of vertical prism can be prescribed in gas-permeable contact lenses, and soft contact lenses can be prescribed with prism up to approximately 4 Δ also. Gravity causes prism contact lenses to rotate so the prism is oriented base-down. Thus prism must be placed in the lens that will be worn on the eye requiring base-down prism. When prism is prescribed in contact lenses, the amount required is often less than that required in spectacle lenses. As a result, when contact lenses are utilized it is necessary to remeasure the vertical associated phoria through the contact lenses to determine the amount of prism to prescribe. Typically about 0.75 Δ less prism than the associated phoria measure through the spectacle lenses is a viable starting power. The final amount should be determined from the associated phoria measurement when a trial prism contact lens is in place.

CASE STUDY 5   *Prescribing Prism in Contact Lenses*

A 16-year-old girl was referred because of transient vertical diplopia and frequent headaches when reading. The refractive findings were similar to her current correction:

OD −1.00 −1.25 × 010 (20/15)
OS −1.00 −1.50 × 175 (20/15)

Her contact lens overrefraction revealed

OD   Plano
OS   +0.25 DS

Cover test and Maddox rod testing performed through the contact lenses revealed 2 Δ of left hyperphoria in all fields of gaze at distance and near. Vertical vergence ranges were

Left supra 5 Δ/2
Left infra 1 Δ/−1 Δ

Associated phoria testing revealed 1.25 Δ of left hyper-associated phoria at distance. There were no changes in associated phoria response as the patient shifted vision into lateral gaze.

Based on the examination findings, she was referred back to her contact lens practitioner for a new gas-permeable contact lens with 1.25 Δ for the left eye and the same diameter, base curve, and power as the previous lens. With this new lens she had clear comfortable binocular vision.

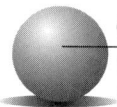

CLINICAL PEARL

When prism is prescribed in contact lenses, the amount required is often less than that needed in spectacle lenses; therefore one should remeasure the vertical associated phoria through the contact lenses to determine the amount of prism to prescribe.

Prism Adaptation

When vertical prism is placed before one eye of a person with normal binocular vision and no vertical heterophoria, remeasurement of the induced vertical deviation after 15 minutes will indicate that the resultant deviation is less than the amount of prism placed before the eye.[34] This adaptation to vertical prism by persons with normal binocularity has been shown by Rutstein and Eskridge[35] and by others,[17,36] and individual differences in the rate and amount of such prism adaptation have also been observed[37,38] (see Chapter 4). Nearly 80% of subjects with normal binocular vision show these adaptive responses to vertical prism.[39] However, since subjects who completely adapt to vertical prism typically have normal binocularity, they seldom report symptoms of binocular distress.[40] Schor[41] has demonstrated that it is the symptomatic patients who do not adapt adequately to prism. These factors, which suggest that patients with reduced ability to adapt to prism are those who have abnormal binocularity *and* manifest symptoms, indicate that the clinician can confidently prescribe prism to correct a vertical deviation when the patient is symptomatic, without concern that there might be unwanted adaptation to the prism.

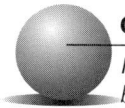

CLINICAL PEARL

Patients with reduced ability to adapt to prism are those who have abnormal binocularity and manifest symptoms; the clinician can confidently prescribe prism to correct a vertical deviation in these individuals, without concern that there might be unwanted prism adaptation.

Clinical reports by Surdacki and Wick[31] suggest that patients may require multiple prism corrections before the deviation is completely compensated. Lie and Opheim[42] used prism to correct heterophoric patients with long-standing severe visual symptoms. They reported that a small vertical deviation was present in most of the cases. Furthermore, in 80% of their cases prism corrections needed to be increased over time before the full deviation was determined.

Basic and clinical research suggests that the prescription of vertical prism for symptomatic patients with vertical heterophorias probably does not lead to prism adaptation. Increases in the prism required are probably not adaptation in the classic sense but rather are similar to clinical observations noted when prescribing plus lenses for patients with latent hyperopia; there is an increase in plus that is not adaptation but occurs because the entire correction was not prescribed initially.

Summary

Symptoms of uncompensated vertical heterophoria may be present in up to 20% of patients.[31] Attention to case history combined with careful examination will usually reveal which patients are likely to benefit from the prescription of vertical prism. Determination of the vertical associated phoria at distance and near (and in downgaze when needed) is probably the most important factor in analyzing the role of vertical heterophoria. Prism prescriptions based on these measures are useful in alleviating symptoms of vertical heterophorias.

References

1. Wick BC: Horizontal deviations. In Amos J (ed): *Diagnosis and management in vision care,* Boston, 1987, Butterworths, pp 472-473.
2. Maddox EE: *Tests and studies of the ocular muscles,* ed 3, Philadelphia, 1907, Keystone Publishing, pp 218-222.
3. Daum KM: Heterophoria and heterotropia. In Eskridge JB, Amos JF, Bartlett JD (eds): *Clinical procedures in optometry,* Philadelphia, 1991, Lippincott, pp 72-90.
4. Hansell HF, Reber W: *The ocular muscles,* Philadelphia, 1913, P Blakiston's Son, p 144.
5. Emsley HH: *Visual optics,* vol. 2, ed 5, London, 1953, Hatton Press, p 111.
6. Maddox EE: Discussion on heterophoria, *Trans Ophthalmol Soc UK* 49:2-17, 1929.
7. Giles GH: *The practice of orthoptics,* ed 2, London, 1949, Hammond, pp 325-326.
8. Duke-Elder S: *Text book of ophthalmology,* vol 6, St Louis, 1973, Mosby, pp 553-554.
9. Peter LC: *The extra-ocular muscles,* Philadelphia, 1941, Lea & Febiger, pp 118-119.
10. Hugonnier R, Clayette-Hugonnier S, Veronneau-Troutman S: *Strabismus, heterophoria, ocular motor paralysis,* St Louis, 1969, Mosby, p 675.

11. Krimsky E: *The management of binocular imbalance,* Philadelphia, 1948, Lea & Febiger, pp 360-361.
12. Tait EF: *Textbook of refraction,* Philadelphia, 1951, WB Saunders.
13. Borish IM: *Clinical refraction,* ed 3, Chicago, 1975, Professional Press, pp 872-874.
13a. Borish IM: *ibid,* pp 866-872.
14. Morgan MW: Clinical aspects of accommodation and convergence, *Am J Optom Arch Am Acad Optom* 21:301-313, 1944.
15. Ellerbrock V, Fry GA: The after-effect induced by vertical divergence, *Am J Optom Arch Am Acad Optom* 18:450-454, 1941.
16. Ellerbrock VJ: Tonicity induced by fusional movements, *Am J Optom Arch Am Acad Optom* 27:8-20, 1950.
17. Ogle KN, Prangen A: Observations on vertical divergences and hyperphorias, *Arch Ophthalmol* 49:313-334, 1953.
18. North RV, Sethi B, Owen K: Prism adaptation and viewing distance, *Ophthalmic Physiol Opt* 10:81-85, 1990.
19. Eskridge JB: Flip-prism test for vertical phoria, *Am J Optom Arch Am Acad Optom* 38:415-419, 1961.
20. Henson DB, Dharamski BG: Oculomotor adaptation to induced heterophoria and anisometropia, *Invest Ophthalmol Vis Sci* 22:234-240, 1982.
21. Sheedy JE: Acutal measurement of fixation disparity and its use in diagnosis and treatment, *J Am Optom Assoc* 51:1079-1084, 1980.
22. Sheedy JE, Saladin JJ: Association of symptoms with measures of oculomotor deficiencies, *Am J Optom Physiol Opt* 55:670-676, 1978.
23. Eskridge JB, Rutstein RP: Clinical evaluation of vertical fixation disparity. II, Reliability, stability, and association with refractive status, stereoacuity, and vertical heterophoria, *Am J Optom Physiol Opt* 62:579-584, 1985.
24. Daum KM: The stability of the fixation disparity curve, *Ophthalmic Physiol Opt* 3:13-19, 1983.
25. Rutstein RP, Eskridge JB. Studies in vertical fixation disparity, *Am J Optom Physiol Opt* 63:639-644, 1986.
26. Petito T, Wick B. (Unpublished observations, 1992.)
27. Morgan MW: The Turville infinity binocular balance test, *Am J Optom Arch Am Acad Optom* 26:231-239, 1949.
28. Elvin FT: The results of prescribing vertical prisms from the Turville test, *Am J Optom Arch Am Acad Optom* 31:308-314, 1954.
29. Tubis RA: An evaluation of vertical divergence tests on the basis of fixation disparity, *Am J Optom Arch Am Acad Optom* 31:624-635, 1954.
30. Sucher DF: Use of horizontal prism to correct vertical fixation disparity, *Am J Optom Physiol Opt* 56:504-508, 1979.
31. Surdacki M, Wick B: Diagnostic occlusion and clinical management of latent hyperphoria, *Optom Vis Sci* 68:261-269, 1991.
32. Bannon RE: Diagnostic and therapeutic use of monocular occlusion, *Am J Optom Arch Am Acad Optom* 20:345-358, 1943.
33. Marlow FW: The technique of the prolonged occlusion test, *Am J Ophthalmol* 15:320-323, 1932.
34. Henson DB, North R: Adaptation to prism-induced heterophoria, *Am J Optom Physiol Opt* 57:129-137, 1980.
35. Rutstein RP, Eskridge JB: Clinical evaluation of vertical fixation disparity. III, Adaptation to vertical prism, *Am J Optom Physiol Opt* 62:585-590, 1985.
36. Carter DB: Fixation disparity and heterophoria following prolonged wearing of prisms, *Am J Optom Arch Am Acad Optom* 42:141-152, 1965.
37. Eskridge JB: Adaptation to vertical prism, *Am J Optom Physiol Opt* 65:371-376, 1988.

38. Eskridge JB, Rutstein RP: Clinical evaluation of vertical fixation disparity. IV, Slope and adaptation to vertical prism of vertical heterophoria patients, *Am J Optom Physiol Opt* 63:662-667, 1986.

39. Allen DC: Vertical prism adaptation in anisometropes, *Am J Optom Physiol Opt* 51:252-259, 1974.

40. North R, Henson DB: Adaptation to prism-induced heterophoria in subjects with abnormal binocular vision or asthenopia, *Am J Optom Physiol Opt* 58:746-752, 1981.

41. Schor CM: The relationship between fusional vergence eye movements and fixation disparity, *Vision Res* 19:1359-1367, 1979.

42. Lie I, Opheim A: Long-term acceptance of prisms by heterophorics, *J Am Optom Assoc* 56:272-278, 1985.

Self-Assessment Questions

1. The vertical fixation disparity graph is typically linear for about how many of the patients tested.
   a. 85%
   b. 55%
   c. 35%
   d. 15%

2. The associated phoria measure
   a. is the amount of prism that reduces the fixation disparity to zero
   b. can be determined using a Maddox rod
   c. can be determined using a disparometer, Wesson card, or AO vectographic adult slide
   d. only a and c

3. Vertical vergence testing can be performed with
   a. rotary prisms, a prism bar, or the Risley prisms of the phoropter
   b. the patient observing a horizontal line of letters as vertical prism power is slowly increased using base-down prism over one eye (supravergence) until diplopia is reported; subsequently, the prism is reduced until fusion is recovered
   c. any kind of prism since neither the type of prism nor the rate of change in prism power influence the findings
   d. only a and b

4. When fixation disparity data are being graphed
   a. diplopia or suppression marks the end point of the curve
   b. and the patient reports difficulty with the observations because of instability of the nonius lines, it helps to cover one line and present it briefly ("flash" it) for a number of times at each setting until the patient reports alignment
   c. occassionally there will be diplopia for base-up vergence demands when the patient can still fuse base-down vergence demands (or vice versa). If diplopia occurs prematurely, vergence demands are alternated between the appropriate base-up and base-down values that the patient can just fuse
   d. all of the above are correct

Answers: 1. a. 2. d. 3. d. 4. d.

7

The Use of Prism in the Surgical Management of Acquired Esotropia

---

David G. Kirschen

Key Terms

prism adaptation	strabismus surgery	vision therapy
esotropia	suppression	peripheral fusion
prism adaptation study	anomalous correspondence	monofixation syndrome
orthoptics	sensory fusion	

The importance and efficacy of prisms in the diagnosis and management of strabismus and heterophoria are evident from numerous chapters in this volume. Prism glasses and orthoptics are mainstays in the nonsurgical treatment of strabismus. The use of prism presurgically, however, as part of the *surgical* treatment of strabismus has been slow in gaining acceptance.

The phrase *prism adaptation* is used by many authors to describe a patient's motor or sensory response when prisms are placed before the eyes. Depending upon the doctor's experience and training, prism adaptation has been considered in both a positive and a negative light for the functional treatment of strabismus.

Prism adaptation is a process that occurs in both nonstrabismic and strabismic patients. For nonstrabismic patients it can be demonstrated by measuring the phoria and then having him/her wear a relatively small amount of prism for some time (a few days) and then measuring the phoria again through the prism. If the patient adapts fully, the same phoria will be measured through the prism as was measured before the prism was put in place (see Chapter 4). This phenomenon is also called "eating prism." When the prism is removed and a few minutes or hours have elapsed, the phoria returns to its original value.

For strabismic patients, several mechanisms have been proposed to explain why prism adaptation occurs.

Suppression is one that could be responsible. As illustrated in Figure 7-1, A, if a strabismic patient has normal correspondence and suppression of the image point (T'_L) in the deviating eye, no diplopia will be seen under normal viewing conditions. If a partially correcting prism is placed before the deviating eye (OS), the image of the fixated target (T') will fall outside the suppression zone, resulting in diplopia (Fig. 7-1, B). In response to this prism, the patient's eyes will verge so the image point (T'_L) falls again within the suppression scotoma, eliminating the diplopia (Fig. 7-1, C). The fusion movement to reutilize the suppression scotoma may be responsible for this prism adaptation.

Anomalous correspondence also has been proposed as a mechanism for prism adaptation. In a fashion similar to the analysis for suppression, when correcting prisms are placed before the eyes a vergence movement occurs to reestablish T'_L on the anomalous point corresponding to the fovea of the normally fixating eye, thus maintaining haplopia with anomalous fusion. In this way many patients with anomalous correspondence are able to maintain their angle of anomaly in the presence of vergence stress.

Prism adaptation also may foretell a latent deviation that is not manifested initially. This phenomenon is common in exophoria/intermittent exotropia in which a certain angle of deviation (exo) is measured and then one eye is patched (or alternate patching is done) and the exo angle is measured a week later and found to be significantly larger (latent deviation). In a similar way, if an esotropic patient has a positive response to prism adaptation which leads to stabilization at a larger angle of deviation, the process may be uncovering the larger latent angle of esotropia (that is, the true angle).

Prism adaptation is a rather confusing term that has had multiple meanings and uses by different authors. For the purpose of explaining the prism adaptation test (PAT) in this chapter, *prism adaptation* is defined as the increase in the angle of deviation while a person wears a correcting prism. A positive PAT occurs when the angle of deviation increases and then stabilizes at a larger angle and gross sensory fusion develops. A negative PAT occurs when the angle of deviation keeps increasing with each correcting prism added and does not stabilize (>60 Δ) or when motor stability does occur but gross sensory fusion fails to develop.

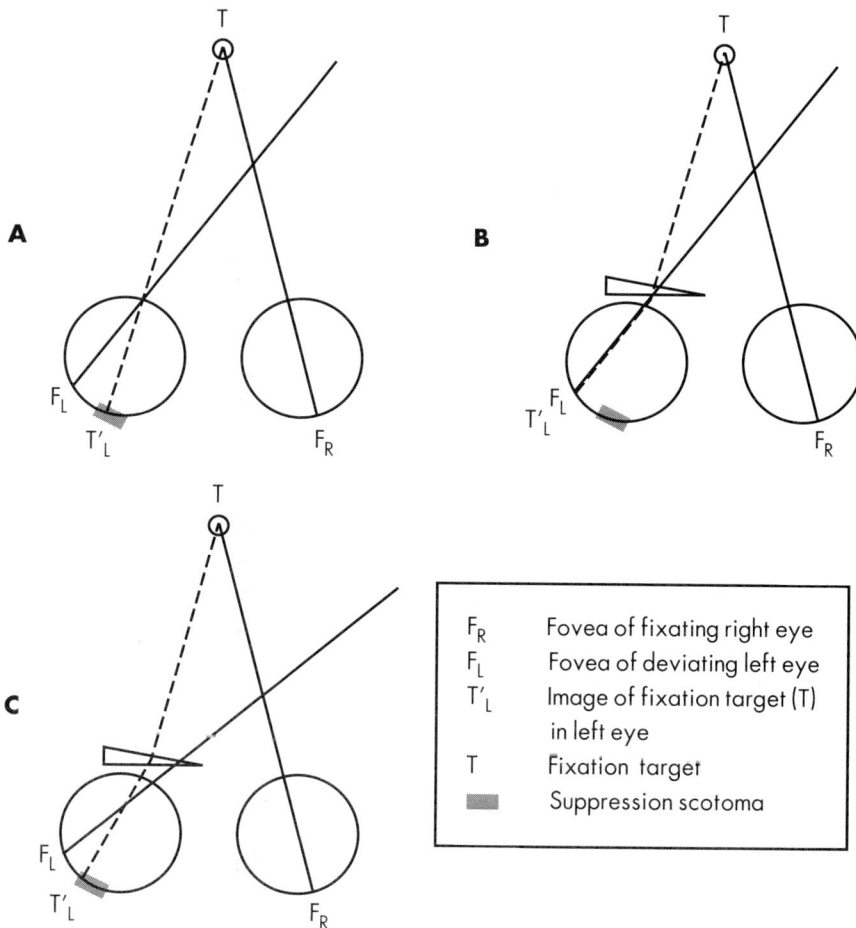

FIGURE 7-1 Suppression as a possible mechanism for prism adaptation. **A,** The image point (T'_L) is suppressed to eliminate diplopia in an esotrope with normal correspondence. **B,** Placing a partially correcting prism base-out before the left eye *(OS)* moves the image (T'_L) out of the suppression scotoma. **C,** The patient responds with a convergent eye movement to reestablish the image point (T'_L) within the suppression scotoma.

    The first systematic study of presurgical prism therapy was reported by Aust and Welge-Lussen[1] in 1971. It had been observed that in some cases of esotropia the angle recurred after the operation. This postsurgical drift was thought to be caused by anomalous correspondence. It was hoped that wearing prism presurgically could identify those patients most likely to drift after surgery. In this initial paper, 84% of the 88 cases changed their angle of strabismus as a result of wearing the prism. Some 85% increased the angle, and 15% decreased it. For the patients whose esotropia increased with prism wear (angle increased), the surgery amount was guided by the increased angle of squint rather than by the presenting angle. Postoperative results indicated no increase in the overcorrection rate as a result of operating for the larger angle.

In 1971 Jampolsky,[2] at the New Orleans Symposium on Strabismus, first described the prism adaptation test developed by his orthoptist Fletcher Woodward. This test was able to predict presurgically which patient would develop a significant postsurgical residual esotropia. Jampolsky recommended that the patient wear an overcorrecting prism (the alternate cover test demonstrating an exotropic deviation with the prism in place) for approximately 1 hour in the office. A favorable reaction (prism acceptance) would be a stable exodeviation or a slight convergence movement to attain bifoveal fixation (no movement on the unilateral cover test through the prism). Patients with either of these favorable reactions, he believed, would have a fully corrected stable surgical result. If the patient converged to the overcorrecting prism, becoming esotropic by unilateral cover test with the overcorrecting prism in place, Jampolsky maintained that this individual was telling the doctor that the surgical result would be poor and would create a postsurgical residual esotropia.

Stella[3] modified the PAT as described by Jampolsky by recommending that if the patient converged to the initial overcorrecting prism the angle be "chased" (that is, more base-out prism be added to correct the new angle until a stable small exotropia could be maintained).

Scott[4] and Scott and Thalacker[5] analyzed a series of patients in whom the PAT technique was used presurgically. They examined their data for surgical success 6 months after surgery and found that 82% of 41 patients who wore prisms presurgically and prism adapted had a successful surgical result at 6 months postoperative. Only 51% of the non–prism-adapted patients were successful by the same criteria. When the PAT was used and a patient adapted and stabilized to the prism at a larger angle of deviation with peripheral fusion, Scott operated for the larger prism-adapted angle. (For example, if a patient with a pre-PAT angle of 20 Δ esotropia stabilized during PAT at 30 Δ esotropia, Scott would operate for the 30 Δ of esotropia.) Significantly, there were no overcorrections in the PAT response group despite the increased amount of surgery performed. For patients who adapted to greater than 60 Δ or who did not obtain a stable angle with peripheral fusion, he operated for the original angle of deviation.

The PAT Study

In the last 20 years the use of prisms presurgically as part of the surgical treatment for acquired esotropia has taken many forms.

Although the indications were that it would be helpful, studies varied significantly in almost all their parameters (the power and direction of prism worn, the definition of prism adaptation, the amount of surgery performed, the criteria of successful treatment etc.). In an attempt to evaluate the true effectiveness of prism adaptation, a prospective randomized multicenter clinical trial[6] was conducted with the support of the National Eye Institute. It attempted to answer the following two questions: (1) Does the overall effect of prism adaptation increase the chances of a good postsurgical alignment of the eyes? (2) Are patients who demonstrate fusion after a period of wearing prisms more likely to have successful alignment if they undergo surgery for their presenting angle of esotropia or for their prism-adapted angle of esotropia?

Investigators at 14 clinical centers screened 3574 patients who met three criteria. They had to be at least 3 years of age, to have had no previous eye surgery, and to have had an esotropia between 12 and 40 Δ. Of these, 333 (approximately 10%) were eventually randomized into the study. The remaining patients were excluded for a variety of reasons (Table 7-1). Before entry into the study, all patients underwent two cycloplegic refractions (two drops of 1% cyclopentolate 5 minutes apart) and had to wear their proper spectacle correction for at least a month. Visual acuity had to be at least 20/40 in each eye, and patching therapy was done in advance to achieve this acuity and maintain it during the study. Motor alignment was measured by means of the unilateral cover test (with prism estimation) and alternate cover test

TABLE 7-1
Exclusion Criteria and Number of Screenees Reporting

Exclusion criteria	Screenees reporting (criterion*)
Unwilling to participate	168 (4.7)
Onset of esotropia before 6 months	462 (12.9)
Dissociated vertical deviation	190 (5.3)
Manifest nystagmus	151 (4.2)
Latent nystagmus	168 (4.7)
Vertical strabismus >3 Δ	599 (16.8)
A/V pattern	552 (15.4)
Incomitance	245 (6.9)
Visual acuity worse than 20/40	943 (26.4)
Inability to assess visual acuity	497 (13.9)
Distance and near deviation differential >10 Δ	514 (14.4)
Inability to do Worth dot test	311 (8.7)
Fusion on red filter test	393 (11.0)
Not a surgical candidate	760 (21.3)
Other reason for exclusion	484 (13.5)

*More than one reason for exclusion may have been reported. The total number of patients screened was 3574; 333 patients were randomized.

with prism neutralization at both 6 m and 33 cm. Sensory tests were performed at the time of entry into the study and at each of the pre- and postoperative follow-up examinations. These tests included the Worth dot at distance and near, stereotesting at distance and near (AO vectographic slide and Titmus stereo fly), Bagolini striated lenses, and the red filter and light.*

A patient was classified as a prism adaptation responder (PAR) if when wearing the prism the unilateral cover test was between 0 and 8 Δ of esotropia at distance and near and one of the following applied: (1) A fusion response occurred on the Worth dot test at near. (2) Diplopia was reported on the Worth dot test at near but a stereo response of 2 out of 3 animals or 2 of 9 circles occurred on the Titmus test at near.

A patient was classified as a prism adaptation nonresponder (PANR) if any of the three following conditions developed: (1) Exotropia was manifested during the wearing of prisms along with suppression on the Worth dot test. (2) Motor stability was achieved between 0 and 8 Δ of esotropia with no fusion on the Worth dot test with up to 30 days of prism wear. (3) The prism adaptation process was so large that the angle adapted to was greater than 60 Δ.

The primary end point of the study was defined as the angle of deviation at distance measured by a masked examiner at the 6-month postoperative examination. A successful outcome was defined as a deviation of 8 Δ or less of esotropia or exotropia.

For the data analysis, four main study groups were categorized according to their randomization assignments (Fig. 7-2). Non-PA/ES referred to those subjects who did not undergo prism adaptation and had surgery for their entry angle of esotropia. PANR/ES referred to subjects who underwent prism adaptation and were nonresponders who had surgery for their entry angle of esotropia. PAR/ES referred to those subjects who underwent prism adaptation and were responders but had surgery for their entry angle of esotropia. Finally, PAR/PS referred to subjects who underwent prism adaptation and were responders who had surgery determined by their prism-adapted angle of esotropia.

Figure 7-3 illustrates the major question answered by the PAT study. The highest success rate, 89%, was achieved in the PAR/PS group. Success rates were lowest in the non-PA/ES group, 72% (92/127 patients). Prism-adapted nonresponders had a similar success rate, 73% (49/67 patients). The overall rate of success for patients who underwent the prism-adaptation process was estimated, from a weighted average of the success rates in the PAR/PS and PANR/ES groups, to be 83%. The difference between the success rates of the prism-adapted and the non–prism-adapted groups was statistically significant (p = 0.04).

*See Appendix for a full description of the patient selection criteria, methods of randomization, prism application, response or non-response criteria, etc.

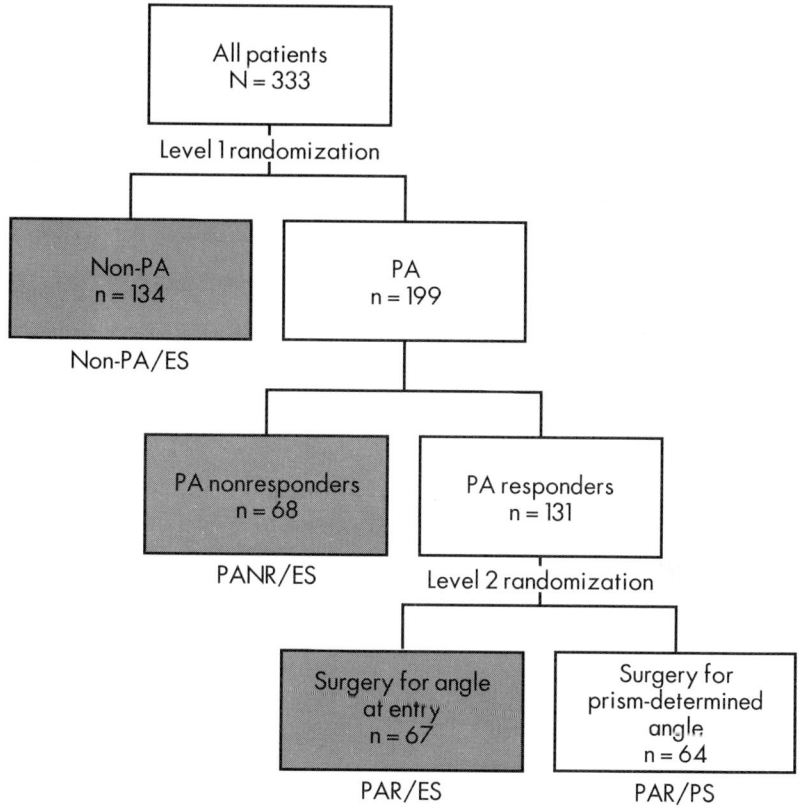

FIGURE 7-2 Prism adaptation (*PA*) trial and numbers of patients in each treatment group. *Non-PA/ES,* Non-PA patients who underwent surgery for the entry angle of esotropia; *PANR/ES,* PA nonresponders who underwent surgery for the entry angle of esotropia; *PAR/ES,* PA responders who underwent surgery for the entry angle of esotropia; *PAR/PS,* PA responders who underwent surgery for the prism-determined angle of esotropia.

The second major question of the study concerned the differences in success rates between the prism responders who had surgery determined by their prism-adapted angle of estropia and those who had surgery for their entry angle of estropia. The success rates were higher in the PAR/PS group, 89% (54/61 patients) than in the PAR/ES group, 79% (59/67 patients). This difference, although important, was not statistically significant (p = 0.23).

Figure 7-3 illustrates also that the best sensory results, as measured by the Worth dot test at near, were achieved in the PAR/PS group. The lowest rate for motor alignment and sensory fusion was in the PANR/ES group, 34%.

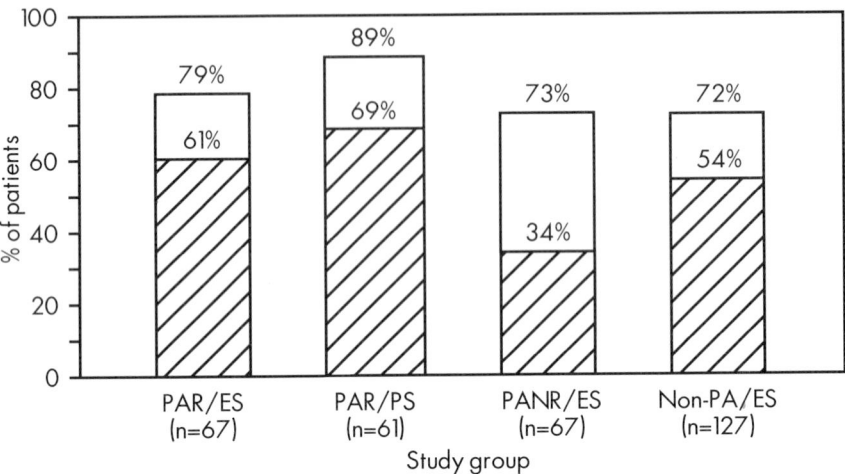

FIGURE 7-3 *Open bars* indicate the percentages of patients with deviations of 0 to 8 Δ by study group, measured 6 months after surgery by the unilateral cover test with prism estimation at 6 m. The overall prism adaptation (PA) motor success rate was 83%. *Shaded bars* indicate the percentages of patients with motor success plus fusion on the Worth dot test at near. *PAR/ES,* PA responders who underwent surgery for the entry angle of esotropia; *PAR/PS,* PA responders who underwent surgery for the prism-determined angle of esotropia; *PANR/ES,* PA nonresponders who underwent surgery for the entry angle of esotropia; *Non-PA/ES,* non-PA patients who underwent surgery for the entry angle of esotropia.

The data for the prism-adapted groups were analyzed further and divided into those whose angles built up to between 0 and 9 Δ and those with angles greater than 10 Δ. Patients whose angles built up very little had essentially the same surgery as the PAR/ES group; therefore we would expect similar success rates, and in fact the success rates were 86% and 88% respectively (Fig. 7-4). Those who built up to a greater angle (>10 Δ), however, had more millimeters of surgery and their success rates were higher, 70% versus 89% (p = 0.15).

Under- and overcorrection rates were also examined by group. There was real concern that the augmented amounts of surgery in the PAR/PS group might produce a greater overcorrection rate than normal. The opposite was true. A total of 7 overcorrections (exotropic deviations >8 Δ) occurred out of 322 operations performed. Five were in the non-PA/ES group, one was in the PANR/ES group, and one in the PAR/PS group.

Undercorrection rates were also examined (esotropia >8 Δ) and were found to be 21% to 25% in the groups having esotropia surgery for their entry angle but only 10% in the PAR/PA group.

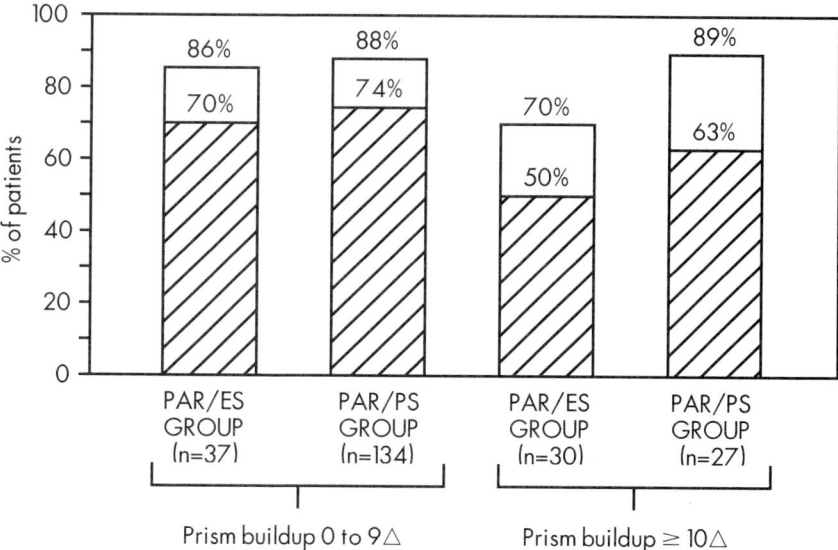

FIGURE 7-4 *Open bars* indicate the percentages of prism responders with deviations of 0 to 8 Δ by prism buildup and study group, measured 6 months after surgery by the unilateral cover test with prism estimation at 6 m. *Shaded bars* indicate the percentages of patients with motor success plus fusion on the Worth dot test. *PAR/ES*, PA responders who underwent surgery for the entry angle of esotropia; *PAR/PS*, PA responders who underwent surgery for the prism-determined angle of esotropia.

Figure 7-5 illustrates the final eye alignment as measured by the unilateral cover test (with prism estimation) at distance at the 6-month postoperative examination. The PAR/PS group had the highest percentage of orthotropic patients, 49%. Only 24% of the PANR/ES group were orthotropic and 31% of the non-PA/ES.

Clinical Significance

What have we learned from this 5-year, prospective randomized, multicenter clinical trial on acquired esotropia? The wearing of prism presurgically that neutralizes the angle of deviation, along with waiting a sufficient time for rudimentary sensory fusion to develop, offers the patient and the doctor the best hope of attaining a stable angle postsurgically and sufficient sensory fusion to maintain that eye alignment. In the study, 89% of the patients who wore prism and had surgery for the prism-adapted angle achieved a stable angle at the

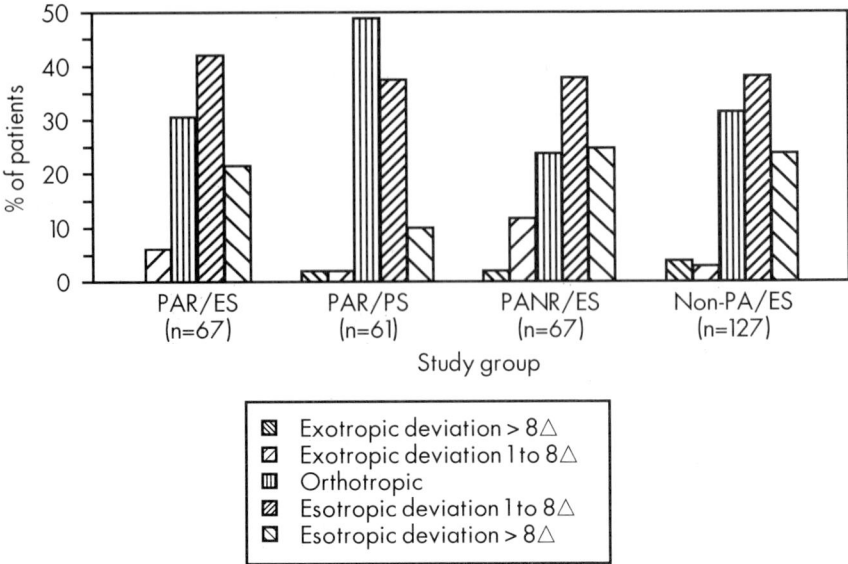

FIGURE 7-5 Percentage of patients in deviation categories by study group, measured 6 months after surgery by the unilateral cover test with prism estimation at 6 m. *PAR/ES,* PA responders who underwent surgery for the entry angle of esotropia; *PAR/PS,* PA responders who underwent surgery for the prism determined angle of esotropia; *PANR/ES,* PA nonresponders who underwent surgery for the entry angle of esotropia; *Non-PA/ES,* non-PA patients who underwent surgery for the entry angle of esotropia.

6-month postoperative examination. Additionally, 69% of those who had stable angles also attained rudimentary sensory fusion. This is a clinically and statistically significant improvement over the 72% success rate achieved when no prism was worn and the surgical target angle was the initial presenting angle.

Vision literature has supported the notion that sensory fusion enhancement before surgery increases the chances of attaining fusion after surgery,[7,8] and the PAT study supports that position. The use of prisms in orthoptic treatment can be passive, active (with vision therapy), or both. In this study Fresnel prisms that neutralized or almost neutralized the angle of deviation were worn by the patients for several weeks. No active orthoptics to break down suppression or enhance fusion was permitted. If gross fusion at near occurred, as tested by the Worth dot test, no further treatment was given and the patient simply wore the prism until surgery. If fusion did not occur, the prisms were worn for an additional 30 days to see if it would develop over time. No orthoptic treatment to establish fusion was permitted.

It is believed[9,10] that peripheral fusion is one of the essential elements needed to hold the eyes in motor alignment. Loss of the peripheral visual field in some pathological diseases can precipitate a strabismus, just as the lack of fusion can lead to a postsurgical drift following strabismus surgery. This point was borne out in the study also, because in cases in which fusion could not be established presurgically (PANR) only 34% of the cases demonstrated gross fusion after surgery. This compares to 61% and 69% when fusion was demonstrated before surgery.

If peripheral sensory fusion is the "glue" for motor alignment postsurgically, it would follow that every attempt should be made presurgically to establish sensory fusion. The PAT study made the first attempt at this by having patients wear prisms (passively, no orthoptic treatment permitted) to see if fusion would develop (presumably by magic). The next logical step would be for patients whose angles had been neutralized with prism to undergo active orthoptics to try to establish peripheral sensory fusion. Depending on the patients' needs, any or all of the following kinds of training could be used: (1) antisuppression therapy, (2) sensory fusion training with vergence demand (to build up motor fusion ranges around the angle of strabismus), (3) stereoawareness (third-degree fusion training). If successful, these techniques would enhance a patient's binocular sensory status presurgically and thus increase the chances of sensory fusion and long-term motor alignment postsurgically.

CLINICAL PEARL

If peripheral sensory fusion is the "glue" for motor alignment post-surgically, it should follow that every attempt should be made presurgically to establish sensory fusion.

The definition of a successful outcome from the PAT study was motor alignment between 8 Δ of esotropia and 8 Δ exotropia at the 6-month postoperative examination. This end point was chosen somewhat arbitrarily, although there is precedence for it in the literature. Parks[11] has described a phenomenon called monofixation syndrome in which patients generally have a small-angle strabismus (0 to 8 Δ), some central suppression, gross fusion at near, limited fusional vergence, and gross stereopsis. Parks[12] mentioned that when this condition occurs postsurgically the prognosis for long-term alignment stability is good. The postsurgical clinical profile of the PAT patients seems to parallel Parks' description of patients who would have a stable motor angle over time. Seventy-nine percent of the prism-adapted responders had an angle of esotropia 8 Δ or less at the 6-month examination. This certainly would fulfill the criteria of a good cosmetic result and perhaps a stable motor angle over time, but it often falls short of an acceptable functional result. If success was defined with a sensory component as well as motor alignment, however, the surgical success as reported in the PAT study[6] does not look as impressive. For those subjects who had their surgery determined by the entry angle of esotropia, there was only about a 37% chance that they would have a postsurgical angle less than 8 Δ and some rudimentary sensory fusion. If the prism-adapted angle was used to determine the amount of surgery, the patient had only a slightly better than 50% chance of achieving gross sensory fusion after surgery (61%). It would appear from these statistics that, although the amount of surgery performed helps determine the short-term stability of the angle, there are other more important factors determining the postsurgical sensory status. The most obvious is the presurgical sensory status.

Conclusions

If the goal in surgically treating an acquired esotropia is cosmetically straight eyes with functional binocular vision, then patching, prisms, and orthoptics must be used in the overall treatment both before and after surgery. The treatment sequence that follows illustrates how they can be used to achieve a successful motor *and* sensory result.
1. Full correction of the refractive error
2. Patching and orthoptics/pleoptics to equalize the visual acuity (if possible) when amblyopia is present
3. Prism adaptation until the motor angle stabilizes (if anomalous correspondence is *not* present)
4. Orthoptics to break down suppression and to enhance sensory and motor fusion, and stereopsis (if possible)
5. Surgery for the prism-adapted angle
6. Neutralization of any postsurgical deviation with prism to maintain bifoveal stimulation
7. Postsurgical sensory and motor fusion training to cement the surgical result

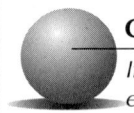

CLINICAL PEARL
If the goal in surgically treating an acquired esotropia is cosmetically straight eyes with functional binocular vision, then patching, prisms, and orthoptics must be used in the overall treatment both before and after surgery.

The prism adaptation study has demonstrated that prisms are definitely an integral part of the successful *surgical* treatment of acquired esotropia.

Appendix

All participating investigators were trained in and tested on the study protocol and were certified to ensure the uniformity of testing skills. Each of the 14 centers was provided with standardized equipment, and site visitations were conducted to verify adherence to the study protocol.

The prism prescribed for each patient was determined based on prism neutralization of the alternate cover test at distance. Fresnel prisms, necessary to neutralize this deviation, were mounted on the patient's spectacles. The prism power was divided as equally as possible between the two eyes. If unequal prisms were necessary, the higher value was placed before the fixating eye. The patient wore the prism prescription for 10 minutes while waiting in the office, and then the unilateral cover test was repeated. The unilateral cover test through the prism had to be within 0 to 8 Δ of esotropia at near. If it was not, the prism values were readjusted until this criterion was met. The patients wore their prism prescription for 1 week and then were retested to determine their response. If the angle was greater than 8 Δ of esotropia through the Fresnel prisms and no fusion with the Worth dot test at near was elicited, the prisms were removed and larger prisms were applied to neutralize the greater deviation. If the motor alignment was stable but sensory fusion on the Worth dot test could not be demonstrated, the same prisms were worn for 4 more weeks to see if sensory fusion could be established. This adjustment procedure was followed weekly until the patient could be classified as a prism responder or nonresponder.

The study involved two levels of randomization of 333 patients:

The first level was based on whether a patient was randomly selected to undergo prism adaptation. Figure 7-2 shows that 199 patients were assigned to prism adaptation and 134 did not wear prisms but had surgery based on their presenting angle of esotropia as measured by the alternate cover test at distance.

Of the 199 prism-adapted patients, the study classified 68 as nonresponders and 131 as responders. For the *nonresponders,* prisms were removed from the glasses and the angle of deviation was allowed to return to the entry level value. These patients received conventional amounts of surgery based on their presenting angle as measured by the alternate cover test at distance. For the *responders* (that is, whose angle of strabismus increased somewhat and then stabilized at the higher value, with some fusion demonstrated) a second level of randomization occurred. Sixty-seven of 131 had surgery amounts determined by their presenting angles of esotropia before prism adaptation. (Effectively, the prism adaptation information was not used to determine the amount of surgery.) For example, if a patient presented initially with 20 Δ of esotropia and was prism adapted and stabilized at 30 Δ, the surgery was performed for 20 Δ of esotropia (3.5 mm bimedial recession versus 4.5 mm bimedial recession). Sixty-four of 131 had amounts of surgery determined by their prism adapted-angle of esotropia.

Tables and figures are from Prism Adaptation Study Research Group: Efficacy of prism adaptation in the surgical management of acquired esotropia, Arch Ophthalmol *108:1248-1256, 1990.*

References

1. Aust W, Welge-Lussen L: Pre-operative and post-operative changes in the angle of squint following long-term, pre-operative prismatic compensation. In Fells P (ed): *The First Congress of the International Strabismological Association,* St Louis, 1971, Mosby.
2. Jampolsky A: A simplified approach to strabismus diagnosis. In *Symposium on Strabismus, Transactions of the New Orleans Academy of Ophthalmology,* St Louis, 1978, Mosby, pp 66-75.
3. Stella S: Prism adaptation in nonaccommodative esotropes. Presented at the Western Regional Orthoptic Meeting, Snowmass, Colo, 1974.
4. Scott WE: Office use of prisms. In *Symposium on Strabismus, Transactions of the New Orleans Academy of Ophthalmology,* St Louis, 1978, Mosby, pp 91-103.
5. Scott WE, Thalacker JA: Preoperative prism adaptation in acquired esotropia, *Ophthalmologica* 189:49-53, 1984.
6. Prism Adaptation Study Research Group: Efficacy of prism adaptation in the surgical management of acquired esotropia, *Arch Ophthalmol* 108:1248-1256, 1990.
7. Lyle TK: Orthoptic training. Oxford Ophthalmology Congress, *Trans Ophthalmol Soc UK* 59:491, 1939.
8. Berens C, Elliot AJ, Sobacke L: Orthoptic training and the surgical correction of strabismus, *Am J Ophthalmol* 24:1418-1422, 1941.
9. Burian HM: Fusional movements: role of peripheral retinal stimuli, *Arch Ophthalmol* 21:486-491, 1939.
10. Kertesz AE: Effect of stimulus size on fusion and vergence, *J Opt Soc Am* 71:289-293, 1981.
11. Parks MM: The monofixation syndrome. In *Symposium on Strabismus, Transactions of the New Orleans Academy of Ophthalmology,* St Louis, 1978, Mosby, p 127.
12. Parks MM: Monofixation syndrome. In Tasman W, Jaeger EA (eds): *Duane's clinical ophthalmology,* vol 1, Philadelphia 1989, JB Lippincott, pp 1-10.

Self-Assessment Questions

1. The Prism Adaptation Test is most useful in
   a. congenital esotropia
   b. acquired esotropia
   c. intermittent exotropia
   d. constant exotropia

2. A responder to the prism adaptation process would have a stable angle between 0 and 8 Δ of esotropia while wearing prisms and
   a. two out of four circles correct on the distance Titmus stereo test
   b. only moderate suppression on the red light test
   c. a fusion response on the Worth dot test at near
   d. at least 20/40 vision in one eye

3. The highest surgical success rate was reported for which group?
   a. prism-adapted responders undergoing prism-determined surgery
   b. prism-adapted responders undergoing entry angle–determined surgery
   c. prism-adapted nonresponders undergoing prism-determined surgery
   d. prism-adapted nonresponders undergoing entry angle–determined surgery

4. What are the four treatment steps recommended prior to the surgical correction of strabismus (in their correct order)?
   a. fully correct the refractive error, treat the anomalous correspondence, patch for amblyopia, and increase the base-in vergence ranges
   b. fully correct the refractive error, patch for amblyopia, prism adapt to stabilize the motor angle, and institute a program of orthoptics to enhance binocularity
   c. fully correct the refractive error, prism adapt to stabilize the motor angle, patch for amblyopia, and institute a program of orthoptics to enhance binocularity
   d. fully correct the refractive error, increase the base-in vergence ranges, treat anomalous correspondence, and prism adapt to stabilize the motor angle

---

Answers: 1. b.   2. c.   3. a.   4. b.

8

Prescribing Prisms for Strabismus

Elizabeth E. Caloroso
Susan A. Cotter

Key Terms

strabismus	yoked prism	muscle contracture
esotropia	sector prism	suppression
relieving prism	inverse prism	penalization
vision therapy	corrective prism	cosmetic prism
amblyopia	fusion prism	titration
eccentric fixation	noncomitant	
diplopia	strabismus	

The decision to prescribe prisms for strabismic patients is made after a diagnostic profile is determined by taking a complete history, performing tests to evaluate sensory and motor processing, and summarizing the key factors leading to a reasonable prognosis for binocular vision. Prisms are most often prescribed to establish or stabilize efficient binocular vision, but they may also be used to diagnose masked oculomotor deviations, disrupt sensory anomalies, treat sensorimotor dysfunction, eliminate diplopia, and improve cosmesis in some nonresolvable cases.

Prism therapy for heterophores has been advocated for years,[1-10] and prism-prescribing criteria for symptomatic patients has been investigated in many later studies.[11-17] Strabismic patients also benefit from prism therapy, but they exhibit different sensorimotor processing from heterophores, and this influences the choice of goals to achieve and the type of prisms prescribed to accomplish these goals.[18-24] Heterophores have binocular vision for all waking hours and exhibit a strong propensity to maintain binocular vision even when binocular visual skills are inefficient. If a binocular vision dysfunction is present, it most frequently occurs in the vergence system controlling the oculomotor deviation or in the accommodative convergence system in an effort to assist a deficient vergence system. Sensory skills may appear to be reduced but often will be normal if testing is done without contamination by the motor system (for example, a stereopsis test performed with corrective or relieving prisms). Although active vision therapy (orthoptics or vision training) is recommended as additive therapy when accommodative, sensory, and motor dysfunctions are present, prisms that optically decrease the demand to fusional vergence may quickly eliminate subjective symptoms and restore efficient binocular vision for many heterophores whose primary problems lie in the vergence system (see Chapters 5 and 6).

Strabismic patients, however, often present with multiple sensory anomalies as well as motor anomalies and exhibit a low to moderate propensity toward obtaining or maintaining binocular vision. If relieving prisms are prescribed before sensory anomalies are eliminated, the results may be poor and prism therapy may appear to be contraindicated. Actually, prism therapy may be very successful if delayed until the sensory anomalies are corrected. While prisms do not replace other needed treatment options (Table 8-1) for a given strabismic patient, many patients can be successfully managed by prism therapy alone. More often, prisms are an important tool within the overall binocular vision treatment plan[25] (Table 8-2) and are used in combination with other treatments.

Prisms are not a substitute for the optical correction of a significant ametropia. First, lenses are prescribed that both correct the ametropia

TABLE 8-1
Common Treatment Options for Strabismus

Passive	Active
Lenses	Active vision therapy
Prisms	
Occlusion	
Surgery	

TABLE 8-2
Sequential Binocular Vision Treatment Plan

Phase	Goal	Technique
1	Establish initial optical correction	Prescribe optimum lenses Consider relieving or training prisms Consider occlusion therapy
2	Improve monocular visual functioning	Improve amblyopia to 20/80 Improve accommodative functioning Improve ocular motilities, eye-hand coordination
3	Establish normal peripheral fusion	Eliminate peripheral suppressions Eliminate anomalous correspondence Stabilize normal peripheral sensorimotor fusion skills
4	Establish normal central/foveal fusion	Eliminate central/foveal suppressions Improve shallow amblyopia Stabilize efficient central/foveal sensorimotor fusion skills
5	Obtain binocular vision in open space	Consider need for relieving prisms Consider need for strabismic surgery Stabilize accommodative and vergence efficiency
6	Prescribe at-home maintenance program	Prescribe active therapy for fitness maintenance Reevaluate health and refraction at needed intervals Reevaluate visual skills at needed intervals

From Caloroso EE, Rouse MW: *Clinical management of strabismus,* Boston, 1993, Butterworth-Heinemann, p 69.

and reduce the strabismic angle maximally. Then a decision is made to prescribe prisms, either for establishing binocular vision or for achieving a specific visual goal. When treating a strabismic patient sequentially, one prescribes relieving prisms initially as long as the patient has normal sensory skills and motor skills that are sufficiently high to permit binocular vision in open space viewing most of the time (80%) (that is, strabismus 20% or less of the time). Improved visual skills should occur through passive stimulation (habitual environmental viewing) or active stimulation (active vision therapy with specific target parameters). If binocular vision for most open space viewing time cannot be expected, relieving prisms should be postponed until sensory skills are corrected by active vision therapy and motor skills improved by active therapy or surgery.

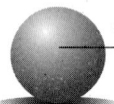

CLINICAL PEARL

When treating a strabismic patient sequentially, one prescribes relieving prisms initially as long as the patient has normal sensory skills and motor skills that are sufficiently high to permit binocular vision in open space viewing most of the time (80%).

Prism Applications

Many types of prism application[26] with different optical actions and goals (Table 8-3) are available for clinical use, the most frequently prescribed being relieving prisms. A prism bends the incident light toward its base while moving the image of the viewed target toward its apex.[27] Relieving prisms reduce, but do not eliminate, the demand for fusional vergence to control the deviation and thus are effective when the strabismus is intermittent and some motor fusion skills exist (Fig. 8-1). The facilitation of efficient motor control of an oculomotor deviation (objective angle) by relieving prisms should lead to improved vergence skills and sensory fusion stabilization and should also eliminate the subjective symptoms associated with attempts to achieve or maintain motor fusion without prism.

TABLE 8-3

Prism Therapies

Type	Goal	Action
Corrective	Stabilize normal sensory fusion	Neutralize demand for controlling fusional vergence
Inverse, binocular	Increase fusional vergence ability	Increase demand for controlling fusional vergence
Inverse, monocular	Disrupt eccentric fixation	Change retinal location of viewed targets
Overcorrective	Disrupt anomalous correspondence	Reverse demand for controlling fusional vergence
Relieving	Stabilize sensorimotor fusion	Reduce demand for controlling fusional vergence
Rotating, binocular	Disrupt anomalous correspondence	Change sensorimotor stimulation in time sequence
Rotating, monocular	Disrupt eccentric fixation	Change monocular sensorimotor stimulation in time sequence
Sector	Stabilize binocular vision in one or more gaze positions	Reduce demand for controlling fusional vergence in one or more gaze positions
Yoked prisms	Stabilize binocular vision in noncomitancy or dampen nystagmus	Direct eyes into specific gaze position

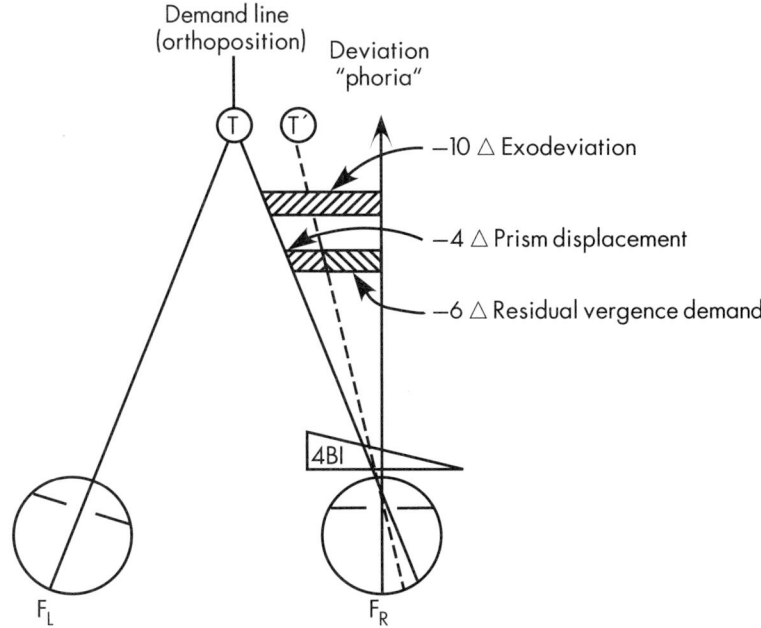

FIGURE 8-1 Binocular prism viewing. The target (*T*) is optically displaced (*T'*) by a 4 Δ base-in prism, reducing the vergence demand to 6 Δ. The fusional convergence response to obtain bifoveal fixation is reduced from 10 to 6 Δ. F_L, Fovea of the left eye; F_R, fovea of the right eye. (From Caloroso EE, Rouse MW: *Clinical management of strabismus*, Boston, 1993, Butterworth-Heinemann.)

A single-powered relieving prism is generally all that is needed for a comitant horizontal deviation, although a multi-powered prism (that is, one power for far and another for near) may be necessary for patients with a high or low AC/A ratio. A common example is the patient who has a divergence insufficiency esodeviation that is greater at far than at near[28] and who typically needs a prism power at distance that is intolerable at near. When a noncomitant deviation exists, multi-powered relieving, yoked, or sector prisms must also be considered.

Other prism therapies for strabismus are designed to achieve specific binocular goals by changes in prism power and base directions as well as laterality. Corrective prisms neutralize the strabismic angle and should produce normal sensory fusion for a constant strabismus if other sensory anomalies (such as suppression, amblyopia, or anomalous correspondence) are not present. Overcorrective prisms are designed to change habitual visual stimulation from the nasal to the temporal hemiretina and to disrupt habitual anomalous correspondence in esotropias (see Chapter 9). Inverse prisms may disrupt eccentric fixation when prescribed for monocular viewing by

an amblyopic eye. When prescribed binocularly, inverse prisms increase the demand for controlling fusional vergence and thus stimulate an expansion of vergence ranges (Fig. 8-2).

Prism therapies for strabismus may be prescribed in lieu of or
combined with an orthoptic vision therapy program. Whenever
prisms are used, the practitioner must check the patient at

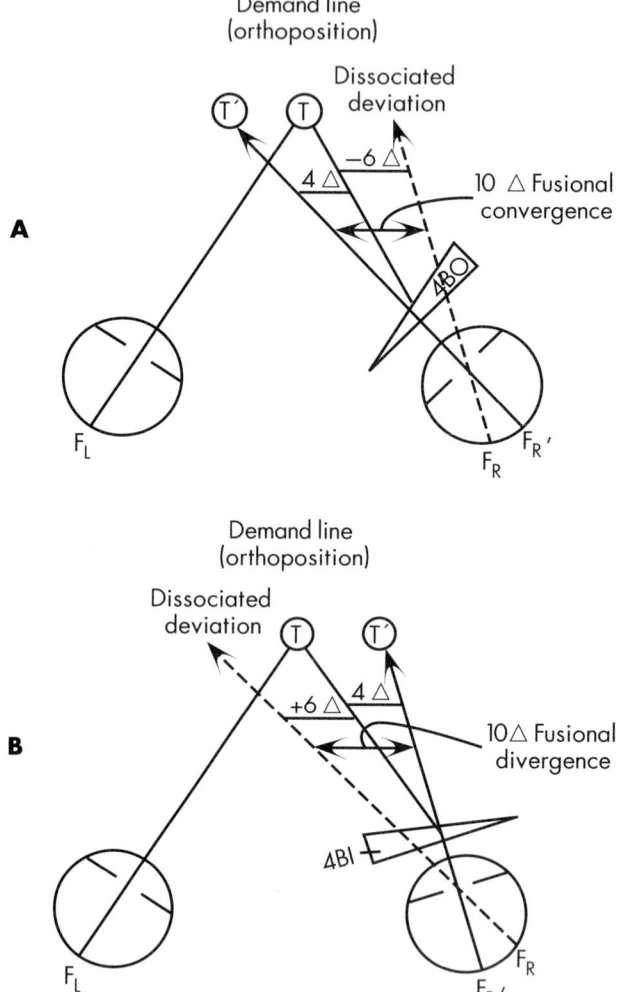

FIGURE 8-2 Inverse prism with binocular viewing. The image (T')
of the target (T) is optically displaced toward the apex of the prism,
stimulating an increased vergence response to maintain bifoveal
fixation. **A,** A 6 Δ exophore with 4 Δ increase in fusional convergence resulting from an added 4 Δ BO prism. **B,** A 6 Δ esophore
with 4 Δ increase in fusional divergence from an added 4 Δ BI
prism. F_L, F_R, Foveas of the left and right eyes.

appropriate intervals to see that the visual goals of therapy are being achieved and must be prepared to modify the prism power as needed. If unexpected or undesirable results occur,[29-32] (such as prism adaptation), it may become necessary to reevaluate the diagnostic data and modify the therapy program. However, many strabismic patients do respond to prisms as theoretically predicted and these individuals can progress to efficient binocular vision with one or more prism applications during the therapy program. The appropriate type and power of prism must be selected to accomplish the desired goal within the framework of the total treatment sequence; and when binocular vision is the goal, changes in prism type and prism power are to be expected as progress is made.

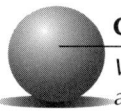

CLINICAL PEARL

Whenever prisms are used, the practitioner must check the patient at appropriate intervals to see that the visual goals of therapy are being achieved and must be prepared to modify the prism power as needed.

Prognostic Guidelines

The diagnostic profile of a strabismic patient will determine the type of prism therapy to prescribe. However, other factors should be considered when attempting to predict the success of this treatment option. Although the patient's attitudes (motivation, understanding, perseverance, compliance) are crucial, some predictions can be made based on the age of onset and the duration of the strabismus before instituting prism therapy.

Early Onset and Long Duration Strabismus

Patients in whom strabismus occurred before 7 years of age can be expected to have the most profound sensory anomalies and generally increased resistance to the reestablishment of binocular vision. A "long" duration, however, may be a relatively short time interval for infants and a relatively longer time interval for older patients. Although time periods for the development of sensory anomalies after a strabismic onset are currently unknown, our clinical observations suggest the following: 1 to 3 months for infants, 3 to 6 months for toddlers, and 6 months to 1 year for preschoolers and children to age 7 years.

Patients with a constant strabismus of long duration typically do not respond well to relieving prism until normal sensory processing has been reestablished and motor skills improved to a maximal level by either active vision therapy or other types of prism treatment. A common mistake in long-duration strabismus is to prescribe relieving prisms too soon, often when peripheral fusion is possible but central suppression or amblyopia remains. In addition, peripheral vergence skills may be absent or minimal. Typically, the result is a fragile binocular system with regressions of visual skills or the continuing need for higher amounts of prism. The best prismatic results occur when (1) normal central and foveal sensory fusion skills are present and (2) motor fusion skills have improved to a maximal level before the patient starts wearing relieving prisms designed to stabilize binocular vision in open space.

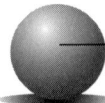

CLINICAL PEARL

Patients with a constant strabismus of long duration typically do not respond well to relieving prism until normal sensory processing has been reestablished and motor skills improved to a maximal level.

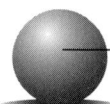

CLINICAL PEARL

The best prismatic results occur when (1) normal central and foveal sensory fusion skills are present and (2) motor fusion skills have improved to a maximal level before the strabismic patient starts wearing relieving prisms designed to stabilize binocular vision in open space.

Recent Onset and Short Duration Strabismus

Patients who are treated soon after the onset of strabismus usually respond well to prism therapy. Adults who present with a recent onset have usually had many years of normal binocular vision before the onset; they therefore typically present with a motor deficit but no sensory anomalies. Consequently, their chief complaint is diplopia in all or certain fields of gaze. Relieving, yoked, or sector prisms may be all that are needed to improve motor functioning and reestablish binocular vision in primary and other affected gazes. For patients with transitory motor anomalies (such as recovery from stroke or closed head trauma), changes in the power or type of prisms can be expected during the treatment plan.[33-36]

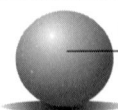

CLINICAL PEARL

Patients who are treated soon after the onset of a strabismus usually respond well to prism therapy.

Successful prism therapy can also occur in children with a recent strabismic onset. Although infant and early childhood strabismus may quickly result in multiple sensorimotor anomalies, treatment performed within critical time periods can lead to fast recovery.[37-38] Prism therapy applied quickly after the onset of a strabismus may prevent sensory anomalies from developing and may stabilize normal sensorimotor responses. Changes in prism power can be expected to be made as improvement in binocular visual skills occur.

Prism Therapies for Amblyopia

Strabismic patients with a unilateral deviation typically have functional amblyopia of the deviating eye that can range from a deep to a shallow loss of visual acuity. In many cases the monocular fixation pattern shows an eccentricity in the retinal site used for fixation of a target; and in other cases, foveal fixation may be present despite reduced visual acuity. Uncorrected anisometropes, with or without an associated strabismus, also may have amblyopia with either eccentric fixation (EF) or foveal fixation (FF). A plan combining occlusion and active vision therapy is the preferred treatment modality, with direct occlusion (that is, patching the preferred eye) for patients with either foveal or unsteady EF and inverse occlusion (patching the amblyopic eye) for patients with steady EF. However, alternative prism therapies can be considered for patients unable or unwilling to participate in the preferred program.

The method of monocular inverse prism wear[39-40] is designed to disrupt EF of an amblyopic eye and has been used the most extensively. Other treatment methods for amblyopia with either EF or FF combine prisms with passive treatment options such as filters, penalization lenses, and medication. These methods, typically, allow some level of binocular visual stimulation while forcing the transfer of fixation to the amblyopic eye (by degrading visual input to the preferred eye). Thus improvement of visual acuity of the amblyopic eye can occur as binocular skills are established or improved. Patients responding best to these binocular methods are nonstrabismic anisometropes, heterophores, and small-angle strabismics with latent vergence skills, the latter activated as acuity in the amblyopic eye improves. For many other strabismic patients, additional procedures to obtain binocular vision must be added after amblyopia treatment goals have been obtained. Our discussion of two prismatic methods—monocular inverse prism for amblyopia with EF and binocular corrective prisms combined with penalization for amblyopia with EF or FF—illustrates some of the goals and methodologies of current prism therapies proposed for the treatment of amblyopia associated with strabismus or anisometropia.

Monocular Inverse Prism

A prism with its base in the direction of the EF is prescribed for full-time wear over the amblyopic eye, BI for nasal EF and BO for temporal EF, while the nonamblyopic eye is totally occluded. The power of this prism equals or exceeds the size of EF by about 2 prism diopters (Δ), and in cases of unsteady EF the largest position is selected. The goal is to displace the target viewed by the amblyopic eye to a retinal site other than the habitual EF site, thus altering the sensorimotor input (Fig. 8-3, *A* and *B*). The apparent target is displaced by an amount equal to the prism power and in the direction of the prism apex. A duction movement of the amblyopic eye occurs to compensate for the apparent displacement of the target and maintain the habitual EF pattern (Fig. 8-3, *C*), thus moving the amblyopic eye into primary gaze. By reaching out and touching objects in the environment, the patient becomes aware of the error between the real and apparent target locations and the mismatch existing between visual and kinesthetic inputs. In a period of 1 to 4

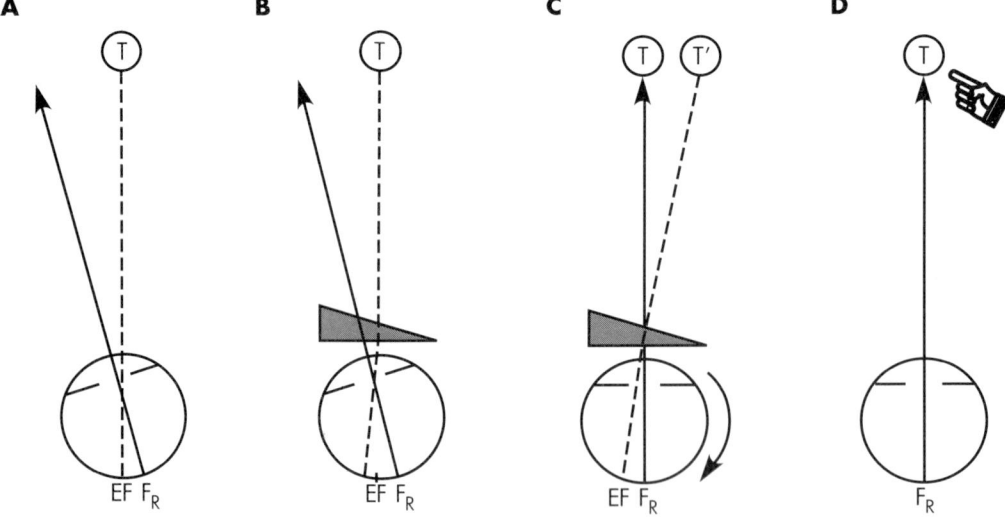

FIGURE 8-3 Inverse prism with monocular viewing. **A,** The patient's right eye shows nasal EF. **B,** The addition of base-in prism displaces the image of the target (*T'*) toward the nasal retina, beyond the EF point. **C,** The right eye makes an abduction movement in response to the base-in prism, aligning the EF point with the image *T'*. **D,** Foveal fixation stimulated by the combined visual/kinesthetic input is established, and EF is eliminated. (Modified from Caloroso EE, Rouse MW: *Clinical management of strabismus,* Boston, 1993, Butterworth-Heinemann.)

months, EF should change to foveal fixation and visual acuity should improve to 20/50 or better[39,40] (Fig. 8-3, D).

Inverse prism therapy may be prescribed for all magnitudes of EF, although the results seem most favorable for magnitudes between 3 and 20 Δ. For amblyopes with an eccentricity of 3 Δ or less, this may be improved by adding monocular amblyopia therapy (such as form recognition, accommodative training, eye-hand activities and visual activities with decreasing target sizes). The addition of active vision therapy generally results in a shorter treatment time for all amblyopes; however, it is possible for some patients to attain success in all the monocular treatment goals of amblyopia with only habitual viewing through the inverse prism.

After completion of inverse prism therapy, the amblyope should have steady foveal fixation and normal visual acuity of the amblyopic eye when tested monocularly. If acuity regression is to be prevented after the occluder and prism are removed, stabilization of binocular vision must then be undertaken. Suitable binocular prisms or other treatment options (Table 8-1) are added to establish efficient and stable binocular vision. In those cases in which binocular vision is not possible, a visual acuity–maintenance program[41] using part-time monocular visual stimulation of the amblyopic eye or a penalization lens for the nonamblyopic eye is prescribed.

Corrective Prisms and Penalization

A prism whose magnitude is equal to the strabismic angle at near and whose base direction is such that the amblyopic eye turns synergistically into primary gaze[42] is applied before the nonamblyopic eye. Because EF is manifested only under monocular conditions, the amblyopic eye turns an amount equal to the oculomotor deviation, which is generally larger than the amount of EF (for instance, a 15 Δ basic constant right esotrope with amblyopia of 20/200 and an unsteady 2 to 3 Δ nasal EF of the right eye) (Fig. 8-4, A). In this example a 15 Δ BO prism would be placed before the preferred left eye and would cause an adductive movement to maintain fixation on the apparently displaced target (Fig. 8-4, B). Based on Hering's law, the amblyopic eye would turn the same amount and in the same direction. Thus its fovea would now be in line with the real target, although a left esotropia would remain.

The preferred eye wears the distance retractive correction and continues to fixate distant targets. The amblyopic eye wears an overcorrection of +3.00 DS (a fogging or "penalization" lens), which creates an optical blur for distance while becoming an add for near. Alternation of fixation should occur; in other words, the nonamblyopic eye should be used for distant objects and the amblyopic eye for near objects (as visual acuity improves). In certain cases it is expected that the EF will decrease and be eliminated as foveal fixation is stimulated over time or as a result of the altered motor innervation to the amblyopic eye. Gross

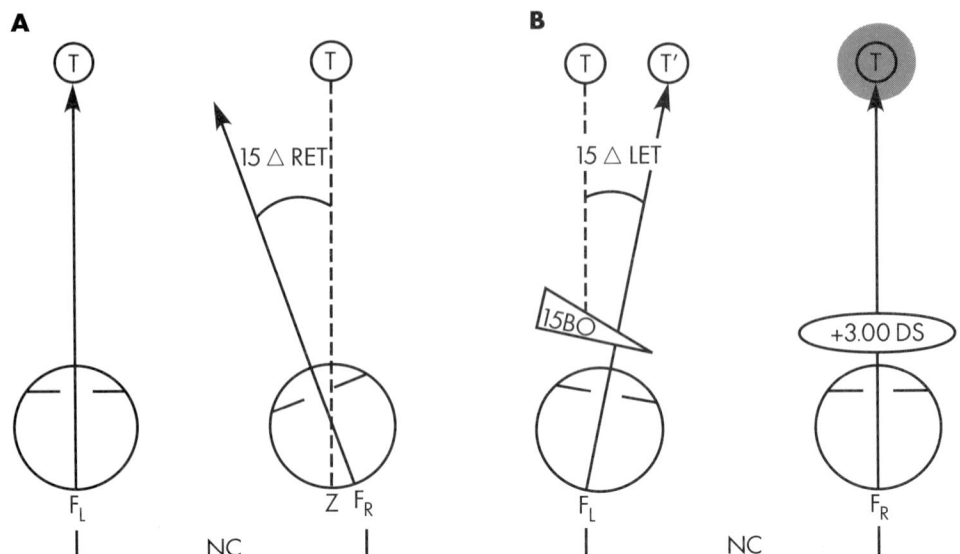

FIGURE 8-4 Corrective prism and penalization therapy for amblyopia. **A,** The retinal image of the target (*T*) is habitually centered at the fovea of the left eye and the zero measure point (*Z*) of the esotropic right eye. **B,** A corrective 15 Δ base-out prism is placed before the left eye, and a +3.00 fogging lens before the right eye. At distance, the OS retinal image is clear but the OD is blurred. *RET,* Right esotropia; *NC,* normal correspondence; *LET,* left esotropia.

peripheral sensorimotor fusion may also be established simultaneously with amblyopia improvement because objects are being viewed binocularly at the objective angle in open space (because the patient is wearing corrective prism). A higher level of binocular fusion is not expected due to the induced optical anisometropia (a 3.00 D difference in the ametropic correction). Correspondence and alternation of fixation must be carefully monitored during the therapy.

Although this prism method is not commonly used and needs further study, it may serve as an alternative procedure for patients resistant to occlusion or when occlusion is contraindicated (as in latent nystagmus) and can be prescribed for amblyopes with either foveal or eccentric fixation. Likewise, it may be useful for very young children or difficult-to-treat small-angle esotropes in whom the goal of rapidly maintaining or reestablishing binocularity is important to the ultimate restoration of efficient binocular vision.

Prism Therapies for Intermittent Strabismus

Strabismic patients are classified as intermittent when normal binocular alignment is present part of the time and an eye turn is present at other times. For this discussion, patients who present with a constant strabismus but who can achieve binocularity with added prism in all or needed fields of gaze will also be considered as intermittent strabismics.

Relieving Prisms

Relieving prisms are prescribed to eliminate subjective symptoms and stabilize efficient binocular vision in open visual space. The intermittent strabismic, who is capable of achieving motor fusion and bifixation of a viewed target for limited periods (such as a minimum of 80% of the time), can be treated in a manner similar to the heterophoric patient, the major difference being that higher prismatic powers are prescribed for the strabismic patient. Strabismics typically have an oculomotor deviation larger than that of heterophores; thus relatively large amounts of prism are needed so the patient can maintain bifoveal fixation using fusional vergence.

Although the common rule for prescribing relieving prisms (that is, give the minimal amount that will achieve comfortable binocular vision) applies to strabismics as well as to heterophores, the minimal amount for strabismics may be moderate to high (Table 8-4). If too little prism is given, binocular vision will not be attained or maintained. When binocular visual skills and the propensity to maintain binocular vision have improved, prism power can be decreased (in small steps, such as 2 or 4 Δ). The general rule for strabismics is to prescribe as much relieving prism as necessary to stabilize normal sensorimotor fusion in open space and then decrease the power over time as either motor fusion skills improve or the size of the deviation decreases.

CLINICAL PEARL

The general rule for intermittent strabismic patients is to prescribe as much relieving prism as necessary to stabilize normal sensorimotor fusion in open space and then decrease the power over time as either motor fusion skills improve or the size of the deviation decreases.

TABLE 8-4

Prism Power Classification

	(Δ)
Minimal	1 to 2
Low	3 to 10
Moderate	11 to 20
High	21 and higher

Many guidelines have been proposed to aid the practitioner in arriving at the direction and power of relieving prism to prescribe, but the most popular are Sheard's criterion, the fixation disparity curve (FDC), and fixation disparity neutralization (FDN) (that is, associated phoria). (See Chapter 5.) The first of these, Sheard's, considers the size of the oculomotor deviation and the compensating fusional vergence range available to control it. The FDC considers the stability of the fixation disparity as vergence is stimulated. The FDN considers the direction and power of relieving prism needed to eliminate this vergence error (that is, the fixation disparity) when bifoveal fusion is present. Although some intermittent strabismics can achieve efficient binocular vision using the prism prescribed from these criteria, others cannot because of an inability to bifixate and fuse the test target or because suppression prevents a binocular response.

When sensorimotor skills have been improved to maximal levels in instruments but the patient is unable to achieve binocular vision in open space, Caloroso's *residual vergence demand* (RVD) may be used to prescribe prismatic power. This criterion considers the deviation size that can be expected to be controlled efficiently and comfortably through normal sensorimotor fusion skills based on longitudinal observations of treated patients.[43] The residual ocular deviation desired after adding relieving prisms would be an esodeviation demand of 4 to 6 Δ, an exodeviation demand of 10 to 15 Δ, or a vertical deviation of 2 to 4 Δ. Prism power is calculated by subtracting the desired deviation size from the dissociated deviation size; for example, 16 Δ of esodeviation would have 10 Δ BO prescribed, leaving a residual demand of 6 Δ. This criterion can be used only for certain sizes of strabismic deviations (Table 8-5), and for cases in which the maximum vergence ranges have been obtained before wearing the prism. For strabismic patients who can achieve a higher than expected vergence range (comfortably and with accommodative accuracy), prism power may be reduced and other criteria (such as fixation disparity or Sheard's) should provide a more appropriate prism power to prescribe.

TABLE 8-5
Residual Vergence Demand (RVD) Criterion Guidelines

Direction	Magnitude (Δ)	RVD (Δ)
Esodeviation	6 to 20	4 to 6
Hyperdeviation	3 to 10	2 to 4
Exodeviation	20 to 30	10 to 15

Modified from Caloroso EE, Rouse MW: *Clinical management of strabismus,* Boston, 1993, Butterworth-Heinemann, p 104.

The preferred sequence for successfully prescribing relieving prisms to stabilize efficient binocular vision is to (1) correct accommodative and sensory anomalies by lenses, occlusion, and active vision therapy, (2) prescribe active vision therapy to increase vergence ranges and facility, and (3) prescribe relieving prisms to optically reduce the size of the oculomotor deviation to a controllable level. When binocular goals are to be achieved through a prism therapy–only approach, the best lens prescription correcting the ametropia and reducing the strabismic deviation, together with the prisms that will achieve binocular vision in open space, are prescribed.

Fusion Prisms

Prisms that change a diplopic or suppression response to a normal binocular response are called "fusion prisms" and are either corrective or relieving in the base and power prescribed. For example, a patient fixates a white light with the preferred right eye while a red filter is placed before the left eye to monitor suppression. Prism is placed before the left eye and the prism power that results in a normal sensorimotor fusion response (one pink light) is the prism that is prescribed. It provides a starting place for the intermittent strabismic to obtain binocular vision. Later, when sensorimotor skills improve, a stereopsis or fixation disparity test can be performed to modify prism power under conditions stimulating accuracy in accommodation and vergence. It should be noted that patients having either poor sensory skills or a masked larger deviation are likely to need different prism powers over time, less if visual skills improve and more if visual skills are inefficient or deteriorate.

Strabismics with either a horizontal or a vertical deviation can be treated with relieving prisms[44-47] that are generally a single power for all distances and gazes. However, it is the patient with a combined horizontal and vertical deviation who is the most difficult to treat and who frequently responds best to tests determining fusion prism power. Although this person is nearly always noncomitant, the difference in angle size at different gazes may be minimal so that a single prism power (either horizontal and/or vertical prism) can stabilize binocular vision. The prescribing prism criteria will be similar to those used for an intermittent comitant strabismic patient. However, the patient with a moderate to marked noncomitancy frequently needs more than one prism power to achieve fusion. In addition, many noncomitant patients require more than one type of prism application—a combination of relieving, yoked, and/or sector prisms.

Combined horizontal and vertical strabismus

A useful means of measuring and prescribing for both horizontal and vertical deviations at once has been described by Jampolsky,[48] the Tanganelli vector prism measure. To begin, the patient wears his or her best lens correction in a trial frame and fixates a transilluminator light. A single Bagolini striated lens, oriented at any axis, is placed in the trial frame before the fixating eye and a red lens is placed before the strabismic eye (Fig. 8-5, *A*). The patient should see a white light (fixating eye), a red light (strabismic eye), and a white streak of light (fixating eye) produced by the Bagolini lens. The patient is asked to fixate the white light while noting the position of the red light. The Bagolini lens then is rotated until the white streak crosses through the middle of the red light (Fig. 8-5, *B*). At this point, the orientation of the white streak (as well as the orientation mark on the Bagolini lens) denotes the axis of the correcting prism. Prism in increasing amounts with its base perpendicular to the Bagolini streak indicator and its apex pointing in the direction of the red light is placed over the Bagolini lens until the patient reports fusion of the white and red lights (Fig. 8-5, *C*). This value determines the single prism power that neutralizes the horizontal and vertical components of the deviation.

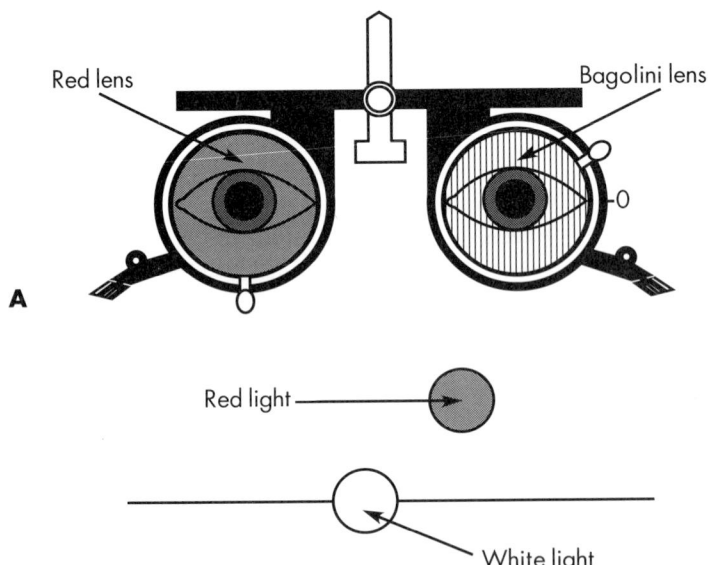

FIGURE 8-5 The Tanganelli vector prism measure. **A,** The patient wears a trial frame with red lens OD and Bagolini lens OS arbitrarily oriented at an axis of 180°. Through the Bagolini lens the red light appears above and to the right of the white light (from the patient's perspective). The vertical striations on the lens create a horizontal streak of light. **B,** The Bagolini lens is rotated to an axis of 135°, at which point the streak intersects the red light. **C,** A prism placed with its base perpendicular to the 135° indicator and its apex pointing up and in, and gradually increased in power until the patient reports fusion of the lights. (From Cotter SA, Frantz KA: In London R: Prescribing prism for vertical deviations, *Probl Optom* 4:629-645, 1992.)

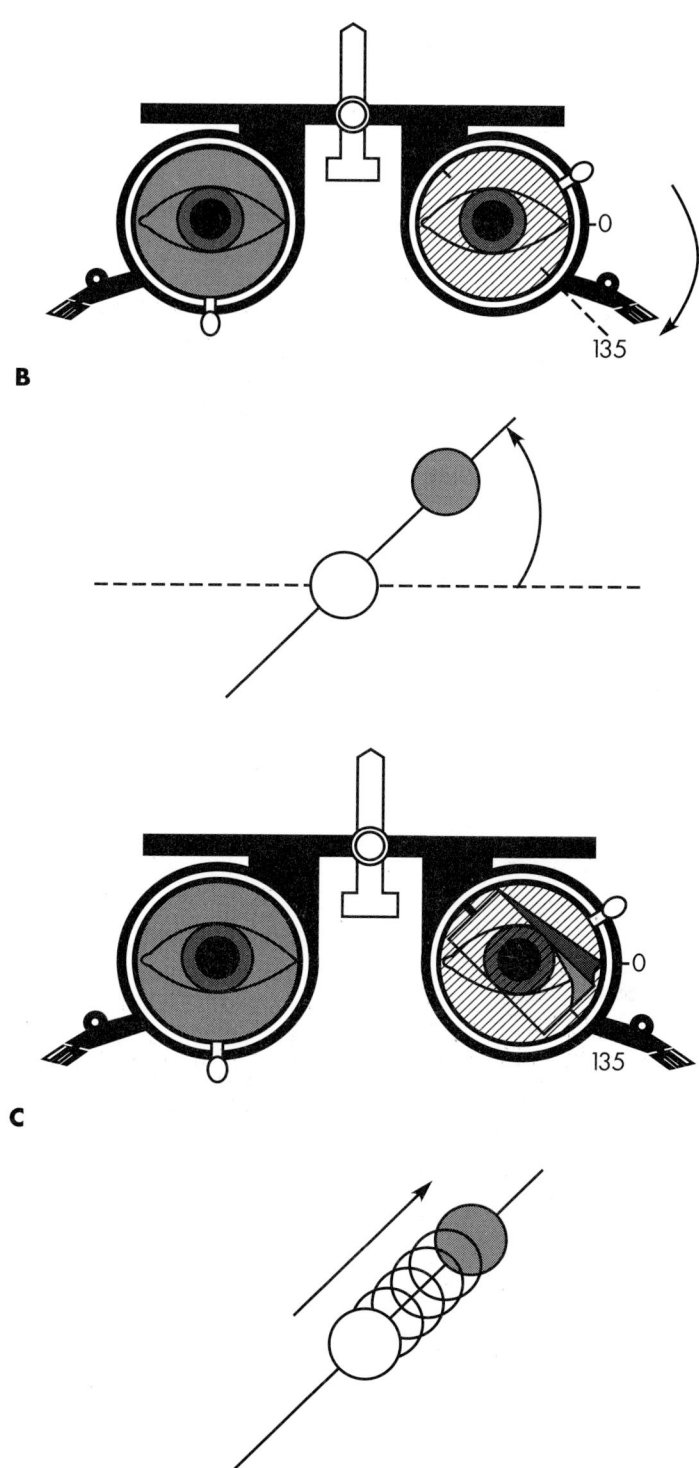

B

C

FIGURE 8-5, Cont'd.

An alternative method of prescribing for combined horizontal and vertical deviations is described by Moradiellos and Parrish.[49] A red Maddox rod trial lens is placed in a trial frame before one eye (that is, the eye with poorer acuity). The patient should notice a red line (seen by the eye with the Maddox rod) and a white transilluminator light (seen by the other eye). If both the red line and the white light are seen simultaneously, the Maddox rod is rotated until the patient reports the red line crossing through the center of the white light (Fig. 8-6, A). The doctor notes the axis at which this occurs and rotates the Maddox rod 90° from this position. The red line and white light are now separated and the axis of the Maddox rod specifies the axis of the correcting prism. To neutralize the oculomotor deviation, prism with its base perpendicular to this axis is placed before the eye with the Maddox rod in increasing increments until the red line once again passes through the white light (Fig. 8-6, B). At this point, both the axis and the amount of prism fully neutralizing the deviation have been measured. To determine the magnitude of prism to prescribe, the prism and Maddox rod should be removed and a smaller amount of prism introduced at the appropriate axis. Prism power is increased 1 Δ at a time until the patient is able to fuse the target comfortably.

A 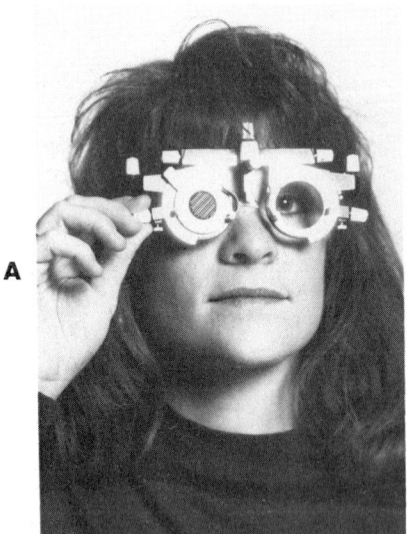   B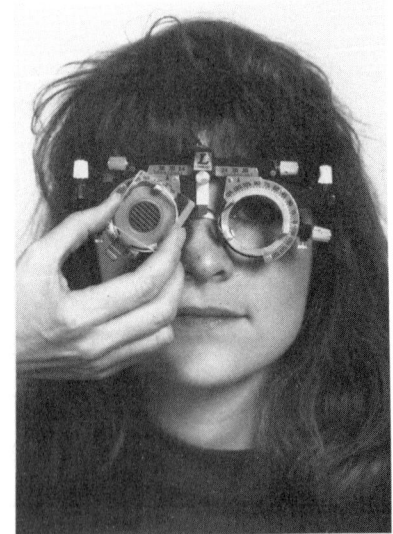

FIGURE 8-6 A, The Maddox rod in a trial frame is rotated by the patient. B, A prism is placed before the Maddox rod with its base perpendicular to the axis of the Maddox rod until the patient reports that the red line intersects the white light. (From Cotter SA, Frantz KA: In London R: Prescribing prism for vertical deviations, *Probl Optom* 4:629-645, 1992.)

Either of the above two methods for prescribing horizontal-vertical prism may be used with heterophoric patients as well as those with strabismus. It is important that prism prescribed at an oblique axis be specified carefully to the optical laboratory; power and base direction as well as which eye is to wear the prism should be clearly noted (for instance, 8 Δ base-out and down axis 135° OS). If one desired to split the prism between the eyes, this prescription would become 4 Δ base-out and up axis 135° OD, 4 Δ base-out and down axis 135° OS.

Noncomitant strabismus

Prescribing prism for noncomitant strabismus requires additional considerations. Obviously, the diagnosis and management of under-lying systemic or neurological conditions for any noncomitant strabismus must first be addressed. However, even if the strabismus is expected to resolve or is in the process of resolving, symptomatic patients (such as with diplopia in one or more positions of gaze, asthenopia, headache, or neck and back pain due to an anomalous head position) often benefit from a prism prescription that may be only temporary. This is especially true when the deviation is not so long standing that muscle contractures or sensory adaptations (suppression or anomalous correspondence) have developed.

Because the magnitude of the noncomitant deviation will vary in different positions of gaze, the optimal prismatic prescription also will vary. The goals are usually to eliminate any abnormal head posture and provide single binocular vision in the most important fields of gaze (that is, primary gaze for distance vision and inferior gaze at near point). As with other forms of strabismus, the smallest amount of prism needed to achieve one's goals should be prescribed. When the cause of noncomitancy is a muscle underaction (for instance, a paresis), however, there are special considerations. In cases of marked restriction, less prism will be needed to attain fusion if most or all of it is placed before the eye with the underacting muscle.[50] To keep the prism power to a minimum, therefore, it should *not* be split equally between the eyes but should be divided so the greater amount is before the affected eye. The more significant the restriction, the more of the total prism power should be placed before the affected eye. If there is a completely paralyzed muscle, all of the correcting prism may be placed before the affected eye.[50,51]

CLINICAL PEARL

When the cause of noncomitancy is a muscle underaction (for instance, a paresis), less prism will be needed to attain fusion if most or all of it is placed before the eye with the underacting muscle.

The reasons for these guidelines are two: First, by placing the prism before the affected eye, the practitioner allows the nonaffected eye to remain in primary position while the underacting eye deviates. Thus, the smaller primary (rather than the larger secondary) angle of deviation is manifested.[47,51] Second, if the prism were to be placed before the nonaffected eye, this eye would turn toward the prism's apex to fixate and (due to Hering's law) the eye with the underacting muscle would turn into its involved field of gaze, further increasing the size of the deviation and requiring more prism for fusion.[50] By placing the prism over the affected eye, however, one avoids movements in the direction of the underacting muscle. For example, consider a patient with a moderate paresis of the left lateral rectus, a habitual head turn to the left, and eyes turned to the right (where fusion is possible because of a decreased esodeviation in right gaze). When base-out prism is placed before the nonstrabismic right eye, both eyes will be directed into left gaze. Because the angle of deviation is larger in left gaze, part or all of the effect of the prism will be negated. When base-out prism is placed, instead, before the left eye, both eyes will be directed into right gaze (where the ocular deviation is smaller), permitting bifoveal fusion with a lesser amount of prism. Therefore, if one wishes to prescribe the least amount of prism that will allow bifoveal fusion, as much of the necessary prism as possible must be placed before the nonaffected eye so the eyes are not directed into the field of action of the affected muscle.

It should be noted, however, that in cases of recent-onset paralytic strabismus it may be wiser to place prism over the *non*affected eye[52,53] in an effort to prevent a secondary contracture of the ipsilateral antagonist of the paretic muscle (which can occur in a matter of weeks).[57] For example, placing base-out prism over the nonaffected eye of a patient with a left lateral rectus paresis will cause the eyes to turn left, forcing the left eye out of its adducted position and producing relaxation of the left medial rectus rather than a continual state of contraction. The affected muscle thus will be stimulated and the chances of an opposing muscle contracture minimized.[54] Alternatively, monocular ocular motility activities or part-time alternate occlusion can be prescribed to prevent secondary contractures.[55]

CLINICAL PEARL

In cases of recent-onset paralytic strabismus, consider placing prism over the nonaffected eye in an effort to prevent a secondary contracture of the ipsilateral antagonist of the paretic muscle; alternatively, monocular ocular motility activities or part-time alternate occlusion can be prescribed to prevent secondary contractures.

When prescribing prism, one should consider the patient's habitual head posture. Because the magnitude of a noncomitant deviation changes with various head positions, compensatory head postures often are used as mechanisms to achieve single binocular vision. Therefore, the deviation should be measured with the head both straight and in its habitual position. If the problem is of recent onset, prism can usually be safely prescribed based upon measurements taken when the patient's head is straight. If the problem is long standing, it is important to determine how deeply ingrained the anomalous head posture is.[56] To make this assessment, one can physically straighten the patient's head and assess whether he/she perceives it now as straight or whether the head feels straight when it is actually postured abnormally. A response that the head no longer feels straight when it is physically straightened implies that the abnormal posturing is deeply ingrained. Full prism correction for the head positioned straight may be too disruptive and therefore rejected. In these cases prism that neutralizes the deviation when the head is postured anomalously should initially be prescribed, with the intent of gradually increasing the amount over time. Ultimately, a full prism prescription will be given for the deviation that exists when the head is straight, thereby eliminating the need for any compensatory head posture.[56]

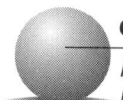

CLINICAL PEARL

In cases of recent-onset noncomitant strabismus leading to a compensatory head posture, one can usually prescribe prism safely based upon measurements taken when the patient's head is straight. However, a full prism correction for a long-standing anomalous head posture may be rejected, and in this situation a prism that neutralizes the deviation present with the anomalous head posture should be prescribed initially.

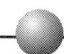

Yoked prisms

Certain noncomitant deviations will need yoked prisms to obtain binocular vision in needed gaze positions. Yoked prisms optically move the apparent images of the fixated target in a parallel direction toward the apex of the prisms.[61] Thus both eyes synergistically turn away from primary gaze and into a different field of gaze. An example of this is yoked base-down prism for a patient with a V pattern esodeviation who has diplopia only in downgaze. The prisms alter the apparent position of objects by shifting them upward (toward the prisms' apices). The eyes then rotate upward with respect to their normal position to view the apparent images of objects, allowing the patient to avoid downgaze (the gaze that produces difficulty in this case).

Relieving prisms can be combined with yoked prisms for patients with noncomitant deviations.[57] While the yoked prisms direct the eyes to the field of gaze where binocularity is possible, the relieving prism reduces the demand for compensating vergence. In this way binocularity can be stabilized in a specific field of gaze. For example, Mende[57] described a symptomatic exophoric patient (headaches, asthenopia, diplopia, and neck pain with reading) who presented with a head turn to the left because fusion was easier to achieve in right gaze. The patient was found to have Duane's retraction syndrome Type III, showing an abduction and adduction deficit of the right eye. Yoked base-left prism allowed the patient to assume a more comfortable head posture (by shifting the apparent position of reading material to the patient's right) and additional base-in relieving prism over the right eye was given for the exodeviation.

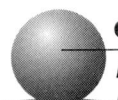

CLINICAL PEARL

Relieving prisms can be combined with yoked prisms for patients who have a noncomitant deviation. While the yoked prisms direct the patient's eyes to a field of gaze where binocularity is possible, the relieving prism serves to reduce the demand for compensating vergence.

Trial framing helps in determining whether a compromise between two or more prism powers (for various gaze directions) is possible. Alternatively, more than one pair of prismatic spectacles for particular gaze needs (for example, separate spectacles for driving and for reading) can be prescribed. Another option[56] is to give a bifocal prescription containing the primary gaze prism correction to allow comfortable distance vision, with brief periods of near viewing and then prescribe a pair of reading glasses that incorporate the optimum prism for downgaze for more lengthy near tasks. Still other possibilities are specially ground lenses incorporating two prism powers or spectacles with sector Fresnel membrane prisms (see Chapter 3). The patient should be informed that monocular diplopia may occur when looking through the demarcation line between the two prism powers and that adjustment of eye position to avoid this zone will be necessary.

Prism Therapies for Constant Strabismus

When the frequency of strabismus is constant, a decision must be made to either establish or not establish binocular vision. This decision is based on the patient's entire diagnostic profile (that is, the summary of all prognostic factors). The strabismus is classified as resolvable (with a good prognosis for achieving binocular vision) or nonresolvable (a poor prognosis). Although final visual goals— singleness and clearness of vision, comfort, good cosmesis—are the same for resolvable and nonresolvable strabismus,[59] the nonresolvable strabismic patient must achieve them with his/her eyes deviated and without the precipitation of diplopia. The resolvable constant strabismic patient must obtain bifoveal fixation on targets of regard and achieve efficient binocular vision not only in-instrument but also ultimately in open visual space.

Management of patients with resolvable constant strabismus starts at the beginning of the binocular vision treatment plan (Table 8-2) and proceeds in sequential steps to achieve sensory and motor processing that results in a stable and efficient binocular vision system.[25] Relieving prisms are prescribed early in the sequence (phase 1) only if sensory skills are good and vergence ability is adequate to control the residual strabismus, conditions that usually exist in constant strabismus with a late onset or short duration. If sensory or vergence skills are poor, relieving prisms are delayed until late in the sequence (phase 5) and are worn after normal sensorimotor skills have been reestablished. Prism therapies designed to eliminate sensory anomalies (such as amblyopia or anomalous correspondence) or to reestablish normal sensory fusion may be prescribed early in the sequence (phase 1) and changed to relieving prisms after sensory and motor skills have improved (phase 5).

The application of prism therapies for constant strabismus is thus based on the diagnostic decision of binocular vision resolvability and generally falls into two categories: (1) corrective prisms for resolvable strabismus and (2) cosmetic prisms for nonresolvable strabismus. Corrective prisms simulate active vision therapy tasks performed in-instrument at the objective angle.[21,23,60,61] Although corrective prism therapy (CPT) is most frequently recommended for constant esotropia, it is theoretically possible to use the same methodology for constant exotropia or vertical strabismus. When binocular vision therapy is not recommended, CPT is contraindicated and cosmetic prisms may then be considered to improve appearance, especially for the constant unilateral small to moderate angle esotrope.[62] Although corrective and cosmetic prisms are limited in use to select patients, they do add another means of care to our prism-management armamentarium.

Corrective Prisms

Prisms with their power equaling the size of the strabismic angle and their base opposite to the eye turn (for instance, BO for esotropia) are called corrective prisms. Corrective prisms move the retinal image on the deviating eye from the zero measure point to the fovea (Fig. 8-7) so visual stimulation of normally corresponding retinal sites occurs

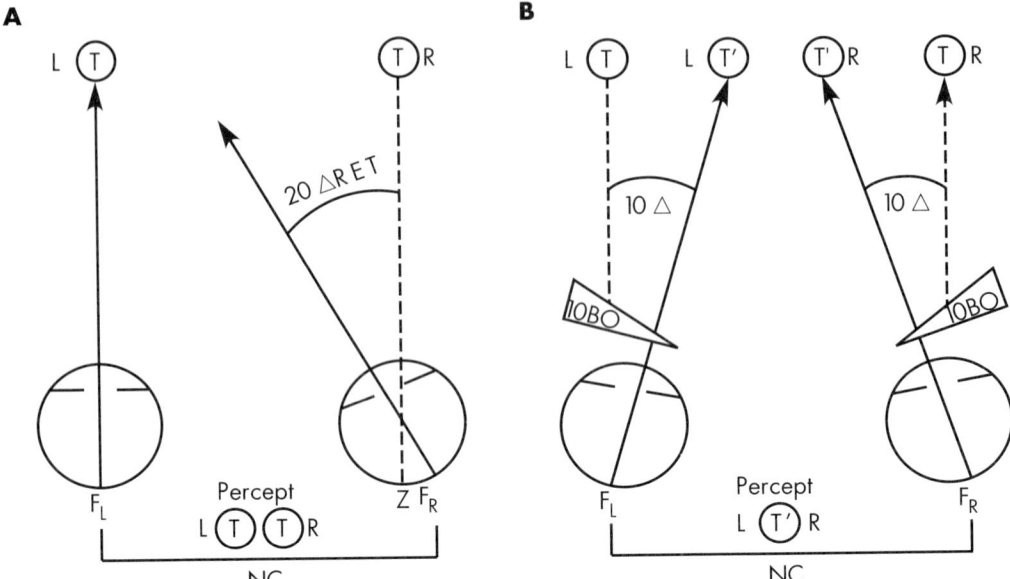

FIGURE 8-7 Corrective prism therapy for a constant 20 Δ right esotropia with normal correspondence (*NC*). **A,** Without prisms, the target viewed by the right eye is centered on the retina at point Z (the zero measure point). Uncrossed diplopia occurs with NC and no suppression. **B,** With 10 Δ BO before each eye, the targets are centered on the foveas. Normal sensory fusion can thus occur.

even though the eyes remain misaligned. Theoretically, binocular neural stimulation of the foveas and other anatomically corresponding retinal sites over time should lead eventually to the establishment of normal sensory fusion. However, sensory fusion may not occur and the strabismic angle may actually increase in size[63-65] if sensory anomalies such as suppression, amblyopia, and anomalous correspondence are present when corrective prisms are applied. Therefore, any anomalous sensory condition should be eliminated by occlusion, active vision therapy, or other prism therapies before corrective prism application.[60,61] Corrective prisms are seldom prescribed in the initial treatment of a constant strabismus unless it is of recent onset and the sensory system remains intact despite the strabismic misalignment. It is best to prescribe CPT when normal correspondence and peripheral sensory fusion have been established and can be maintained with binocular viewing. If central and foveal fusion is also possible, the prognosis for faster progress and more stable fusion responses improves dramatically.

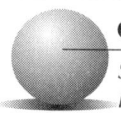

CLINICAL PEARL

Sensory fusion may not occur and the strabismic angle may actually increase, if sensory anomalies such as suppression, amblyopia, and anomalous correspondence are present when corrective prisms are applied.

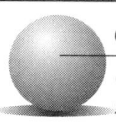

CLINICAL PEARL

Corrective prisms are seldom prescribed in the initial treatment of a constant strabismus unless it is of recent onset and the sensory system remains intact despite the strabismic misalignment.

Corrective prisms are worn bilaterally for comitant or mildly noncomitant deviations so that visual and spatial distortions from high-power prisms are minimized. For moderate to marked noncomitant strabismus, prism may be placed before the affected eye only or divided unequally between the normal and affected eyes. In cases of noncomitancy a specific gaze such as primary (the most commonly used) is selected and prism power is then prescribed that equals the size of the deviation in that gaze. When sensory fusion is stable in this field, other gaze positions are considered and additional applications of relieving or yoked prisms may be prescribed to obtain binocular vision in other fields of gaze.

Patients with high or low AC/A ratios present with different deviation sizes at far and near distances. In most cases the prism power selected is equivalent to the distant angle. A plus add at near for the convergence excess (high AC/A) patient can be selected so that the near angle of deviation is equal to the far deviation. The divergence insufficiency (low AC/A) patient may need CPT prescribed for one distance along with a half patch to prevent binocular viewing for the nonselected distance (such as corrective prisms for near and occlusion therapy for far). Binocularity at all viewing distances may be obtainable later in therapy with a multipowered relieving prism prescription after sensorimotor skills at far and near have been well established. Although some patients with variable magnitudes of strabismus can be treated successfully by CPT, the basic comitant nonaccommodative esotrope whose angle remains essentially the same in all gazes and at all distances is easiest to treat.

The success of corrective prisms is not complete with sensory fusion stability alone but should progress to the restoring of all binocular goals. To do so, the *titration* of prism (TP) (that is, reducing the power in small steps) is added to CPT (CPT-TP). After sensory fusion is stabilized with corrective prisms, the prism power is reduced so that vergence can be stimulated and improved to its normal physiological limits. The usual reduction in prism power is very small (2 to 4 Δ); however, if active vision therapy directed toward improving vergence is added to the treatment plan, larger reductions may be possible. The goal is to prescribe the amount of prism that will stimulate vergence maximally without disrupting sensory fusion or precipitating suppression.

CLINICAL PEARL

The usual reduction in prism power is very small (2 to 4 Δ) when titrating prism during CPT; however, if active vision therapy directed toward improving vergence is added, larger reductions may be possible. The goal is to prescribe the amount of prism that will stimulate vergence maximally without disrupting sensory fusion or precipitating suppression.

The size of the strabismic angle as well as the presence of sensory anomalies must be reevaluated at each follow-up visit. Careful monitoring is important for all patients; but the younger the patient, the more frequent the follow-up visits should be. Infants may continue to be seen on a 2-week schedule while older patients may have longer periods between follow-ups (4 to 8 weeks). The follow-up schedule can be modified for certain patients to allow even longer periods between office visits (for example, when progression is slower than expected or in special cases when a patient's residence is far from the office). However, the preferred schedule for patients other than infants is 2-week intervals for the first month and 1-to-2-month intervals thereafter. If prism adaptation occurs, follow-ups in 2-week intervals should resume until prism adaptation reaches a plateau or is eliminated. At that time, monthly follow-ups can again be scheduled.

Knowing when sensory fusion is stable and when prism titration should begin can be difficult for the clinician, especially if the patient is an infant or very young child who cannot respond to sensory testing. Ideally amblyopia, suppression, and anomalous correspondence should be treated before CPT is started because regressions can occur if normal sensory fusion is not present. When unsure of the frequency of normal sensory fusion, it is best to leave corrective prisms in place as long as motor alignment remains unchanged for an arbitrarily selected period of 3 to 6 months. However, the younger the child or the shorter the strabismic duration, the shorter will be the needed CPT time. For example, if CPT results are as expected (no prism adaptation), infant esotropes may start prism titration after

2 months of corrective prism wear. The successful timing of prism titration can be verified by the patient's divergence responses as corrective base-out prisms are reduced in power to become relieving prisms. If prism adaptation (that is, an increase in size of the esodeviation) occurs with prism wear, an esotropia will again be manifested through the prisms. Corrective prisms with the original power should again be prescribed but worn for a longer period (say, 3 months) before titration is resumed. If the esotropic angle does not stabilize with the original prism power and prism adaptation continues, increasing amounts of base-out prism to equal the new deviation size can be prescribed until stability of the strabismic angle does occur. For example, a 30 Δ esotrope may start with 30 Δ base-out but then need increasing powers until stabilization (that is, no increase in the deviation size) occurs. The process of prism titration can then be started.

The cover test is valuable for assessing the progress of this technique. When corrective prisms are worn successfully, there should be no movement seen on the alternate cover test because the retinal images of the targets are centered on the fovea of each eye. When corrective prisms are reduced, the eye movement visible by alternate cover should be equal to the reduction in prism power. For example, if corrective prisms of 40 Δ BO are prescribed and normal sensory fusion is present for the desired length of time, then the prism should be reduced by 4 Δ to a total of 36 Δ BO, resulting in a divergence demand of 4 Δ. The unilateral cover test should show no movement of either eye (indicating the absence of strabismus) and the alternate cover test should show outward movement of 4 Δ (indicating an esophoria of 4 Δ under prismatic viewing conditions). When this response is stable, the prisms are again reduced and binocular responses are reevaluated following a specified period of prism wear. This process continues until further reduction of the prism power is not possible and divergence improvement no longer occurs.

CLINICAL PEARL

The cover test is valuable for assessing the progress of corrective prism therapy. When corrective prisms are reduced, there should be no movement on the unilateral cover test, and the eye movement visible by alternate cover should be equal to the reduction in prism power.

A reduction in the size of the strabismic angle can also occur during CPT-TP. If it does, the esotropic patient wearing corrective prisms will show an exodeviation by cover test. Prism power is then reduced to equal the size of the new esotropia minus the prism needed to stimulate divergence. This process is repeated until no further reduction in size of the esotropia occurs and divergence is at its maximal level. For some patients a significant decrease in size of the esotropia or a spontaneous recovery (ortho alignment without prisms) will occur. For others the esotropic angle will remain the same or increase. The goals of achieving normal sensory and motor fusion skills should be attainable despite any changes in the magnitude of the esotropic deviation.

The use of corrective prism therapy and prism titration can be slow (3 to 4 years in severe cases)[61]; however, some patients (especially infants, toddlers, and preschoolers) respond quickly and the total time may be less than 1 year. After CPT-TP is completed, the final steps of establishing binocular vision in open visual space (Table 8-2, phases 5 and 6) must be accomplished if the visual skills attained by CPT-TP are to remain. Although elimination of the strabismic angle can occur, it is more common to see the angle remain the same or become reduced in size. If the angle in open visual space remains too large for control of the deviation through fusional divergence and relieving prisms after CPT-TP is completed, surgical reduction will be needed. Because normal sensory and motor fusion are established by CPT-TP, a successful surgical outcome should result in binocular vision. A short postsurgical period of active therapy (1 month) is advisable to ensure that regressions do not occur and that binocular efficiency is present at a reflex level.

Cosmetic Prisms

Prism may be used to improve cosmesis for patients with a constant unilateral strabismus of small to moderate size and who have a poor prognosis for a functional cure.[62] Inverse prism (that is, base in the direction opposite that used to elicit fusion) is placed before the deviated eye—base-in for esotropes, base-out for exotropes. Because an object viewed by an observer through a prism appears to be displaced toward the apex of the prism, a patient's strabismic eye when viewed through a prism will also appear to be displaced toward the apex. For example, an esotropic eye behind base-in prism will appear to be displaced temporally (and thus be less esotropic) approximately 1 mm for each 8 Δ applied.[58]

Cosmetic prism is most appropriate for patients with a constant unilateral deviation whose strabismic eye is blind or deeply amblyopic or has marked suppression. The reason is that displacement of the target's image on the retina will be unlikely to result in a motor fusional movement (that is, the eye will probably not rotate in response to prism) when sensory fusion is unlikely because of the reduced visual acuity or deep suppression of the strabismic eye. Cosmetic prism is also useful in patients with constant strabismus who have fairly good visual acuity and anomalous correspondence. In an effort to maintain the habitual and anomalous sensory relationship, these patients may actually make a slow fusional (albeit anomalous) vergence movement in response to the displacement of the target's image on the retina. Because the strabismic eye verges, the size of the deviation becomes less. Therefore a dual effect—an actual reduction of the associated angle through anomalous fusional vergence and an apparent displacement of the eye because it is viewed through the inverse prism—results in better cosmesis.

CLINICAL PEARL

Cosmetic prism is most appropriate for patients with a constant unilateral deviation whose strabismic eye is blind or deeply amblyopic or has marked suppression. It is also useful in patients with a constant strabismus who have fairly good visual acuity and anomalous correspondence.

• Case Reports

I. Inverse and CPT-TP Prism Therapy for Aniso-Esotropia with Amblyopia and Eccentric Fixation

A 7-year-old boy presented with an uncorrected comitant left esotropia of 20 Δ at far and near. The age of onset was uncertain but was probably about 2 years. Cosmesis was fair. Associated visual conditions were hyperopic anisometropia, normal correspondence, constant left eye suppression in open visual space and in-instrument, and amblyopia of 20/400 with an unsteady nasal eccentric fixation of 2 to 4 Δ. General health history for the patient and his family was unremarkable. Ocular health was negative. Familial esotropia was present.

Initial treatment, directed at eliminating the amblyopia and EF, consisted of (1) spectacle lenses, OD +2.00 DS and OS +4.00 DS, worn full-time; (2) total occlusion with opaque tape covering one lens, worn full-time, OD patched 6 days and OS 1 day; and (3) monocular home vision therapy. A follow-up visit at 4 weeks showed visual acuity OS improved to 20/100 (Snellen line of letters) and 20/80 (Snellen single letters). Eccentric fixation by visuoscopy was 1 to 3 Δ unsteady nasal, and the esotropic angle was 16 Δ. Because the family had moved to another city, a combined program of passive and active treatment was prescribed using monocular inverse prism and daily monocular amblyopia therapy.

A 5 Δ BI Fresnel membrane was placed on the left lens, and the right eye was totally occluded full-time each day. Although occlusion amblyopia is not likely to occur after age 7, the upper age limit for amblyopia onset is unclear so a patch was placed on the amblyopic eye for ½ hour 3 days per week. In this way the normal eye received weekly central/foveal visual stimulation by TV watching or reading. Monocular amblyopic activities were prescribed (without the inverse prism) for 30 minutes once a day; smaller-size targets were used as visual acuity improved.

The follow-up visit at 8 weeks showed that the amblyopia had improved to 20/40 with 1 to 2 Δ of unsteady nasal eccentric fixation. Prism was changed to a Fresnel 3 Δ BI OS. The occlusion and home vision therapy remained the same, but smaller foveal-sized targets were now used. At the next follow-up visit, at 12 weeks, fixation of the left eye was unsteady foveal and visual acuity had improved to 20/30 (line of letters) and 20/20 (single letters). The refractive error was unchanged, correspondence was normal, the esotropic angle (through his spectacles) was 16 Δ, and diplopia was present whenever the patch was removed. The Fresnel inverse prism and the occluder were then discontinued, and corrective prisms (8 Δ BO before each eye) were prescribed for binocular viewing. Thus diplopia was eliminated and sensory fusion established by the corrective prism therapy. Monocular home vision therapy with foveal-sized targets was continued, but binocular peripheral and central activities were added to eliminate any suppressions and stabilize sensory fusion.

When the patient returned 1 month later (having completed 5 months of therapy), fixation of each eye was steady foveal and visual acuity OS was 20/20 Snellen line of letters. Sensory fusion was normal and stable, and random dot stereopsis was present. Fresnel prism power was then reduced by 2 Δ in each eye so that the new total prism power worn was 12 Δ BO, leaving a divergence demand of 4 Δ. Monocular home vision therapy was discontinued, but binocular activities stressing bifoveal fusion was continued on a daily basis.

At the next visit (completion of 6 months), foveal fixation and 20/20 acuity were present in each eye; the dissociated esotropic angle (through his hyperopic spectacles) showed a decrease from the initial 20 Δ to an angle of 10 Δ. Vergence ranges were 15/25/20 BO and 5/10/2 BI, measured from the objective angle in a major amblyoscope. Prisms were again reduced by 2 Δ BO before each eye to a total power of 4 Δ BO (leaving a residual divergence demand of 6 Δ). Home vision therapy using a Brewster stereoscope with binocular central and foveal-sized targets continued but was reduced to three times per week.

The diagnostic results at the next follow-up visit (completion of 7 months) showed a comitant intermittent alternating basic esotropia of 10 Δ through habitual lenses. Fixation disparity neutralization (that is, the associated phoria) showed that 4 Δ BO was needed to eliminate a small eso fixation disparity and obtain a stereopsis level of

40 seconds at near (Randot stereotest). A prescription with ground-in prism, 2 Δ BO OD and 2 Δ BO OS, was ordered for full-time wear. Binocular home vision therapy continued on a three-times per week schedule for maintenance care. Follow-ups scheduled in 3 months and then in 6 months showed efficient and comfortable binocular vision with 20/20 OU. Regression of amblyopia and esotropia did not occur.

II. Relieving Prisms for Intermittent Vertical Strabismus

A 35-year-old businessman presented with the complaint of fatigue while reading that had been present for several years but had become more bothersome recently. He denied having spontaneously occurring diplopia but did note that if he wished to see double he could easily do so. More significant than the asthenopia, however, were chronic neck and back problems (neck tension and back muscle spasms). He reported that these were caused by his habitual head posture (tilt to the right shoulder, Fig. 8-8, *A*) and that he had been under the care of a chiropractor for the previous 7 years.

Ocular history revealed that a "lazy eye" had been diagnosed at age 13; however, no treatment was ever recommended or implemented. The patient had worn a myopic correction since that time and, as far as he was aware, his glasses had never contained a prismatic correction. There was no history of head trauma. Medical history was unremarkable except for the neck and back difficulties. The patient was not taking any medication, and his family's ocular and medical histories were unremarkable.

Current spectacle prescription and distance visual acuities

OD $-2.00 -0.50 \times 167$ (20/20)
OS $-3.00 -0.50 \times 060$ (20/25)

Subjective refraction and distance visual acuities

OD $-2.00 -0.50 \times 165$ (20/20)
OS $-3.00 -0.50 \times 040$ (20/20)

Cover testing through habitual spectacle prescription

With head straightened: Constant left hypertropia of 27 Δ
With habitual head tilt: Intermittent left hypertropia of 15 Δ

Comitancy testing (Park's three-step test and versions)

Left superior oblique paresis

Stereopsis (Randot stereotest) with habitual spectacles

With head straightened: none
With habitual head tilt: 100 seconds

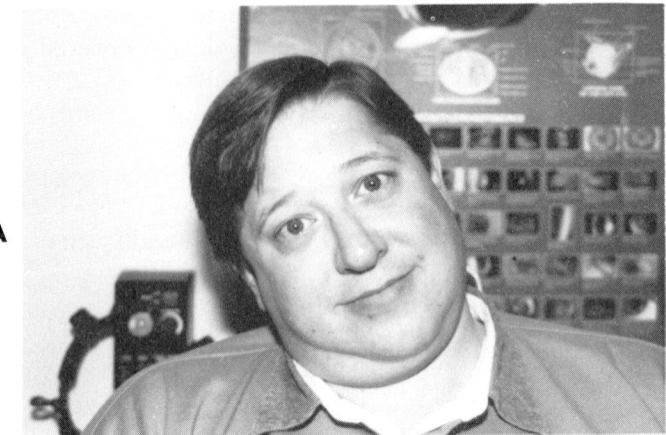

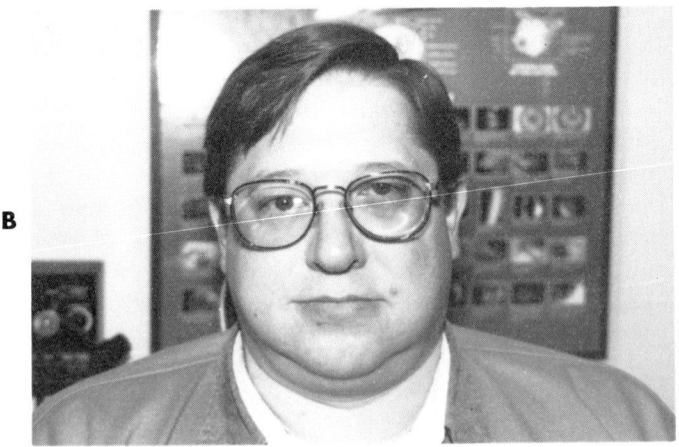

FIGURE 8-8 **A,** Habitual posture of a man with a left superior oblique paresis. The obvious head tilt has been adopted to compensate. **B,** Head posture when a total of 18 Δ (8 Δ BUOD, 10 Δ BDOS) is being worn.

Ocular health

Unremarkable

A diagnosis of left superior oblique paresis, probably congenital in nature, was made. The most appropriate treatment options were a prism correction or muscle surgery. The patient chose to try the prism. After trial framing various magnitudes of prism and evaluating the patient's ocular deviation and head tilt through the prisms, we determined empirically that 18 Δ would be appropriate. The following spectacle prescription was ordered:

OD   −2.00 −0.50 × 165   8 Δ BU
OS   −3.00 −0.50 × 050   10 Δ BD

The patient was seen for follow-up 1 month after he received his new spectacles (Fig. 8-8, *B*). He reported that he had had some adaptation problems with the new glasses initially but had adapted fairly quickly. Examination revealed a small left hyperphoria and 50 seconds of stereopsis (Randot stereotest). The asthenopic complaints were essentially eliminated, and (more important to him) the tension in his neck was gone and he no longer experienced back spasms. He has been wearing this prescription with no complaints for the last 3 years.

III. Relieving Prisms for Constant Noncomitant Hyper-Esotropia

A 35-year-old woman police candidate presented with the chief complaint of an inability to meet the vision standards for securing a law enforcement position. Although she had passed the written, general physical, and psychological examinations, she could not pass the vision screening. She had met the standards for visual acuity, color vision, visual fields, and night vision but had not met those for binocular vision and stereoacuity. The standards required were "clear, comfortable binocular vision with good stereopsis (80 seconds) at all normal working distances and viewing angles with correction."

The patient's ocular history revealed full-time wear of a spectacle prescription since age 14, with the left eye having "weaker vision." She reported that this eye "crossed" when she was young but then straightened as she became older. No treatment was ever recommended or implemented for it. She denied any ocular symptoms, including diplopia, although, when questioned, acknowledged that she was aware she tilted her head to the left shoulder and she had done this for as long as she could remember.

The medical history was unremarkable, and she was not taking any medications. Family eye and health histories were also unremarkable. The patient was currently a full-time mail carrier and worked part-time as a plainclothes security guard for a large department store.

Current spectacle prescription and distance visual acuities

OD −0.75   DS   (20/25−)
OS −3.00   DS   (20/25−)

Subjective refraction and distance visual acuities

OD −0.75 −0.50 × 090   (20/20)
OS −2.75 −0.25 × 060   (20/25+)

Cover testing through the habitual spectacle prescription

6 m: Constant alternating right hyper-esotropia
            OD fixating: 25 Δ BUOS, 3 Δ BO
            OS fixating: 18 Δ BDOD, 3 Δ BO
40 cm: Constant alternating right hyper-esotropia
            OD fixating: 16 Δ BUOS, 3 Δ BO
            OS fixating: 20 Δ BDOD, 3 Δ BO

Comitancy testing

Three-step test with prism neutralization revealed a right superior oblique paresis.
Versions showed underaction of the right superior oblique and overaction of the right inferior oblique.

Stereopsis with habitual spectacles

Random Dot E: None
Lang: No appreciation

Stereopsis with 7 to 10 Δ BUOS (least prism to obtain a response) over habitual prescription

Random Dot E: 4/4
Lang: Identified all 3 forms
Randot: Identified all forms and obtained 20 seconds on circles

Ocular health

Unremarkable

A diagnosis of right superior oblique paresis, probably congenital in nature, was made. Options for treatment included a prism correction or muscle surgery. It was recommended that a prism prescription would probably be the best initial treatment. Relieving prism of 8 Δ was prescribed based on the positive stereoacuity response achieved with 7 to 10 Δ BUOS. The following spectacle prescription was ordered:

OD   −0.75 −0.50 × 090, 4 Δ BD
OS   −2.75 −0.25 × 060, 4 Δ BU

The patient was seen for follow-up 2 weeks after she received her new spectacle prescription. She reported no adaptation problems with the new glasses and that she could see just fine. Examination, however, revealed an 8 Δ right hypertropia that was constant at distance and intermittent at near. An associated esodeviation of 5 Δ was also found. Stereopsis measured at 40 cm through the prism correction was 4/4 correct responses on the Random Dot E and 25 seconds on the Randot stereotest circles.

It was obvious that 8 Δ was not sufficient to adequately compensate for the vertical deviation so the patient could meet the required vision standards. Therefore varying amounts of additional vertical prism were trial-framed and then cover testing and stereopsis testing were performed. An additional 8 Δ of vertical prism was found to eliminate the strabismus at distance and near in primary gaze. Alternate cover testing revealed only a small esophoria; no vertical component was seen. Based on these measurements the following new lenses were ordered:

OD −0.75 −0.50 × 090, 8 Δ BDOD
OS −2.75 −0.25 × 060, 8 Δ BUOS

The patient was examined 1 week after receiving her new lenses. She had no strabismus at distance or near by cover testing. Alternate cover test measurements revealed 4 Δ BDOD and 7 Δ BO, indicating a small phoria only. Stereopsis with the Randot test was 30 seconds. She was now able to meet the required vision standards for the law enforcement position for which she had applied. In addition, spectacle cosmesis was quite good (a frame with a small eye size was chosen). It was possible that if a greater amount of prism (>8 Δ) had been applied before the paretic right eye less total prism (<16 Δ) would have been needed. However, we did not evaluate this clinically because we believed we were already close to the upper limit of cosmetically acceptable ground-in prism with the 8 Δ before the right eye.

IV. Sector Prism for Constant Noncomitant Esotropia

A 42-year-old woman reported horizontal diplopia of sudden onset that had begun the previous month. It was constant in nature, with the images farther apart when she looked to her left. She had a history of vertical diplopia subsequent to treatment for a benign brain tumor and was currently under the care of a neuroophthalmologist, who had performed a neurological evaluation and an MRI 1 week after the onset of the horizontal diplopia. Her MRI results were unremarkable, and the physician was of the opinion that the diplopia was unrelated to the brain tumor. His plan was to follow the patient carefully. If the diplopia did not remit in a couple of months, he was going to perform muscle surgery. Until that time, he instructed the patient to wear a patch to eliminate the bothersome diplopia.

Other than the brain tumor, the patient's medical history was unremarkable; she was not taking any medications. Family eye and health histories were also unremarkable. She was wearing a spectacle prescription that contained ground-in vertical prism.

Current spectacle prescription and visual acuities at distance and near

OD −2.25 DS, 6 Δ BU/+1.00 add (20/20)
OS −3.50 DS, 6 Δ BD/+1.00 add (20/20)

Cover testing through the habitual spectacle prescription

6 m: Constant left esotropia
         Primary gaze: 35 Δ BO
         Right gaze: 10 Δ BO
         Left gaze: 50 Δ BO
40 cm: Constant left esotropia of 20 Δ in primary gaze

Comitancy testing

Noncomitant deviation; left lateral rectus paresis

Stereopsis

None

Ocular health and visual fields

Unremarkable

A diagnosis of a left lateral rectus paresis of unknown etiology was made. Because the magnitude of the deviation was different in right, left, and primary gazes, we prescribed sector prism. A 30 Δ BO Fresnel prism was applied so that it covered the center and left half of the spectacle lens of the left eye. A 10 Δ BO sector Fresnel was then applied to cover the remaining right portion of the left spectacle lens. The magnitude of this prism was based on alternate cover test measurements (corrective prism for primary and right gazes) and the patient's subjective responses to elimination of the diplopia (fusion prism). The exact placement of the sector prisms was determined by where the alternate cover test measurements changed as the eye rotated laterally and by the patient's subjective responses. The patient currently wears this sector Fresnel design on her prescription lenses. It has worked quite satisfactorily for the last 4 months. In addition, monocular active vision therapy was prescribed to prevent a contraction of the left medial rectus.

V. Relieving Prism for Intermittent Exotropia with Diplopia

A 34-year-old man was referred by his ophthalmologist for a strabismus consultation and possible vision therapy. He had presented with chief complaints of (1) intermittent horizontal diplopia at distance and near and (2) headaches and eyestrain associated with reading. The diplopia was intermittent in nature and more frequent when he was tired. The patient, a pilot, was particularly concerned about the diplopia because runways would sometimes "double" when he was attempting to land.

The ocular history was significant for a pseudomonas corneal ulcer of the right eye that occurred 6 months previously and one of the left eye 5 weeks earlier. The patient was currently using Muro 128 and Tobrex qid. He reported that the pseudomonas infection had resulted in a corneal scar of the right eye with a subsequent decrease in vision from 20/15 to 20/20. He was aware that he had a long-standing tendency for one eye to wander out, especially when he was tired. This tendency had become more frequent in the last 2 years, although he had not received any treatment for it.

The medical history was unremarkable, and he was taking no medication other than the Tobrex. Family eye and health histories were also unremarkable.

Refractive error and distance acuities

OD   Plano   (20/20−)
OS   Plano   (20/15)

Cover test

Comitant intermittent right exotropia
   6 m: 15 Δ BI,   2 Δ BDOD
   40 cm: 28 Δ BI,   2 Δ BDOD

Vertical associated phoria (disparometer)

2 Δ BDOD

Stereopsis (Randot stereotest)

50 seconds

Ocular health

Unremarkable except for a small corneal scar OD

The intermittent exotropia was present at both distance and near with a considerably larger magnitude at near than at distance. Although vision training would have been the preferred treatment, this patient was unable to participate in an active vision therapy program because of time constraints. Therefore relieving prisms were prescribed. The vertical prism component of this prescription was based on the associated phoria measure (see Chapter 6), and the horizontal prism magnitude was based on Caloroso's residual vergence demand criterion for exodeviations—reduce the demand to 10 or 15 Δ. We used the magnitude of the larger near deviation (28 Δ) as the guiding factor. A spectacle prescription of plano with 6 Δ BI, 1 Δ BD for the right eye and plano with 6 Δ BI, 1 Δ BU for the left eye was ordered. At a 1 month follow-up visit the patient reported he no longer had diplopia when landing his plane and he did not have headaches, eyestrain, or diplopia when reading. His goal is to return for active vision therapy so he can reduce the magnitude of or eliminate the need for relieving prism entirely. He is due to return for follow-up as soon as his schedule allows; but until then, the relieving prism has seemed to eliminate his complaints satisfactorily.

VI. Corrective Prisms for Basic Nonaccommodative Infant Esotropia

A 7-month-old infant presented with a comitant constant nonaccommodative right esotropia of 40 Δ at far and near that had begun at

3 months of age. Cycloplegic retinoscopy was +2.00 DS for each eye. The health history was unremarkable. Diagnostic test results suggested that amblyopia was present in the esotropic eye; suppression, correspondence, and sensory fusion were nontestable. Although the potential for binocular vision was unpredictable and the prognosis for a functional cure (based on the early onset) was low, the decision (made together with the parents) was to attempt to obtain normal binocular vision.

The first step in treatment consisted of spectacle lenses of +2.00 DS for both the right and the left eye. Binasal occlusion[66] with opaque tape blocking the fovea and the zero measure point of each eye when deviated was then prescribed. In this way, full-time occlusion could be prescribed and there would be less probability of occlusion amblyopia in the left (nonamblyopic) eye than might occur with the more commonly used total full-time occlusion. Suppression, assumed to be present, could thus be eliminated with binasal occlusion therapy while alternation of fixation was simultaneously stimulated. Because the infant could fixate environmental objects visible in the temporal field with the eye nearer the object—that is, right temporal objects by the right eye, left temporal objects by the left—foveal fixation and good visual acuity should remain in the nonamblyopic eye and foveal fixation and better visual acuity should be stimulated in the amblyopic eye.

After 2 months of spectacle lens and binasal occlusion therapy, the visual responses of fast alternation, foveal fixation in each eye, and equivalent visual acuities (20/100 as measured by forced-choice preferential looking) were present. Although it was still not possible to directly test for suppression, it was assumed that 2 months of occlusion at this age might result in the elimination of suppression, with a diplopic response occurring when the child was esotropic. The next step, applying corrective prisms to establish normal sensory fusion, was attempted. Occlusion was discontinued, and Fresnel membranes of 20 Δ BO OD and OS were added to the spectacle lenses to be worn for 3 months. Careful monitoring of the esotropic angle, monocular fixation patterns, and visual acuities was done at 2-week intervals for the first month and at 1-month intervals for the next couple of months. Daily 15-minute monocular activities supervised by a parent (for example, closely looking at and touching toys) were performed by each eye, without prisms and with the fellow eye totally occluded. A reduction in prism power was attempted, but the divergence was not definitive and corrective prisms were retained for full-time viewing.

Esotropic surgery was performed at age 12 months, with good cosmetic results. Spectacle wear, despite the low amount of hyperopia, was continued since a small esodeviation appeared to be present without the prescription. Follow-up visits were scheduled at 3, 7, and 14 days postsurgically and then on a 2-week basis for 1 month and at 3-month intervals thereafter until age 2 years. Test results suggested no strabismus or amblyopia; however, the status of binocular vision remained inconclusive.

Subsequent visits at 6-month intervals showed little change in the esotropic angle or test results, and no subjective or objective symptoms were reported by the child or parents. A diagnostic examination that tested both sensory and motor processing was performed at age 3 years and confirmed previous assumptions. Binocular vision was present as evidenced by the following key visual conditions: (1) 5 Δ of basic esophoria without lenses and orthophoria with lenses, (2) normal sensory fusion with random dot stereopsis, (3) accommodative accuracy and facility, and (4) vergence ranges of normal amplitudes. Visual acuities as measured by Lighthouse cards and Broken Wheel cards were 20/20 for each eye. Follow-up visits at 6-month intervals from ages 3 to 4 years showed no change, and the child was then placed on annual recall.

Summary

Prisms are an indispensable tool for the practitioner who treats strabismus in his or her practice. They can be used in various ways and for the achievement of various goals in the sequential binocular vision treatment plan. Most often, they are used to establish or stabilize binocular vision; however, they may also be used to eliminate diplopia or anomalous head postures, disrupt eccentric fixation or anomalous correspondence, increase fusional vergence ability, and improve cosmesis in some nonresolvable cases. Many strabismic patients can be managed by prism therapy alone, but more often prisms are an important tool within the overall binocular vision treatment plan to be used in combination with other treatments (for example, lenses, occlusion, surgery, active vision therapy).

Although prisms can be a powerful tool, they should not be prescribed indiscriminately; rather, the decision to prescribe should be based on a complete diagnostic profile (including an evaluation of sensory fusion and motor fusion) and should be made after lenses that both correct the ametropia and reduce the strabismic angle maximally are prescribed. After this, the decision is made to prescribe prisms (for establishing binocular vision or for achieving a specific visual goal) or to delay prescribing until later in the sequential binocular vision treatment plan. Patients with intermittent strabismus and strabismus of recent onset and short duration usually respond well to prism therapy, and one's goals may be achieved merely by prescribing prism. Prism therapy designed to establish or stabilize normal binocular vision in patients with constant strabismus of early onset and long duration, however, is most successful when the prisms are prescribed after sensory anomalies (that is, amblyopia, suppression, and anomalous correspondence) are eliminated.

REFERENCES

1. Percival AS: *The prescribing of spectacles,* Bristol, 1928, J Wright & Sons, p 125.
2. Sheard C: Zones of ocular comfort, *Am J Optom Arch Am Acad Optom* 7:9-25, 1930.
3. Borish IM: Prismatic prescriptions: a clinical report on 147 cases, *Am J Optom Arch Am Acad Optom* 25:579-592, 1948.
4. Morgan MW: The prescribing of prisms, *California Optometrist* 22(4):142-145, 1954.
5. Eskridge JB: Criteria for determining the need and amount of ophthalmic prism corrections, *Am J Optom Arch Am Acad Optom* 40:332-343, 1963.
6. Carter DB: Effects of prolonged wearing of prism, *Am J Optom Arch Am Acad Optom* 40: 265-273, 1963.
7. Mallett RFJ: The investigation of heterophoria at near and a new fixation disparity technique, *Optician* 148(3844):547-551, 1964.
8. Carter DB: Fixation disparity and heterophoria following prolonged wearing of prisms, *Am J Optom Arch Am Acad Optom* 42:141-152, 1965.
9. Carter DB: Effects of prolonged wearing of prism, *Am J Optom Arch Am Acad Optom* 40:265-273, 1963.
10. Worrell BE, Hirsch MJ, Morgan MW: An evaluation of prism prescribed by Sheard's criterion, *Am J Optom Arch Am Acad Optom* 48:373-376, 1971.
11. Sheedy JE, Saladin JJ: Phoria, vergence, and fixation disparity in oculomotor problems, *Am J Optom Physiol Opt* 54:474-478, 1977.
12. Sheedy JE, Saladin JJ: Association of symptoms with measures of oculomotor deficiencies, *Am J Optom Physiol Opt* 55:670-676, 1978.
13. Sheedy JE: Actual measurement of fixation disparity and its use in diagnosis and treatment, *J Am Optom Assoc* 51:1079-1084, 1980.
14. Saladin JJ, Carr LW: Fusion lock diameter and the forced vergence fixation disparity curve, *Am J Optom Physiol Opt* 60:933-943, 1983.
15. Lie I, Opheim A: Long-term acceptance of prisms by heterophorics, *J Am Optom Assoc* 56:272-278, 1985.
16. Wick B, London R: Analysis of binocular visual function using tests made under binocular conditions, *Am J Optom Physiol Opt* 64:227-240, 1987.
17. Despotidis N, Petito GT: Fixation disparity: clinical implications and utilization, *J Am Optom Assoc* 62:923-933, 1991.
18. Guibor GP: Some uses of ophthalmic prisms. In Allen JH (ed): *Strabismus ophthalmic symposium II,* St Louis, 1958, Mosby pp 244-260.
19. Maraini G, Pasino L: Development of normal binocular vision in early convergent strabismus after orthophoria, *Br J Ophthalmol* 49:154-158, 1965.
20. Pigassou R: Prisms in strabismus, *Int Ophthalmol Clin* 6:519-541, 1966.
21. Pigassou-Albouy R: Use of prisms in pre- and post-operative treatment. In Fells P (ed): *The First Congress of the International Strabismological Association,* St Louis, 1971, Mosby, pp 235-242.
22. Pigassou-Albouy R: Prisms in strabismus management: past, present, and future, *J Pediatr Ophthalmol Strabismus* 17:325-303, 1980.
23. Berard PV: Prisms: their therapeutic use in the child. Instrumentation: indications and management, *J Pediatr Ophthalmol* 5:53-65, 1968.
24. Berard PV: The use of prisms in pre- and post-operative treatment of deviation in comitant squint. In Fells P (ed): *The First Congress of the International Strabismological Association,* St Louis, 1971, Mosby, pp 227-234.

25. Caloroso EE: A sequential strategy for achieving functional binocularity in strabismus, *J Am Optom Assoc* 59:378-387, 1988.

26. Caloroso EE, Rouse MW: In *Clinical management of strabismus,* Boston, 1993, Butterworth-Heinemann, pp 94-112.

27. Keating MP: *Geometric, physical, and geometrical optics,* Boston, 1988, Butterworth, pp 355-377.

28. Scheiman M, Gallaway M, Ciner E: Divergence insufficiency: characteristics, diagnosis, and treatment, *Am J Optom Physiol Opt* 63:425-431, 1986.

29. Bagolini B: Sensory anomalies in strabismus, *Br J Ophthalmol* 58:313-318, 1974.

30. Bagolini B: Part II: sensorio-motorial anomalies in strabismus (anomalous movements), *Doc Ophthalmol* 41:23-41, 1976.

31. Schor C: Fixation disparity: a steady state error of disparity-induced vergence, *Am J Optom Physiol Opt* 57:618-631, 1980.

32. Schor CM: Fixation disparity and vergence adaptation. In Schor CM, Ciuffreda KJ (eds): *Vergence eye movements: basic and clinical aspects,* Boston, 1983, Butterworth, 476-494.

33. Rutkowski PC, Burian HM: Divergence paralysis following head trauma, *Am J Ophthalmol* 73:660-662, 1972.

34. Cohen AH, Soden R: An optometric approach to the rehabilitation of the stroke patient, *J Am Optom Assoc* 52:795-800, 1981.

35. Krohel GB, Tobin DR, Hartnett ME, Barrows NA: Divergence paralysis, *Am J Ophthalmol* 94:506-510, 1982.

36. Cohen AH: Optometric management of binocular dysfunctions secondary to head trauma: case reports, *J Am Optom Assoc* 63:569-575, 1992.

37. Christenson GN, Rouse MW: Management of a young esotrope using vision therapy and prismatic prescription, *J Am Optom Assoc* 58:592-596, 1987.

38. Christenson GN, Rouse MW, Adkins DA. Management of infantile-onset esotropia, *J Am Optom Assoc* 61:559-572, 1990.

39. Pigassou R, Toulouse JG: Treatment of eccentric fixation, *J Pediatr Ophthalmol* 4:35-43, 1967.

40. Pigassou-Albouy R, Garipuy MJ: The use of overcorrecting prisms in the treatment of strabismic patients without amblyopia or with cured amblyopia, *Albrecht von Graefes Arch Klin Exp Ophthalmol* 186:209-226, 1973.

41. Caloroso EE, Rouse MW: *Clinical management of strabismus,* Boston, 1993, Butterworth-Heinemann, pp 196-197.

42. Brack B: Penalization and prism: new results with the method of treating squint amblyopia with eccentric fixation. In Moore S, Mein J, Stockbridge L (eds): *Orthoptics: past, present, and future,* New York, 1976, Grune & Stratton, pp 99-103.

43. Caloroso EE, Rouse MW: *Clinical management of strabismus,* Boston, 1993, Butterworth-Heinemann, p 104.

44. Mallett RFJ: The use of prisms in the treatment of concomitant strabismus, *Ophthalmic Optician* 19:793-798, 1979.

45. Wick BC: Horizontal deviations. In Amos JF (ed): *Diagnosis and management in vision care,* Boston, 1987, Butterworth, pp 461-510.

46. Bixenman WW: Vertical prisms: Why avoid them? *Surv Ophthalmol* 29:70-78, 1984.

47. Amos JF, Rutstein RP: Vertical deviations. In Amos JF (ed): *Diagnosis and management in vision care,* Boston 1987, Butterworth, pp 515, 565-566.

48. Jampolsky A: Addendum to Chapter 17, Surgical leashes and reverse leashes in strabismus surgical management. In *Transactions of the New Orleans Academy of Ophthalmology. Symposium on strabismus,* St Louis, 1978, Mosby, pp 266-268.

49. Moradiellos DP, Parrish DE: A clinical technique for correcting diplopia with prism, *J Am Optom Assoc* 57:740-743, 1986.

50. Flom MC, Wick B: A model for treating binocular anomalies. In Rosenbloom AA, Morgan MW (eds): *Principles and practice of pediatric optometry,* Philadelphia, 1990, JB Lippincott, pp 245-273.
51. Apers RC, Bierlaagh J: The use of prisms in paralytic squint, *Am Orthopt J* 27:53-60, 1977.
52. Moore S, Cohen RL: Prism management of acquired incomitant esotropia, *Am Orthopt J* 34: 63-67, 1984.
53. Guibor GP: *Squint and allied conditions,* New York, 1959, Grune & Stratton, pp 247-250.
54. O'Connor R: Contracture in ocular-muscle paralysis, *Am J Ophthalmol* 26:69-71, 1943.
55. Griffin JR: *Binocular anomalies: procedures for vision therapy,* ed 2, Chicago, 1982, Professional Press, pp 275-280.
56. Birnbaum MH: Noncomitant strabismus: evaluation and management, *J Am Optom Assoc* 55:758-764, 1984.
57. Mende S: Duane's retraction syndrome and the relief of secondary torticollis and near point asthenopia with prism, *J Am Optom Assoc* 61:556-558, 1990.
58. Flom MC, Adams AJ: Fresnel optics. In Tasman W, Jaeger EA (eds): *Duane's clinical ophthalmology,* Vol II, Chapter 52, Philadelphia, 1990, JB Lippincott, pp 1-15.
59. Caloroso EE, Rouse MW: *Clinical management of strabismus,* Boston, 1993, Butterworth-Heinemann, pp 3-5.
60. Berard PV: Prisms: their therapeutic use in concomitant strabismus with normal correspondence. In *The First International Congress of Orthoptists,* St Louis, 1968, Mosby, pp 77-82.
61. Pigassou-Albouy R: A discussion of prism therapy for strabismus, *J Ophthalmic Nurs Technol* 7:18-25, 1988.
62. Hirsch MJ: Prism in spectacle lenses for cosmesis, *Am J Optom Arch Am Acad Optom* 45:409-413, 1968.
63. Hofstetter HW: Certain variations in the angle of deviation in concomitant squint, *Am J Optom Arch Am Acad Optom* 24:463-471, 1947.
64. Alpern M, Hofstetter HW: The effect of prism on esotropia: a case report, *Am J Optom Arch Am Acad Optom* 25:80-91, 1948.
65. Birnbaum MH: Adverse response to prism therapy in strabismus, *J Am Optom Assoc* 47:1195-1199, 1976.
66. Caloroso EE, Rouse MW: *Clinical management of strabismus,* Boston, 1993, Butterworth-Heinemann, pp 117-118, 123-124.

Self-Assessment Questions

1. Which of the following statements is *incorrect* regarding the prescription of prism for a patient with a noncomitant strabismic deviation?
    a. Yoked base-down prism would be appropriate for a patient with an A-pattern esodeviation and diplopia in upward gaze.
    b. A secondary contracture of the ipsilateral antagonist of a paretic muscle is less likely to occur in cases of recent-onset paralytic strabismus if the prism is placed over the nonaffected eye.
    c. Prism is often prescribed to eliminate an abnormal head posture in noncomitant strabismic deviations.
    d. When the noncomitant deviation is due to an underacting muscle, less prism will be needed to obtain fusion if most or all of it is placed before the eye with the underacting muscle.

2. Your patient has a constant right esotropia of 30 Δ at distance and near that is cosmetically displeasing. Diagnostic testing reveals that harmonious anomalous correspondence is present and the prognosis for treatment with vision therapy is poor. Which of the following prism corrections would be most appropriate to prescribe as cosmetic prism for this patient?
    a. 8 Δ BI over the right eye
    b. 8 Δ BO over the right eye
    c. 30 Δ BI over the right eye
    d. 30 Δ BO over the right eye

3. Which of the following statements concerning monocular inverse prism designed to eliminate eccentric fixation is *incorrect?*
    a. This specific therapy technique seems most favorable when prescribed for magnitudes of eccentric fixation between 3 to 20 Δ.
    b. Base-out prism is prescribed for patients with nasal eccentric fixation, and base-in prism for patients with temporal eccentric fixation.
    c. The power of the prism prescribed equals or exceeds the size of eccentric fixation by approximately 2 Δ.
    d. The prism is prescribed for full-time wear over the amblyopic eye while the nonamblyopic eye is occluded.

4. Which of the following descriptions of prism prescribed for strabismus is *incorrect?*
    a. A fusion prism changes a diplopic or suppression response to a normal binocular vision response.

    b. Prisms with power equaling the size of the strabismic angle and with the base in the same direction as the eye turn are called corrective prisms.

    c. Prisms with power less than the strabismic angle and with the base in the opposite direction to the eye turn are considered relieving prisms.

    d. Inverse prism is placed before the strabismic eye of a patient with a small to moderate constant unilateral strabismus and a poor prognosis for a functional cure.

5. Which of the following statements describing corrective prism therapy with prism titration (CPT-TP) for strabismus is incorrect?

    a. The initial corrective prism prescription should be prescribed only if normal peripheral sensory fusion is present.

    b. Corrective prisms are usually worn bilaterally so any prismatic distortion is minimized.

    c. Patients treated soon after the onset of a strabismus usually respond well to this type of prism therapy.

    d. After stable sensory fusion is achieved, the prism is gradually reduced in power by 5 to 10 Δ at a time.

Answers: 1. a.   2. a.   3. b.   4. b.   5. d.

9

Overcorrecting Prism Therapy for Anomalous Correspondence

Michael W. Rouse

Key Terms

anomalous correspondence (AC)	anomalous vergence adaptation (AVA)	prism adaptation test (PAT)
overcorrecting prism	disruptive prism	progressive prism adaptation test
anomalous motor fusion	strabismus	
	esotropia	surgery

Sensory anomalies associated with strabismus can have a serious impact on its successful functional treatment. While suppression and amblyopia may have negative effects on the prognosis, anomalous correspondence (AC) is a far greater barrier to establishing normal binocular vision.[1,2] The relative impact of AC varies depending on the frequency of the strabismus, with AC being much more common in constant strabismus than in intermittent cases. In cases of intermittent strabismus with AC, the AC will be present only when the deviation is manifested. When fusional vergence is sufficient to compensate for the deviation and the patient is able to bifixate, the angle of anomaly becomes zero through a phenomenon called *covariation.*[3]

In the case of exotropia, AC has relatively little impact on the prognosis for establishing normal binocular vision.[4] This is based on the fact that exotropias are typically intermittent (~80%) and it is relatively easy to improve convergence and subsequently have the patient covary from anomalous to normal correspondence (NC). The one exception is when the exotropia is created postoperatively in the treatment of esotropia, often referred to as *consecutive* exotropia. These patients generally present with a constant strabismus and paradoxical AC that significantly reduce their prognosis for obtaining normal binocular vision.

About 75% of all esotropias are constant, so the incidence of AC is relatively high (~50%) in this group. Consequently, AC has a greater impact on the prognosis for establishing normal binocular vision in esotropia than in exotropia. Flom[2] reported only a 3% cure rate in a sample of 33 patients. Some authors have reported higher success rates; but, in general, the cure rate for esotropia with AC rarely exceeds 25% and is on the order of 5 times worse than if NC is present. Flom[4] later summarized 12 studies that reported functional correction of strabismus according to the type of correspondence present before treatment. If all the reported subjects were combined, the overall success rate for functional correction of esotropia with AC was only about 14%. The literature suggests that AC represents a significant deterrent to the functional correction of esotropia.

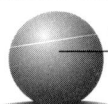

CLINICAL PEARL

With anomalous correspondence present, the cure rate for esotropia is about 5 times worse than if normal correspondence is present.

There are a number of methods that have been reported to treat AC. They typically fall into three broad categories—sensory stimulation, motor stimulation, and disruptive prism. Sensory methods attempt to reestablish the underlying normal sensory system by stimulating corresponding retinal sites. For example, first- or second-degree targets are placed in the major amblyoscope at the patient's objective angle of deviation and a rapid flash pattern is created. The treatment sessions are repeated until the patient reports normal superimposition or fusion of the targets.[5-7] This technique is recommended for esotropes with deviations greater than 15 prism diopters (Δ) and constant exotropes who cannot learn to converge.[8] Motor stimulation methods attempt to increase the compensating vergence ability so the patient is able to align his/her eyes motorically, and thus covariation of correspondence occurs. This is a very effective method if the patient has intermittent exotropia,[4,9] but significantly less so if esotropia,[10] and thus is usually reserved for esotropic deviations of less than 15 Δ.[11]

The sensory and motor stimulation methods are active treatment procedures, requiring participation and effort by the patient. Prism therapy, however, attempts to change or "break up" the habitual incoming sensorimotor information simply by having the patient wear prisms for a specified time and is considered a passive treatment approach. A variety of prism types—rotating-base, inverse, correcting, and overcorrecting—have been reported in the treatment of AC. The technique receiving the greatest attention has been the one that utilizes overcorrecting prisms. Based on an anticipated dramatic change from anomalous to normal sensory processing, these prisms have also been referred to as "disruptive prisms." Sometimes prism therapy is combined with active vision therapy for maximum effectivity, but often it is used in isolation.

Types of Disruptive Prism Therapy

Rotating-base Prisms

Rotating-base prisms provide a method of changing sensory input for the constant strabismic patient, with the intent of precipitating a change from anomalous to normal processing.[12,13] The method involves applying random combinations of prism—base-in, base-out, base-up, and base-down—in an attempt to introduce variation into the angle of anomaly. An example would be prescribing a 10 Δ BO round Fresnel prism before the right eye and each week, or even daily, changing it to BU, BI, and BD. The size of the prism may vary, but 10 Δ seems most popular. On the day that the base-out prism is worn the esotropic angle may increase as the patient prism-adapts. On the day the base-in prism is worn the esotropic angle may decrease. The procedure, which eventually results in diplopia and thus appears to disrupt both sensory and motor patterns, is continued until other tests demonstrate NC.[14] Rotating-base prisms are a form of disruptive prism application that has been mentioned in the literature, but they have received little scientific attention regarding efficacy.

Inverse Prisms

In patients with esotropia, inverse prism therapy involves placing a base-in prism before the fixating eye.[15,16] This encourages divergence and, with increasing amounts of prism, possibly bifixation. The method is analogous to motor stimulation in the major amblyoscope, where the primary goal is to teach the patient to covary by increasing fusional vergence. Although it appears logical and there is some evidence that it may be effective,[15,16] fusional divergence seldom occurs spontaneously and is often difficult to develop even with active therapy. My experience using inverse prisms is limited and, in addition, there appears to have been little investigation into the technique's potential.

Corrective Prisms

The full-time wear of prisms equaling the objective angle has been advocated[17] as a method of treating AC. It involves measuring the size of the deviation with the alternate cover test and then placing the neutralizing amount of prism on the patient. The prism may be divided equally between the two eyes or placed totally before the deviating eye. When it is in place, and as long as the strabismic angle does not change, theoretically the right and left foveas should be stimulated with corresponding information. In many cases, however, the strabismic angle varies with changes in the fixating eye or fixation distance or with the changing fields of gaze. In addition, many authors[3,18-20] have reported that prism adaptation may occur—in which the strabismic angle actually increases after the wearing of a neutralizing prism—with the result that there is no stimulation of the anticipated foveal areas. Thus, in most cases, the use of corrective prisms is not successful. To be successful at disrupting AC when prism adaptation occurs, the overcorrecting prism technique is the method of choice.

Overcorrective Prisms

Overcorrecting prisms have also been advocated[21] as an effective treatment for AC in patients presenting with esotropia. Overcorrective prisms optically change the direction of the oculomotor deviation. The prism power prescribed is larger than the oculomotor deviation and its base is in the direction opposite the eyeturn. The most commonly prescribed power equals the dissociated deviation plus 10 to 15 Δ. In a patient with esotropia and harmonious anomalous correspondence (HAC), the fovea of the fixating eye and point Z of the deviated eye correspond cortically and the patient's percept is anomalous single vision (Fig. 9-1). The overcorrecting prism moves the retinal image beyond the fovea of the viewing eye, and to the opposite hemiretina than previously stimulated (assuming no vergence movements have occurred), resulting in crossed diplopia (Fig. 9-2). The motor fusion demand becomes opposite to that present without the prisms. For example, an esodeviation becomes an *optical exodeviation,* and the patient must now converge rather than diverge to achieve bifixation.

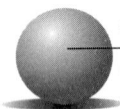

CLINICAL PEARL

Overcorrecting prisms have been advocated as an effective treatment for esotropic patients with anomalous correspondence.

Effectiveness of Overcorrecting Prism Therapy

Whereas rotating-base and inverse prism methods have received little clinical investigation, and corrective prism therapy has been found to

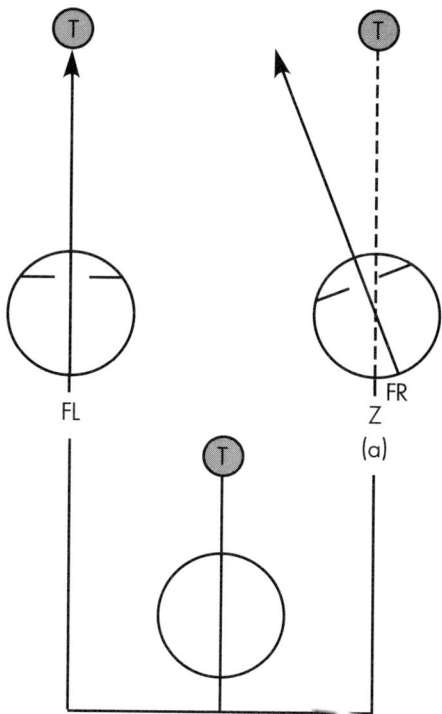

FIGURE 9-1 A patient with constant esotropia and HAC in whom the fovea of the left eye (*FL*) and point Z of the right eye correspond cortically (in this case Z is equivalent to point *a*, which in the strabismic eye corresponds to the fovea of the fixating eye), giving rise to a patient perception of anomalous single vision.

be ineffective because of prism adaptation, overcorrecting prism therapy (OCPT) has received considerable attention and been found to be quite effective.[22] Berard[23] reported successful normalization of AC in 20 of 28 cases using OCPT. Pigassou-Albouy[17] initially reported a 100% success rate in 15 esotropes with AC who underwent OCPT, although Pigassou-Albouy and Garipuy,[21] studying 840 strabismic children less than 8 years of age, found that OCPT normalized correspondence in only 75% to 85%. Wick and Cook[22] reported 53% success in treating 53 patients with esotropia and AC using a combination of occlusion, orthoptics, biofeedback, OCPT, and surgery as needed.

Although OCPT appears to be effective in normalizing correspondence, the technique has been abandoned or ignored by many practitioners primarily because of the time and energy needed.[24] The typical duration of treatment is 6 months to a year. Many practitioners

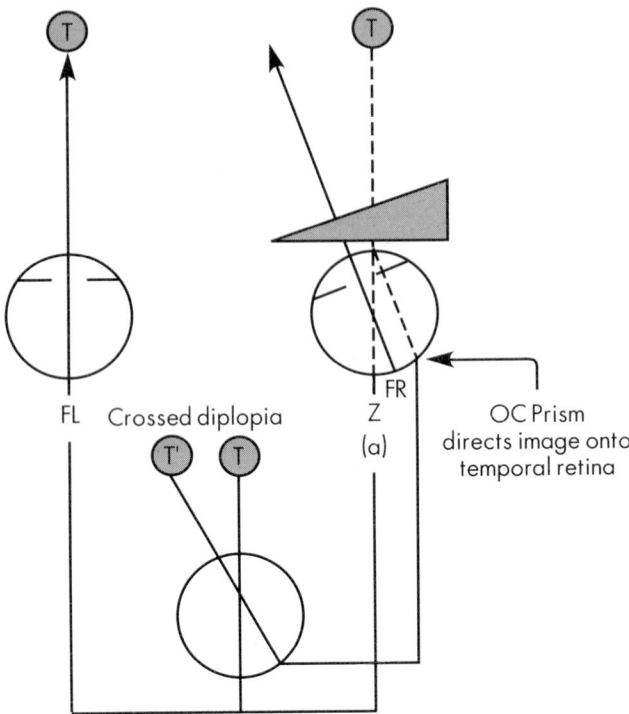

FIGURE 9-2 How OCPT uses a base-out prism (10 to 15 Δ larger than the dissociated angle) to direct the image of the target onto the temporal retina, giving rise to a patient percept of crossed diplopia. *FL,* fovea of the left eye; *FR,* fovea of the right eye; *OC,* overcorrecting prism.

have also been discouraged by treatment failures. Pigassou-Albouy[24] pointed out that failures in treatment are caused mainly by two factors: first, poor patient cooperation and compliance with the treatment instructions and, second, the improper use of prisms (that is, providing insufficient overcorrection at the beginning of therapy and using neutralizing prisms too early). Part of the problem may also lie in the fact that there are no clearly established (step-by-step) clinical guidelines for administering OCPT.

CLINICAL PEARL

Overcorrecting prism therapy failures are caused by either poor patient cooperation and compliance or improper use of the prisms.

Mechanism of Overcorrecting Prism Therapy

Patients with AC, especially esotropes, many times will be found to have very powerful prism-adaptation ability or anomalous motor fusion.[25] Since anomalous fusion is similar to normal fusion, it may be more appropriate to use the term *anomalous vergence adaptation (AVA)*. This condition can be demonstrated by placing a base-out prism equal to the objective angle in front of the fixating eye. Initially it will appear to neutralize the angle of strabismus, but many times (often within just a few minutes) the examiner can begin to measure an esodeviation over the prism. Depending upon the strength of the AVA, the patient may fully adapt to the prism in as little as 30 minutes (that is, the original magnitude of the esotropia will return through the prism). Campos and Catellani[26] have found that some patients can prism-adapt in as short a time as 6 to 9 minutes although others may take longer, with adaptation occurring after a day or even a week. This increase in size of the deviation over the amount of neutralizing prism, often referred to as a positive *prism adaptation test (PAT)*,[27] usually confirms the diagnosis of AC. However, several authors,[26] myself included, have observed that the phenomenon can occur in patients with confirmed NC.

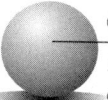

CLINICAL PEARL

Patients may prism-adapt anomalously in as little as 6 to 9 minutes or after a day or even a week of wearing the prism.

The interpretation of AVA is a matter of speculation. Halldén[3] and Bagolini[28] consider AVA to be fusional in nature. Supporting this hypothesis, Campos and Catellani[26] have demonstrated the fusional nature of prism adaptation. AVA shares a common feature with normal fusional (vergence) movements in that, in both cases, there is a variation in muscle tonus when retinal disparity is introduced. However, several important differences exist[29]: (1) AVA is very slow in comparison to normal fusional movements; (2) it also is much less precise, the amount produced often being less than the amount of neutralizing or overcorrecting prism; and (3) it may contain not only a variation in muscle tonus but also a concomitant variation (covariation) in correspondence. AVA can also vary in strength, and the magnitude of that strength may affect surgical outcomes.[30] The practitioner can evaluate the strength of AVA by conducting a progressive PAT, introducing increasing amounts of prism until the patient is no longer able to motor-fuse the target anomalously. At this point an exotropia with crossed diplopia will be produced.

The strength of AVA has been correlated with postsurgical results. For instance, Bagolini[30,31] showed that the stronger the tendency for anomalous fusion the poorer will be the postoperative result (less of the original angle will be eliminated). Thus the initial phase of OCPT for AC involves finding a prism power that the patient can no longer anomalously motor-fuse. This might be considered the point where overcorrecting prism exhausts the patient's AVA. The subsequent phase involves allowing periods of viewing through that prism until AVA decreases and correspondence changes to normal. OCPT is an attractive method because it is a passive treatment approach that simply requires occlusion and intermittent periods of prism wear. Disadvantages include the need for full-time occlusion and reduced visual acuity and contrast sensitivity when viewing through the Fresnel prism. These factors may result in poor compliance.

Overview of Clinical Management Strategy

The general clinical protocol for OCPT that I have found to be effective in normalizing AC is outlined in Figure 9-3. The patient's condition should be carefully assessed, including the frequency and magnitude of the deviation and the status of correspondence. When assessing AC in a patient with amblyopia, the doctor should always evaluate monocular fixation. If eccentric fixation (EF) is found, the measured angle of anomaly (<A) will need to be corrected before one arrives at the final diagnosis of correspondence.[32] The following formula can be used:

<A (measured) + EF (nasal EF is +, temporal EF is −) = <A (true)

The doctor should also reassess the initial treatment decisions, making sure that the patient is wearing his/her best optical correction and the amblyopia is treated to at least a shallow level of 20/40 to 20/50. If the angle of deviation is greater than 20 Δ, the patient and/or parents should be informed about the possible need for its surgical reduction.

The protocol for the OCPT briefly outlined in Figure 9-3 is expanded into a step-by-step procedure in Table 9-1. The first step is to determine the initial overcorrecting prism power. The alternate cover test is conducted, and the magnitude of the deviation is determined by finding the prism power that neutralizes the angle and also the power that creates a small (5 to 10 Δ) exodeviation. The latter prism (in Fresnel form) is applied to the fixating eye's spectacle lens. Magnitudes of Fresnel prism up to 30 Δ are available. Once 30 Δ is

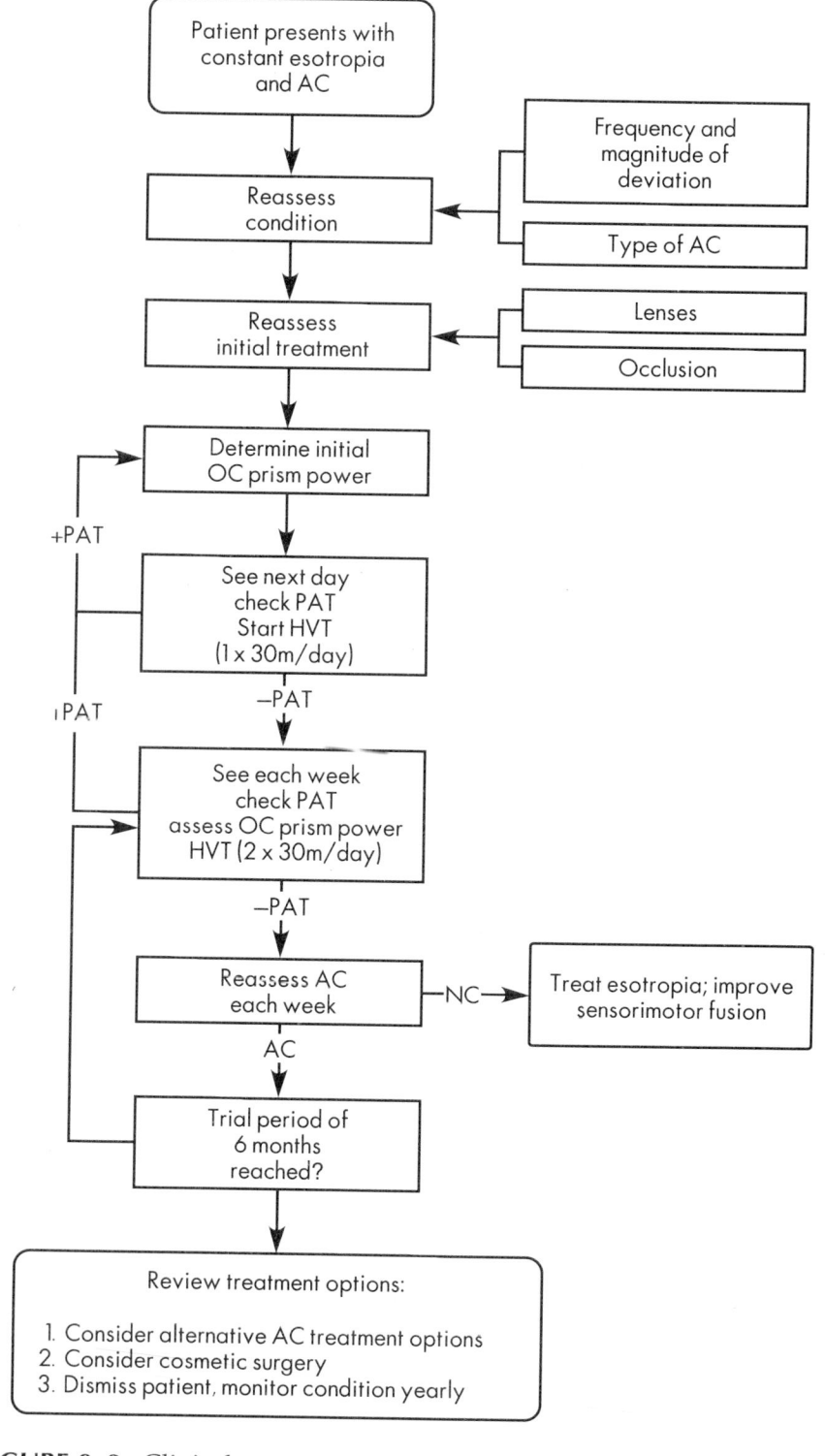

FIGURE 9-3 Clinical management of overcorrecting prism therapy in patients with esotropia and anomalous correspondence (*AC*). *PAT,* prism adaptation test; *HVT,* home vision therapy; *NC,* normal correspondence.

TABLE 9-1
Management Protocol for Overcorrecting Prism Therapy

First Office Visit

Alternate cover test with prism neutralization
Apply prism that produces small (5 to 10 Δ) exodeviation
Monitor prism adaptation (PA) every 10 min for 30 min
If no PA in 30 min, apply a 12 to 15 Δ Fresnel prism overcorrection over fixating eye
If PA in 30 min, repeat steps above

First Day Home Plan

Full-time occlusion
Patient to do one 30 min session of associated viewing (both eyes open) through prism; indoor
    active eye-hand or visual motor activities suggested during this time
Return to office next day

Second Office Visit

Reevaluate PA every 10 min for 30 min
If no PA, continue with first week home plan
If PA, repeat steps for first office visit

First-week Home Plan

Full-time occlusion
One 30 min session each day of associated viewing through prism
Return to office in 1 week

Third Office Visit (1-Week Follow-up)

Reevaluate correspondence
Reevaluate PA every 10 min for 30 min
If no PA, continue with full-time program
If PA, repeat steps for first office visit

Full-time Home Plan

Full-time occlusion
Two 30 min sessions each day of associated viewing with prism
Return weekly to monitor PA and reevaluate correspondence
If weekly visits show no PA, increase number of 30 min sessions or extend time to 1 hr (monitor in-
    office before prescribing)
Consider decreasing power of overcorrecting prism if increase in exodeviation is measured
See flow chart (Fig. 9-3) when NC is present

reached, any additional prism needed is placed over the nonfixating eye. It is convenient to use Fresnel prisms cut 38 to 40 mm round. They can be reused, or, alternatively, an acrylic Fresnel prism can be placed in a Halberg clip over the patient's spectacles.

Two strategies have been proposed for determining the initial overcorrecting prism magnitude. First, Bagolini[33] suggested finding an amount of prism that cannot be adapted to in a convenient period, referred to as "prism temporalization." For example, the doctor would find the amount of overcorrecting prism that created and maintained an optical exodeviation for a period of 30 minutes. The patient would then wear this correction (that is, the minimal prism power that AVA cannot overcome) for sessions of less than 30 minutes. At all other times full-time occlusion would be worn. Second, Adelstein and Cüpper (cited by Bagolini[29]) suggested determining the amount of prism that cannot be adapted to and the patient wears this full time without occlusion. Bagolini's method is preferred because it provides a practical in-office method for determining the initial overcorrecting prism, the patient has to wear the prism for only short periods, and it provides tighter control over whether the patient will adapt to the prism. With Adelstein and Cüpper's technique the patient might slowly adapt to the prism and the doctor would not know until the next office visit.

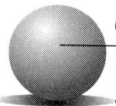

CLINICAL PEARL

The initial overcorrecting prism magnitude is the amount that cannot be adapted to in 30 minutes.

With Bagolini's approach, the doctor monitors the patient for prism adaptation at 10-minute intervals over a 30-minute period. If no prism adaptation is present at 30 minutes, the initial prism power plus a small additional amount is applied so the patient will be 12 to 15 Δ overcorrected.[34] Full prism correction over the fixating eye is preferred. If large amounts of prism are needed it will be necessary to split the prism power between the two eyes. The prism is placed initially over the fixating eye for two reasons: first, it acts as a partial occluder and may help in treating any shallow amblyopia present; second (and more important), a change in correspondence may be caused by changing fixation to the normally turned eye.[17,35-37] The patient should report diplopia through this initial prism power. If prism adaptation occurs within 30 minutes, the prism amount is again increased to overcorrect the deviation by 12 to 15 Δ and the magnitude is reevaluated in 30 minutes. This continues until a power of prism is found that the patient cannot anomalously motor-fuse. Often patients are able to adapt anomalously to prism between 60 and 80 Δ. Greenwald[38] suggested the addition of a blurring lens before the fixating eye. However, this is considered unnecessary because a Fresnel prism in the range of 15 to 30 Δ will significantly reduce visual acuity.[39]

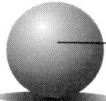

CLINICAL PEARL

The patient should report crossed (exotropic) diplopia during the 30-minute home vision therapy procedures.

Once the initial overcorrecting prism is determined, therapy can begin. The first-day home plan is to use full-time occlusion, except for a 30-minute period of associated viewing (both eyes open) with the prism in place. Why 30 minutes? Because it has been confirmed previously that the patient will not prism-adapt during this time. During the 30 minutes of associated viewing the patient is concentrating on active eye-hand or visual motor activities. There should be crossed (exotropic) diplopia during these activities, which may be distressing, but the patient should be encouraged to continue in spite of it. A red filter and penlight can be given for self-monitoring the direction of diplopia and may be helpful in certain instances when an appointment cannot be kept. The doctor can ask the patient over the phone to check for a crossed diplopia response. If uncrossed diplopia is present, this suggests that AVA has occurred and full-time occlusion should be reestablished until the next office visit. The patient should return the following day for another 30-minute PAT. If no prism adaptation has occurred, a 1-week home therapy plan is started that includes one 30-minute period of associated viewing through the prism combined with eye-hand/visual motor activities, and the patient is scheduled for reevaluation in 1 week. If prism adaptation has occurred, the examiner should repeat the steps of the initial visit to redetermine the overcorrecting prism and proceed as outlined above. If a prism power cannot be found to produce a stable exodeviation at this time, the examiner may want to consider an alternative form of treatment or dismiss the patient.

At the 1-week reevaluation (third office visit) the doctor should again check for prism adaptation. Another PAT will be conducted and correspondence reassessed. Seldom have I seen correspondence change this quickly, but it is important to check on a regular basis. If the patient is still exo through the overcorrecting prism, a full-time OCPT program with monitoring each week thereafter should begin and will include full-time occlusion with two daily 30-minute sessions of associated viewing through the prism. At each weekly office visit the doctor should conduct the alternate cover test over the overcorrecting prism. If an increase in exodeviation is noticed through the prism, this indicates that AVA strength is decreasing. I have seen a rapid decrease in AVA strength over the first 8 weeks of therapy, which indicates it is time to reduce the power of the overcorrecting prism; however, it is critical that a 10 to 15 Δ overcorrection be maintained. The overcorrecting prism will be reduced in a progressive fashion over a period of usually 6 months. Still, I have found[40,41] when using this protocol, which carefully controls the time of prism wear, that between 8 and 20 weeks is necessary for normalizing correspondence. The doctor should be careful to maintain the overcorrecting prism in place until NC is demonstrated consistently over 2 to 3 weeks of testing. At some point in this sequence the patient should demonstrate NC and eventually end up wearing prism that neutralizes the objective angle. Once NC is present, the patient should be scheduled for intensive in-office therapy to establish normal sensory motor fusion at the objective angle.[7]

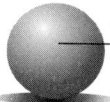

CLINICAL PEARL

Overcorrecting prism is reduced in power when anomalous vergence adaptation decreases, as indicated by increasing exotropia measured through the overcorrecting prism.

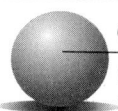

CLINICAL PEARL

Normalization of correspondence often occurs in the first 8 to 20 weeks of treatment.

• Case Study

History

JL, an 8-year-old Hispanic boy, was first evaluated in January 1989 because his parents were concerned that he might be "going blind." Although a right esotropia had been noted since birth, the family was told that nothing could be done until the age of 6, at which time he received his first spectacle correction. No prior treatment for the esotropia was reported. There was a positive family history of esotropia (older brother, aunt, and grandmother). The patient's medical and ocular histories were unremarkable.

Diagnostic Summary

JL was found to have a comitant constant right esotropia of 20 to 22 Δ at 6 m and 24 to 27 Δ at 40 cm through his best distance correction (determined by cycloplegia). The calculated AC/A was 7.2/1. Cosmesis was fair to poor (Fig. 9-4). He also had the following associated conditions: steady central fixation OD, OS; visual acuities of 20/25 OD, 20/20 OS; HAC (major amblyoscope and Hering Bielschowsky afterimage test); and constant OD suppression in open space.

Spectacles

OD: +3.75 − 1.75 × 010   (20/25)
OS: +3.00 DS   (20/20)

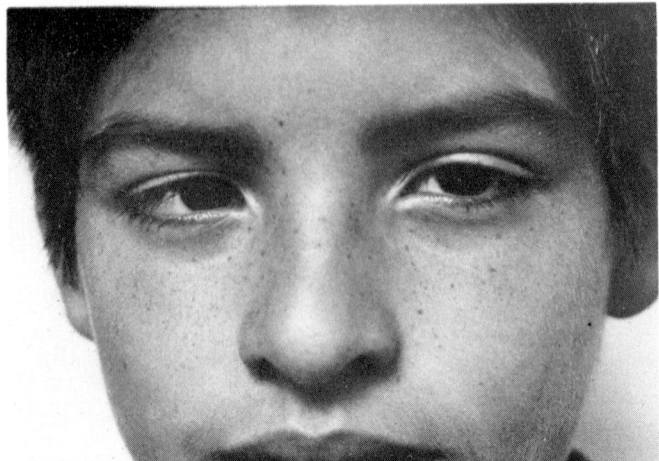

FIGURE 9-4 An 8-year-old patient (JL) presenting with 20 to 25 Δ of constant right esotropia and HAC.

Management

The patient entered into a program of treating the AC with OCPT. The possible need for surgery was discussed with the parents. Spectacles and full-time total occlusion on a direct–one day/indirect–next day schedule were prescribed. The highlights of the therapy program are outlined below, and Figure 9-5 gives an overview of changes in the angle of anomaly.

Therapy Highlights

Week 2	Patient demonstrated strong AVA response; started OCPT with 70 Δ BO, one 30 min viewing session/day, and full-time occlusion all other times
Weeks 2 to 8	Rapid decrease in "strength" of AVA response; continued OCPT with decreasing amounts of prism, two 30 min viewing sessions/day, and full-time occlusion (Fig. 9-6)
Week 20	**Patient demonstrated NC (<A = 0); continued OCPT and full-time occlusion**
Week 20	Break in therapy; patient left country because of family obligations
Week 27	Patient returned; failed to comply with therapy while away, saw HAC again; resumed OCPT and full-time occlusion
Week 36	**Patient demonstrated NC (<A = 0); continued OCPT and full-time occlusion**
Weeks 36 to 53	Worked in-instrument to develop normal sensorimotor fusion at objective angle; continued OCPT and full-time occlusion

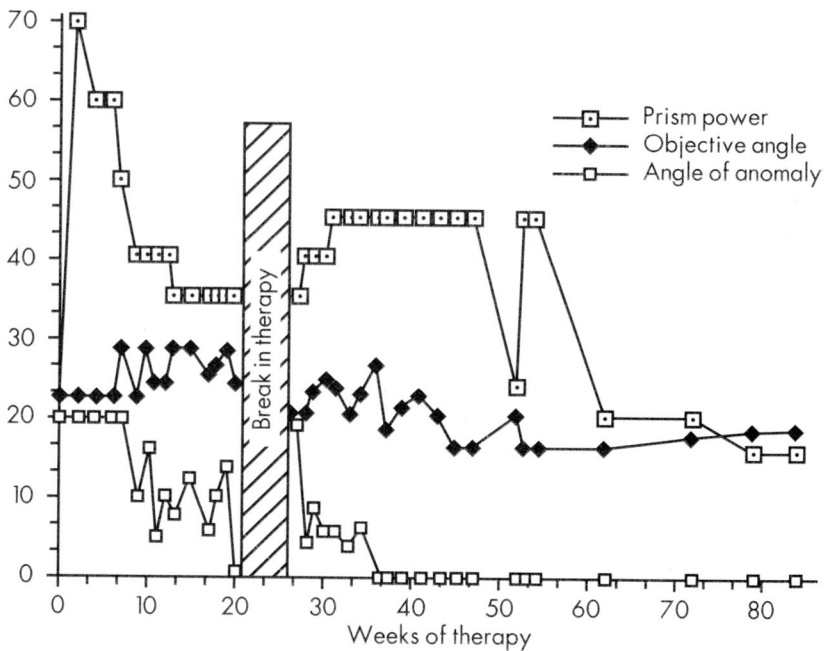

FIGURE 9-5 Changes in the prism power, objective angle, and angle of anomaly (<A) during OCPT.

Week 53   Sensorimotor fusion improved; 24 Δ BO allowed 2° fusion in open space at distance only; applied 24 Δ BO Fresnel prism over patient's spectacles; lower half of left lens was occluded since fusion not present

Week 54   Patient adapted to prism; prism removed, OCPT and full-time occlusion resumed; concentrated on improving in-instrument sensorimotor fusion

Week 62   Patient demonstrated stable 2° fusion (with central suppression) in open space at distance with 20 Δ BO; discontinued OCPT at distance; continued OCPT at intermediate distance and lower half occlusion of left lens

Week 72   20 Δ BO neutralizing Fresnel prism placed on full lens; stable 2° fusion reported at all distances (Fig. 9-7)

Week 79   Spectacles incorporating 16 Δ BO "ground-in" prism and +2.50 add prescribed for full-time wear; stable 2° fusion reported at all distances (Fig. 9-8)

Week 84   Patient showed stable 2° fusion at far and near, no central suppression, and questionable random-dot stereopsis.

Week 89   Patient dismissed from office therapy; progress check in 1 month

In approximately 20 weeks JL demonstrated NC. During the first weeks of OCPT there was a rapid decrease in the AVA response and I

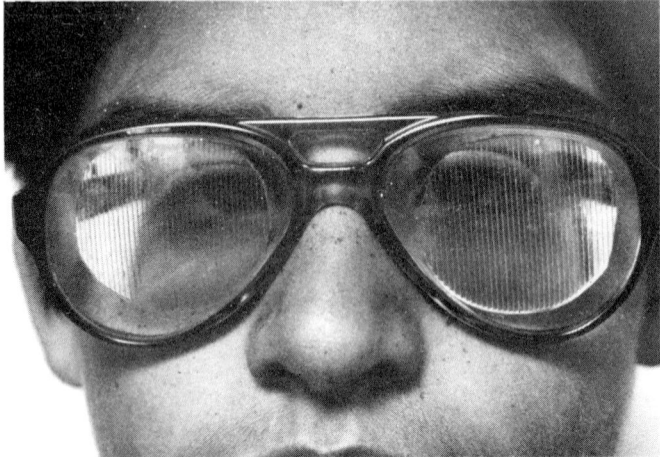

FIGURE 9-6 JL wearing spectacles and 60 Δ of BO prism in the early stages of OCPT (week 3). He reported crossed diplopia.

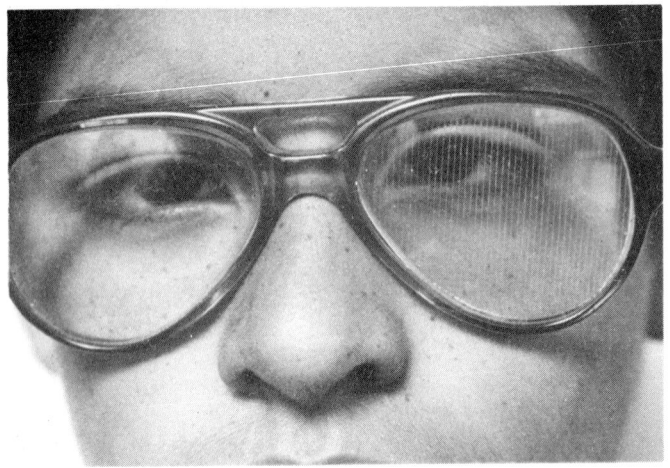

FIGURE 9-7 JL wearing spectacles and a 20 Δ BO Fresnel neutralizing prism, which established bifoveal fixation and normal second-degree fusion at week 72.

subsequently reduced the power of the overcorrecting prism to maintain at 10 to 15 Δ overcorrection. Between 8 weeks and when he demonstrated NC, he reported unharmonious AC in the major amblyoscope and on the Hering Bielschowsky afterimage test. The angle of anomaly was very unstable, varying between 5 and 15 Δ. Some of this variability may have been due to the only fair compliance with full-time occlusion therapy. Unfortunately, about the time JL demon-

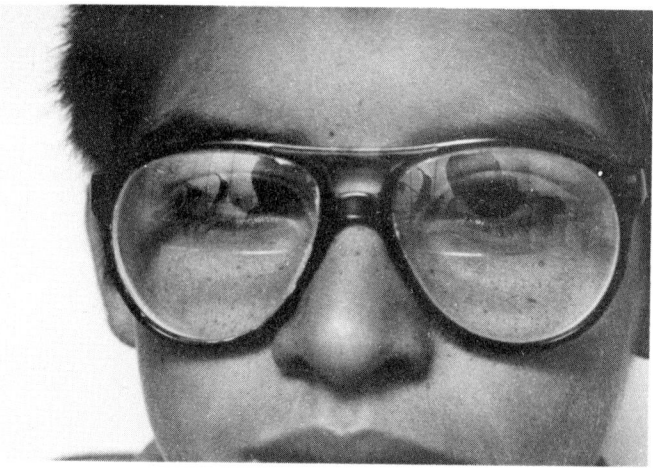

FIGURE 9-8 JL wearing the final correction, which included 16 Δ BO "ground-in" prism and a +2.50 bifocal at week 79.

strated his first NC response he had to leave the country for approximately 7 weeks. During this period he wore his spectacles full time but did not comply with the occlusion or OCPT. Following his return he demonstrated HAC. Once OCPT and full-time occlusion were reestablished, there was a rapid decrease in the angle of anomaly. The change in the angle of anomaly was much more rapid than the 20 weeks necessary to establish the initial NC response. In just 9 weeks JL again demonstrated a stable NC response, and this result was stable over the remaining time of therapy. Subsequent therapy was directed at establishing normal sensorimotor fusion. We maintained the OCPT and full-time occlusion until JL could report stable second-degree fusion in open space testing with neutralizing prisms. An early attempt (54th week) at using neutralizing prism had resulted in prism adaptation. This was attributed to the lack of central and foveal sensorimotor fusion. Therapy was redirected at establishing stable central and foveal sensorimotor fusion in-instrument. The application of neutralizing prism 8 weeks later resulted in stable second-degree fusion in free or open space. There was no further prism adaptation after this point in therapy. Subsequent therapy was directed at establishing normal sensorimotor fusion in open space.

Summary

A review of the literature reveals a number of studies that strongly suggest OCPT can be an effective therapy option for disrupting AC, although the technique has been almost abandoned because of the time and energy needed to achieve successful results. Many practitioners have also been discouraged by treatment failures. Pigassou-Albouy[24] pointed out that treatment failures are caused mainly by two factors: first, poor cooperation and compliance with the treatment instructions and, second, the improper use of prisms. Part of the problem may also lie in the fact that there are no clear, established (step-by-step), clinical guidelines available to assist the practitioner in administering OCPT. The management strategy and case report presented here address the need for a specific protocol, which would also help address the patient's and parents' concerns regarding the time and energy investment by (hopefully) decreasing the therapy time for disrupting AC.

The advantages of OCPT are that it is a passive treatment approach, requiring minimal active therapy and doctor time, and it produces a *relatively* quick decrease in both AVA strength and the angle of anomaly. The disadvantages are that it (1) requires a substantial time commitment on the part of the patient and (2) must be closely monitored by the doctor to detect changes in the patient's visual status. When discussing the treatment of strabismus with the patient (or parent), especially if AC is present, the doctor should remember that "difficult treatment" is not synonymous with "ineffective treatment"[24] and the issue of informed consent regarding available treatment options is an important obligation of the doctor.[42]

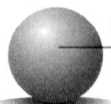

CLINICAL PEARL

Overcorrecting prism therapy represents a passive treatment approach, requiring minimal active therapy and doctor time.

References

1. Burian HM: Anomalous retinal correspondence: its essence and its significance in diagnosis and treatment, *Am J Ophthalmol* 34:237-253, 1951.
2. Flom MC: The prognosis in strabismus, *Am J Optom Arch Am Acad Optom* 35:509-514, 1958.
3. Halldén U: Fusional phenomena in anomalous correspondence, *Acta Ophthalmol Suppl* 37:1-93, 1952.
4. Flom MC: Issues in the clinical management of binocular anomalies. In Rosenbloom AA, Morgan MW (eds): *Principles and practice of pediatric optometry,* Philadelphia, 1990, JB Lippincott, pp 219-244.
5. Gibson HW, Meakin WJ: Symmetrical binocular flicker in the treatment of abnormal retinal correspondence. In *Transactions of the International Optical Congress,* London, 1952, British Optical Association, pp 315-333.
6. Wick B: Home visual therapy for constant esotropia with anomalous correspondence, *Am J Optom Physiol Opt* 55:836-839, 1978.
7. Caloroso EE, Rouse MW: *The clinical management of strabismus,* Boston, 1993, Butterworth-Heinemann, pp. 201-220.

8. Wick B: "Forced elimination" of anomalous retinal correspondence in constant exotropia: a case report, *Am J Optom Physiol Opt* 52:58-62, 1975.

9. Wick B: Visual therapy for constant exotropia with anomalous retinal correspondence: a case report, *Am J Optom Physiol Opt* 51:1005-1008, 1974.

10. Grisham JD: Treatment of binocular dysfunctions. In Schor CM, Ciuffreda KJ (eds): *Vergence eye movements: basic and clinical aspects,* Boston, 1983, Butterworth, pp 637-639.

11. Wick B: Visual therapy for small angle esotropia, *Am J Optom Physiol Opt* 51:490-496, 1974.

12. Ludlam WM: Strabismus/prognosis and treatment results. In Borish IM (ed): *Clinical refraction,* ed 3, Chicago, 1970, Professional Press, pp 1303-1304.

13. Mallett RFJ: Anomalous retinal correspondence: the new outlook, *Ophthalmic Optician* 10:606-624, 1970.

14. Cook DL: Considering the ocular motor system in the treatment of anomalous retinal correspondence, *J Am Optom Assoc* 55:109-117, 1984.

15. Peckham RM: *Squints and heterophorias,* Rochester, NY, 1931, Charles G Lyman, vol 1, pp 137-152.

16. Rubin W: Reverse prism and calibrated occlusion: in the treatment of small angle deviations, *Am J Ophthalmol* 59:271-277, 1965.

17. Pigassou-Albouy R: Use of prisms in pre- and post-operative treatment. In Fells P (ed): *The First Congress of the International Strabismological Association,* St Louis, 1971, Mosby, pp 235-242.

18. Hofstetter HW: Certain variations in the angle of deviation in concomitant squint, *Am J Optom Arch Am Acad Optom* 24:463-471, 1947.

19. Alpern M, Hofstetter HW: The effect of prism on esotropia: a case report, *Am J Optom Arch Am Acad Optom* 25:80-91, 1948.

20. Birnbaum MH: Adverse response to prism therapy in strabismus, *J Am Optom Assoc* 47:1195-1199, 1976.

21. Pigassou-Albouy R, Garipuy J: The use of overcorrecting prisms in the treatment of strabismic patients without amblyopia or with cured amblyopia, *Albrecht von Graefes Arch Klin Exp Ophthalmol* 186:209-226, 1973.

22. Wick B, Cook D: Management of anomalous correspondence: efficacy of therapy, *Am J Optom Physiol Opt* 64:405-410, 1987.

23. Berard PV: The use of prisms in the pre- and post-operative treatment of deviation in comitant squint. In Fells P (ed): *The First Congress of the International Strabismological Association,* St Louis, 1971, Mosby, pp 227-234.

24. Pigassou-Albouy R: A discussion of prism therapy for strabismus, *J Ophthalmic Nurs Technol* 7:18-25, 1988.

25. Bagolini B: Sensorial anomalies in strabismus. I, *Doc Ophthalmol* 41:1-22, 1976.

26. Campos EC, Catellani T: Further evidence for the fusional nature of the compensation (or "eating up") of prisms in concomitant strabismus, *Int Ophthalmol* 1:57-62, 1978.

27. Jampolsky A: A simplified approach to strabismus diagnosis. In *Symposium on strabismus. Transactions of the New Orleans Academy of Ophthalmology,* St Louis, 1971, Mosby, pp 34-92.

28. Bagolini B: Anomalous binocular vision and suppression in strabismic patients, *Ophthalmic Optician* 10:938-947, 949, 1970.

29. Bagolini B: Sensory anomalies in strabismus, *Br J Ophthalmol* 58:313-318, 1974.

30. Bagolini B: Objective evaluation of sensorial and sensorimotorial status in esotropia: their importance in surgical prognosis, *Br J Ophthalmol* 69:725-728, 1985.

31. Bagolini B, Zanasi MR, Bolzani R: Surgical correction of convergent strabismus: its relationship to prism compensation, *Doc Ophthalmol* 62:309-324, 1986.

32. Flom MC, Kerr KE: Determination of retinal correspondence, *Arch Ophthalmol* 77:200-213, 1967.
33. Bagolini B: Postsurgical treatment of convergent strabismus, with a critical evaluation of various tests, *Int Ophthalmol Clin* 6:633-667, 1966.
34. Fleming A, Pigassou R, Garipuy J: Adaptation of a method of prismatic overcorrection, for treating strabismus in children one and two years old, *J Pediatr Ophthalmol* 10:154-159, 1973.
35. Burian HM: Sensorial retinal relationship in concomitant strabismus. III, Clinical picture of anomalous retinal correspondence and its interpretation, *Arch Ophthalmol* 37:504-533, 1947.
36. Brock FW, Folsom W: Binocular methods of investigating amblyopia. I, New test for correspondence. II, New test for foveal integrity, *Am J Optom Arch Am Acad Optom* 41:637-652, 1964.
37. Maraini G, Santori M: Anomalous retinal correspondence and monolateral squint, *Ophthalmologica* 153:179-183, 1967.
38. Greenwald I: *Effective strabismus therapy,* Duncan, Okla, 1979, Optometric Extension Program Foundation, pp 9-19.
39. Veronneau-Troutman S: Fresnel prisms and their effect on visual acuity and binocularity, *Trans Am Ophthalmol Soc* 76:610-653, 1978.
40. Rouse MW, Saldana KK, Horibe FM: Overcorrecting prism therapy for anomalous correspondence, *Optom Vis Sci* 67(Suppl):80, 1990 (abstract).
41. Christenson GN: Treatment of esotropia with anomalous correspondence: a case report, *J Am Optom Assoc* 63:257-261, 1992.
42. Miller PJ: Clinico-legal aspects of infantile strabismus, *Optom Vis Sci* 67:148-149, 1990.

Self-Assessment Questions

1. In which of the following conditions is the prognosis for establishing normal binocular vision most negatively impacted by anomalous correspondence?
   a. constant esotropia
   b. intermittent esotropia
   c. constant exotropia
   d. intermittent exotropia

2. Anomalous vergence adaptation (AVA) that occurs in esotropes with anomalous correspondence is different from normal fusional vergence in which of the following ways?
   a. It is very slow in comparison to normal fusional movements
   b. It is much less precise; the amount produced is often less than the magnitude of the neutralizing or overcorrecting prism magnitude
   c. It is often accompanied by a concomitant variation (covariation) in correspondence.
   d. all of the above

3. The overcorrecting technique recommended by Bagolini, "prism temporalization," involves finding the amount of overcorrecting prism that creates and maintains an optical exotropia over a period of
   a. 10 minutes
   b. 30 minutes
   c. 60 minutes
   d. 1 day

4. During the time the patient wears an overcorrecting prism, he or she should report
   a. uncrossed diplopia
   b. crossed diplopia
   c. no diplopia; the patient should be suppressing the normally strabismic eye
   d. no diplopia; the patient should be anomalously fusing

5. Which of the following alternate cover test measurements (with an esotropic patient wearing overcorrecting prism during OCPT) indicates that the patient's prism should be reduced?
   a. ortho
   b. 12 to 15 Δ BO

c. 12 to 15 Δ BI
d. 20 to 25 Δ BO
e. 20 to 25 Δ BI

10

Prism Use in Vision Therapy

Selwyn Super

Key Terms

behavioral optometry	SILO	intersensory stimulation
vision therapy	strabismus	antisuppression therapy
anomalous correspondence	perceptual system	
	prism saccades	
yoked prism	spatial disruption	perceptuomotor
	spatial orientation	

Vision therapy is an extension of classical orthoptics. Its purpose is to raise the level of a patient's visual efficiency. Because vision influences and, in turn, is influenced by other body functions, vision therapy is also directed toward coordinating and integrating vision with the body's other sensorimotor, perceptual, and cognitive systems.

This chapter provides a rationale for the appropriate use of prism as an integral part of vision therapy. There appear to be sound scientific reasons why prisms should be used as compensatory, remedial, and developmental interventions—not only in problems of strabismus but even more so in the much larger number of nonstrabismic binocular vision disorders that demand attention.

259

My purpose is to suggest, specifically, how prism can be incorporated in vision therapy to benefit general and visual function. In this respect, I plan to go beyond the classical orthoptic use of prisms in compensating for ocular deviations. Prisms are used in vision therapy to develop sensory and motor awareness, to compensate for oculomotor and other visual and perceptual deficiencies, and to improve general and oculomotor postural integration and control.

Effects of Prisms on Intersensory Integration and Perception

How prisms affect intersensory integration and perception has been a subject of considerable interest. It is thought that when the body adapts to prism it then coordinates a rearrangement of the eyes' control over the limbs and objects of manipulation. The interposition of prisms before the eyes affects the kinesthetic, proprioceptive, and vestibular perceptual systems and has more obvious effects on the visual system. Studies in which subjects have interacted with prism-displaced visual environments[1-5] show that these subjects may develop long-term perceptual modifications (referred to as *prism adaptation,* but different than the prism adaptation discussed in Chapters 4–6, 9 and 10) that contribute to spatial appreciation and the degree to which they respond to prism therapy. The bias that occurs when separate systems relay conflicting information to the brain is usually determined by the degree to which an individual is accustomed to trusting one system over another. Systems that threaten to disrupt a person's stable world are therefore suppressed (as much as possible) to avoid confusion. A patient who accepts a certain power of prism may do so because it helps to bring the visual perceptual system into line with other perceptual systems in the combined appreciation of space and of objects within it. However, it is possible that what appears to be acceptance of prism may, in fact, be a rejection of it. In such instances the patient may prefer to ignore the input from the eye with prism before it, and instead rely increasingly on input from the other eye because it agrees more with input from the other perceptual systems contributing to spatial appreciation. The prism adaptation that takes place when individuals accept more prism at each subsequent examination may suggest that the nonvisual perceptual systems have a predominating influence. It is, therefore, important to recognize the effects that prism therapy has in attempting to optimize the integration and coordination of binocular vision with the individual's total perceptual system.

The effects of prism in vision therapy are related in some measure to the degree of plasticity in the various oculomotor control systems that form the basis of prism adaptation. Ebenholtz[6] has created a model to help explain the relationship between perceptual systems and the spatial behavior of the body. He proposes a system of egocentric "head-centered" angular coordinates patterned after Müller's K-system as a basis for encoding spatial orientation and distance in terms of the oculomotor system parameters responsible for controlling disjunctive and conjugate eye movements and their steady states. He provides data to show that adaptation to optical tilt produces a shift in apparent vertical and horizontal target orientations, as well as in the direction of voluntary (self-directed) saccades and the vestibular ocular response (VOR), and he suggests that it is the VOR control system that underlies the adaptation of egocentric target orientation. This is illustrated in Figure 10-1.

The use of prisms in vision therapy may thus be seen as linked to all the perceptual processes (identified by Gibson[7]) that serve to stabilize an individual's space world and help him or her locate, identify, and fixate objects from an egocentric viewing point. It is mainly in answering the questions of what, where, and when that the basic orientating, visual, auditory, haptic/kinesthetic, and olfactory perceptual systems collaborate in stabilizing the individual's space/ time world. The comfort and homeostatic perceptual systems (identified by Bartley[8]) also play an important role in providing comfort and equilibrium, which are attached to stable perception. And it is toward

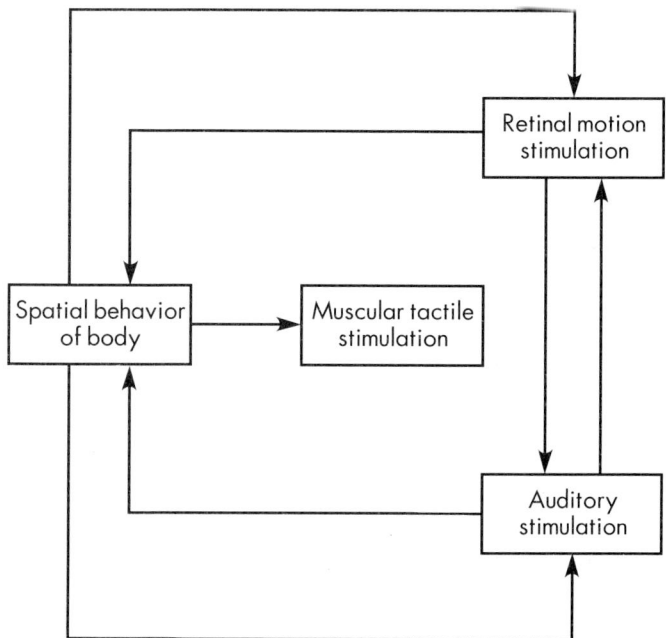

FIGURE 10-1 Relationships between perceptual stimulation systems.

this spatial/temporal balance of the total perceptual system that prism use should be directed as part of vision therapy. Prisms therefore can influence perceptual behavior and function in general and the visual system in particular.

Prisms affect the space of an observer in the following ways[9]:

1. Base-down prism tends to displace space volume upward and away from a person's center of gravity; it also appears to expand the visual space volume.
2. Base-up prism tends to displace visual space downward and closer to a person's center of gravity; it also appears to reduce the visual space volume.
3. Binocular base-in prisms tend to displace the visual space outward and to reduce the tonicity of postural muscles in the upper back and neck (localization); they also appear to expand the visual space volume and to emphasize the ground (as opposed to the figure).
4. Binocular base-out prisms tend to displace visual space inward and to increase the tonicity of postural muscles in the upper back and neck (localization); they also appear to reduce the visual space volume and to emphasize the figure (as opposed to the ground).
5. Yoked prisms (of equal power, with their bases in the same direction) cause spatial shifts that have an effect on body orientation. These changes are represented in Table 10-1.

A person's *orientation* (Where am I?) is altered by the effects of yoked prisms and of prism placed in front of one eye under monocular viewing conditions. Conversely, a person's *localization* (Where is it?) is altered by the effects of binocular base-in and base-out prisms.

The potential to alter the function and behavior of a person through the use of prisms has many ramifications. In the broadest sense it may serve to expand the space world of the centrally postured esophore or to contract the space world of the peripherally postured exophore.

Prisms to Improve and Develop Sensory and Motor Awareness

By virtue of their inherent ability to displace images of objects viewed through them, prisms are eminently suitable for improving and developing visual sensorimotor awareness. A knowledge of the extent of the visual field and of the major actions of the extraocular muscles provides a theoretical basis for the types, powers, and directions of prisms to be used. Such prisms may be square or round; they may be loose, in bars or flippers, or motorized rotatory; they may also be thick

TABLE 10-1

Effects of Yoked Prisms and of Prism Placed Before One Eye Under Monocular Viewing Conditions on Space, Ocular Position, Center of Gravity, and Overall Posture

Base	Space shift	Direction of eye movement	Center of gravity shift	Resultant posture
Up	Down and closer	Down	Forward	On heels
Down	Up and farther	Up	Backward	On toes
Right	To left	Left	Rotate right	Toward right
Left	To right	Right	Rotate left	Toward left

or thin (as in the case of Fresnel membranes). Prisms are sometimes introduced with the viewer and the object of regard both moving or both stationary, or with one stationary and the other moving.

Although research during the last 30 or so years has shed new light on the developmental steps of binocular vision and stereopsis,[10] it is customary in vision therapy to follow Worth's classical theory of binocular development[11] and (therefore) to implement the sequence of monocular, biocular, and binocular therapy procedures.

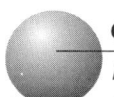

CLINICAL PEARL

It is customary in vision therapy to follow a sequence of monocular, biocular, and binocular therapy procedures.

In monocular prism therapy one eye is open and the other occluded. In biocular prism therapy both eyes are open but prism is used to dissociate the eyes so that equivalent (but not fused) images are seen. In binocular prism therapy a vergence demand is created by introducing prism under binocular viewing conditions.

Monocular, Biocular, and Binocular Prism Therapy

Briefly stated, the following summations apply: monocular prism therapy is directed toward improving monocular sensory awareness and sensorimotor control; biocular prism therapy is usually directed toward eliminating suppression, helping bring about central fixation, and establishing normal correspondence; and binocular prism therapy is directed toward improving the quality and range of binocular vision.

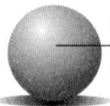

CLINICAL PEARL

Monocular prism therapy is designed to improve monocular sensory aware-ness and sensorimotor control.

Biocular prism therapy is used to eliminate suppression, eccentric fixation, and anomalous correspondence.

Binocular prism therapy is designed to improve the quality and range of binocular vision.

Developing sensitivity to shape changes

Looking at an object through a prism (for example, a white square on a black ground) should cause the object to appear bowed in the direction of the base of the prism. A colored spectral fringe should be noticeable at the edges of the image, with the red end of the spectrum in the direction of the prism base and the indigo end in the direction of the apex. The greater the magnitude of the prism, the more apparent the effect should be.

A basic principle of prism therapy is to start with the lowest power of prism that will consistently elicit a correct response and then gradually reduce the power until the patient is unable to respond correctly. The power of the last prism that can be responded to correctly is then recorded. A threshold-size visual acuity target should be used.

Prisms in Monocular Vision Therapy

Monocular therapy is recommended in all cases of amblyopia and strabismus as well as in other conditions when the sensory and motor abilities of the two eyes are found to differ. The therapy technique should be conducted first on the dominant and habitually fixating eye and then on the nondominant amblyopic or strabismic eye. Monocular vision therapy is administered for purposes of raising the visual efficiency level of each eye separately. It serves to help develop or restore normal eye movements, accommodative function, and visual acuity.

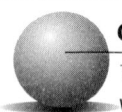

CLINICAL PEARL

The purpose of monocular vision therapy is to develop or restore normal visual acuity, eye movements, and accommodative function.

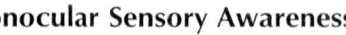

Monocular Sensory Awareness

A prism technique that may be used to develop monocular sensory awareness is as follows: First, occlude the patient's nondominant eye and have him/her look at a centrally placed target some distance away (say, 3 m). Then ask the patient to observe how the target's shape, color, and position in space change when a prism is placed before the open eye. A picture of a white window frame against a black background may be a suitable target with this procedure. The power of the beginning prism and the method of interposition will vary according to the patient's sensory appreciation. When a patient finds it difficult to see any prismatic change with a specific prism, increase the power to the level where changes are noticed. It may be necessary in some instances to have the patient look through both the inside and the outside of the prism simultaneously to compare how the induced double images of the target differ. To achieve this type of monocular double image, place the prism so its outer edge bisects the center of the pupil. It may be necessary to rotate the prism slowly in front of the open eye for prismatic changes to be appreciated.

Prisms in Monocular Motor Therapy

The property of a prism to displace an image toward its apex and make the image appear smaller and closer is used in monocular motor therapy. The technique begins with the nondominant or amblyopic eye occluded. The patient is directed to view a target and to observe what occurs when a prism is placed in front of the unoccluded eye. For this therapy to be successful, the patient must be able to identify the direction in which the image seems to move when the prism is interposed. Responses will depend on the prism power used and on the patient's level of sensory and motor awareness. The power of prism used is determined initially by the magnitude that causes consistently accurate responses. This then is gradually reduced until a difference in directional movement can no longer be perceived. The patient should be able to respond accurately to prism with its base up, down, in, out, or oblique. The prism is held so its base-apex line is parallel to one of the diagnostic action fields of an extraocular muscle (Fig. 10-2).

The therapy should be carried out with the viewer observing near and far point targets, which are placed in the nine cardinal positions of gaze (Fig. 10-3). The lowest power of prism that can be responded to accurately in all the gaze positions should be recorded. The findings for the dominant or nonamblyopic eye may then be compared to findings for the nondominant or amblyopic eye. Theoretically the largest power of prism that can be responded to when performing monocular prism motor therapy will be limited by the extent of the normal visual field (55° superiorly, 60° medially, 75° inferiorly, 100° temporally). However, most loose prism sets do not include powers beyond 45 Δ and therefore deviate the image no more than approximately 25° from the center of the visual field, which proves adequate

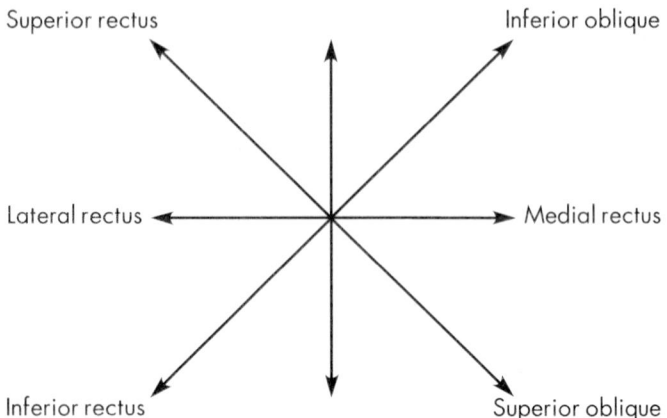

FIGURE 10-2 The different base apex directions for prism interposition (right eye).

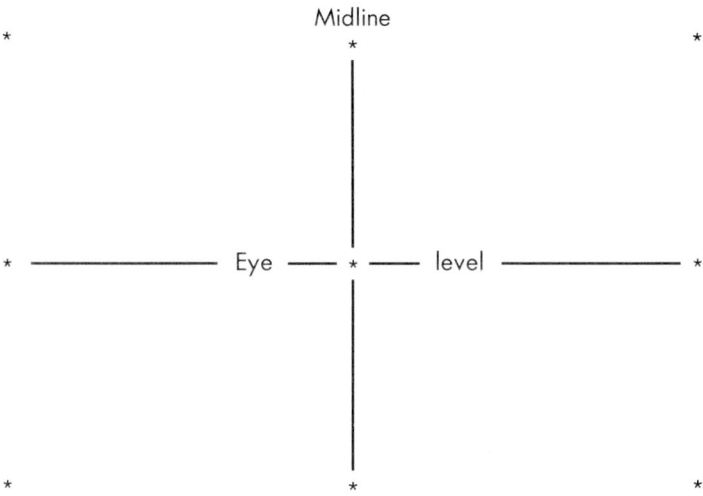

FIGURE 10-3 The nine cardinal positions of gaze.

for the purposes of monocular prism motor therapy. In this therapy the lowest prism power that most patients can respond to with consistent accuracy is between 2 and 4 Δ. (It is possible for trained observers with high visual skills to be accurate in locating directional image changes with prism powers as low as 0.5 Δ.)

CLINICAL PEARL

In monocular prism motor therapy the lowest prism power that most patients can respond to with consistent accuracy is between 2 and 4 Δ.

Monocular motor prism therapy can be performed with the patient stationary or in motion and when viewing stationary or moving targets. The goal of the therapy, ultimately, is to have accurate responses to the lowest prism power in all directions of gaze.

Monocular Prism Saccades

Monocular prism saccade training is often used for amblyopic patients after they have developed adequate fixation, pointing, and pursuit movements. It is used to improve the patient's awareness of his or her eye movements, to enhance the patient's sensitivity to spatial shifts, and to improve saccadic ability. By placing a prism before the amblyopic eye, the examiner displaces both the figure and the ground so that a successful saccadic movement will be evidence of an adequate directional sense. The training should be continued until the patient can reestablish fixation with ease and is able to report movement of the fixated target with prisms as low as 2 Δ.[12] Flax[13] points out that this type of training enhances ocular muscle feedback and integrates the visual sensory and motor systems.

Training Biocular Sensory Awareness

A major purpose of training biocular sensory awareness is to break down the strabismic patient's suppression. The purpose of using prisms in these cases is to move the suppressed image out of the field of suppression so that a diplopic image can be appreciated. In this technique a prism of intermediate power (say, 10 Δ) is placed over the nonstrabismic eye while both eyes are directed at a single target. The target should be placed strategically at the desired far- or near-point working distance in each of the nine cardinal positions of gaze illustrated in Figure 10-3.

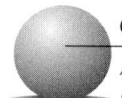

CLINICAL PEARL

A major purpose of training biocular sensory awareness is to break down a strabismic patient's suppression. The purpose of using prisms in these cases is to move the suppressed image out of the field of suppression so that a diplopic image can be appreciated by the patient.

The size of the target must be such that it is visible and discernable to the eye with the poorer visual acuity. If the patient is not able to see the target diplopically in all nine cardinal positions of gaze, prisms of other powers should be tried. It may also be necessary, initially, to degrade the visual acuity (by using filters) of the dominant eye to help break down suppression of the nondominant eye. As soon as the patient is able to maintain biocular diplopic vision in each area of regard, the prism power is increased until one of the images disappears as a result of being displaced outside the field of vision; thereafter the powers of the prisms are gradually reduced until diplopia is again restored. The prism power is then further reduced until the patient no longer sees double, either because the nondominant eye's image has again fallen within the field of suppression or because the patient is now seeing binocularly. This can be confirmed by using Bagolini striated lenses or complementary color anaglyph filters in addition to the interposed prisms.

Biocular Prism Therapy in Anomalous Correspondence

In an attempt to reestablish normal correspondence through training and relearning processes, practitioners have used prisms to disrupt anomalous correspondence. (See Chapter 9.) In his book *Effective Strabismus Therapy*,[14] Greenwald describes how reverse and overcorrecting prisms can be used to create a conscious awareness of diplopia in anomalous corresponders. Reverse prism therapy utilizes the least amount of prism (base in the *opposite* direction from the strabismus) that exceeds the fusional reserve of the patient and causes diplopia. Overcorrecting prism therapy, by contrast, utilizes the least amount of prism (base in the *same* direction as the strabismus) that exceeds the fusional vergence reserve and causes diplopia. According to Greenwald,[14a] clinical experience suggests that the reverse prism technique is useful in small-angle strabismus when anomalous correspondence is not deeply ingrained and amblyopia is moderate (that is, not more than 3 or 4 lines poorer than in the fixating eye). He states that the overcorrecting prism technique is significantly better than the reverse prism technique in cases of large-angle strabismus when anomalous correspondence is deeply ingrained and there is marked amblyopia. He also recommends[14a] that a reverse or overcorrecting prism be placed before the fixating eye in cases of unilateral strabismus and before the preferred eye in cases of alternating strabismus.

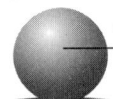

CLINICAL PEARL

Greenwald suggests that reverse prism is more useful for patients with small-angle strabismus and shallow anomalous correspondence whereas overcorrecting prism is better for patients with large-angle strabismus and deeply ingrained anomalous correspondence.

Spatial Disruption and Biocularity

Biocular therapy should be considered beyond its application for disrupting anomalous correspondence. There is also value in considering its use in patients who manifest ocular motility deficiences and/or accommodative inadequacies, whether or not strabismus is present. Essentially, the purpose of such therapy is to deliberately disrupt the patient's balance and test the strength of his or her perceptual and spatial defense mechanisms as a means of maintaining areas of suppression. I find that the introduction of vertical prism is usually effective in dissociating a patient's eyes and creating an awareness of double images. Placing a green filter before one eye and a red filter before the other facilitates the awareness of diplopia.

Spatial disruption techniques

Greenwald[14b] recommends a number of spatial disruption techniques designed to break down embedded suppression. These usually involve wearing dissociating vertical prism and red/green filters. For example, the patient is required to stand on a walking rail and to fixate a Marsden ball (suspended by a string from the ceiling, usually the size of a baseball with black letters printed on it). The patient carries an object (such as a heavy textbook) and walks forward and backward on the rail while fixating the ball and shifting the book from hand to hand every two steps. The disproportionate weight to one side or the other, along with dynamic balancing and walking movements while fixating the Marsden ball, are designed to break the suppression defense mechanism and elicit a diplopia. The reader is referred to Greenwald's book *Effective Strabismus Therapy*[14] for numerous other examples of how prisms in biocular therapy can be used to break down suppression.

Prisms in Binocular Vision Therapy

The major purpose of prisms in binocular vision therapy is to improve the quality, comfort, and range of binocular vision. For more than 50 years prisms have been an accepted mode of developing a patient's fusional vergence reserves. According to Savage[15] the normal size of the fusion area is 8 Δ BI, 25 Δ BO, 3 Δ BU, and 3 Δ BD. This constitutes the range of rectus muscle movements that serve to maintain bifoveal fixation in the median plane and thus maintain single binocular vision (fusion). Prism therapy implemented to improve binocular vision is related to the patient's measured fusional vergence reserves. Fusional vergence reserve at any fixation point is measured by the maximum amount of prism that does not cause diplopia or suppression. Base-out prism is used to measure and train the positive fusional vergence reserve (that is, convergence) whereas base-in prism is used to measure and train the negative fusional vergence reserve (divergence). Base-up prism before the right eye is used to measure right infravergence, and base-down prism before the right eye right supravergence. Prism therapy is not only directed toward extending fusional vergence ability but is also used to improve the speed and point of recovery after the fusion limit has been exceeded. Sheard,[16] a strong advocate of prism therapy, recommended that "prismatic and gymnastic" exercises be given to persons under the age of 40 who presented with exophoria and inadequate positive fusional vergence ability. He divided his exophoric patients into two groups:

1. Those who manifest orthophoria or exophoria at distance and a greater degree of exophoria at near (who would be likely to benefit from prism training or simple "finger toward-the-nose" exercises)
2. Those exhibiting esophoria at distance and considerable exophoria at near (who would likely benefit from combined prismatic and stereoscopic exercises)

Sheard did not place much faith in giving prism therapy to patients found to be esophoric at both far and near—which goes counter to the view expressed by most practitioners conducting vision therapy today, who also do not subscribe to limiting prism therapy to patients under the age of 40 years. Regardless of a symptomatic patient's age, prism therapy should be considered whenever the fusional vergence reserves are found to be substandard and the cause is not a systemic pathological condition.

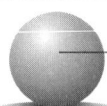

CLINICAL PEARL

Regardless of a symptomatic patient's age, prism therapy should be considered whenever the fusional vergence reserves are found to be substandard and the cause is not a systemic pathological condition.

Many prism or prism-effect techniques have been used to treat patients with heterophorias and inadequate fusional vergence reserves, particularly when asthenopia and symptoms are present. Over the years, this type of treatment has been conducted in instruments such as the stereoscope, amblyoscope, Correct-eye scope, and troposcope. It has also been exploited in space and out of instruments so as to interfere as little as possible with the patient's natural environment.

Base-out prism training, both at far and at near working distances, is recommended for building a patient's positive fusional vergence ability. The patient strives to maintain clear single binocular vision as increasing amounts of base-out prism are introduced before the eyes. Similar base-in prism training is recommended to develop negative fusional vergence ability.

Use of Yoked Prisms

Yoked prisms would seem to be the newest form of prism therapy and have been increasingly applied during the last 20 or so years.[17] They are prisms of equal power with their bases placed in the same direction for both eyes. Their purpose is to shift the patient's binocular field of gaze.

Kaplan[18] states that the use of vertical yoked prisms to correct vergence malfunction "emerges from the need of patients whose asthenopic symptoms cannot be satisfied by current treatment of plus lenses and/or base-in prisms."

> Yoked prisms have a behavioral effect upon patients' asthenopic symptoms. Compression or expansion of observed visual field and change in speed of organizing and controlling the visual field directly relate to each patient's visual condition and affect his vergence malfunction . . . The diagnostic key [to the prescribing of vertical yoked prism] is in the "tight" or "loose" condition of the patient's AC/A ratio.

While one may not necessarily agree with Kaplan's rationale for prescribing yoked prisms (and he concentrates only on the vertical variety), there appear to be sufficient classical and noncontentious anatomical and physiological reasons for at least assessing their effectivity. For example, at the sensory level, persons suffering from homonymous hemianopias or suppression could benefit from a shifting of the nonseeing portions of their visual fields into areas where they do see. (Refer to Chapter 11 for a description of the exact procedure.) Also, at the oculomotor level, persons with noncomitant deviations (for example, oculomotor palsies and AV syndromes) could benefit from a shifting of the eyes to positions where the deviation was less. (See Chapter 8.) Yoked prisms have the effect of helping maintain normal body and head postures, which may be compromised in the interests of maintaining binocular vision and avoiding diplopia. As little as 2 to 6 Δ may be sufficient to direct the eyes of a person suffering from any of these conditions into a position where fusion is obtained.

A brief review of extraocular muscle actions may help demonstrate how yoked vertical prisms can alleviate symptom-inducing vergence and accommodative anomalies. Table 10-2 illustrates the primary, secondary, and tertiary muscle actions.

Training Binocular Sensory Awareness

The same principles apply to the use of binocularly yoked prisms as to the application of monocular prisms. In both instances the goal is to lower the patient's sensory and motor thresholds to optimal levels. The purpose of training binocular sensory awareness is to develop and enhance binocular single vision and to improve the sensory appreciation of differences that occur between monocular and binocular seeing, the objective being to make the patient conscious of binocular fused vision and stereopsis (which contribute to the enriched appreciation of size and the relative positions of objects in

TABLE 10-2
Extraocular Muscle Actions

	Primary	Secondary	Tertiary
Superior rectus	Elevation	Incycloduction	Adduction
Inferior rectus	Depression	Excycloduction	Adduction
Superior oblique	Incycloduction	Depression	Abduction
Inferior oblique	Excycloduction	Elevation	Abduction
Medial rectus	Adduction	—	—
Lateral rectus	Abduction	—	—

space/time). Loose prisms, Risley prisms, the prism bar, and prism flippers (base-in/base-out or base-up/base-down) may be used with a variety of fusional and stereoscopic targets. In binocular fusion training the patient is presented with targets that contain common elements (the same for both eyes) and suppression control elements (unique for each eye). The patient knows that he/she is fusing when a single image is seen that contains the common as well as the different elements presented to each eye. The prisms may be used as a compensatory measure to align the visual axes so that fusion and stereopsis will be stimulated and developed. Prisms may also be used to develop fusional vergence through vergence training, thereby enhancing and extending the range of single binocular vision. The use of prisms to improve stereoscopic awareness is especially valuable when a patient is able to recognize size/space changes as seen with the *SILO* response ("small in, large out"). This phenomenon occurs when a fixated object appears to become smaller and closer in response to a convergence demand and larger and farther away in response to a divergence demand. Prism or prism-effect therapy is most often considered in the treatment of patients with heterphorias and poor fusional reserves. The emphasis of such therapy is directed towards building up the fusional vergence range, but more particularly, the compensating vergence. Patients who have exophoria and poor positive fusional vergence reserves are therefore given base-out (convergence) training. This may be accomplished by increasing the amount of base-out prism as the patient fixates a target. The patient reports when the target starts to blur, when it becomes double, and when it becomes single again as the prism is reduced. Fusional vergence therapy also may be accomplished by using stereograms. These are pairs of drawings or photographs of the same object produced from disparate horizontal angles. One picture is presented to the right eye and the other to the left eye. When the two are fused, the patient should experience binocular vision and stereopsis. A patient's blur, break, and recovery responses related to his or her fusional vergence reserves may be trained using stereograms with different horizontal disparities and at different viewing distances.

Flexibility of divergence and convergence also can be trained by using base-in and base-out flippers of differing strengths. This is known as *jump vergence training.* The same effects can be obtained with stereograms cards that contain pictures with different base-out and base-in disparities, one underneath the other. The accommodation/ convergence flexibility may also be exercised by moving stereograms nearer and farther from the patient. Generally, when the stereograms are brought nearer they stimulate the patient's positive relative accom-modation and negative relative convergence and when moved away they train the negative relative accommodation and positive relative convergence. These procedures are called *tromboning.*

Fusional vergence therapy may be conducted with stationary or moving targets. Instruments like the Correct-Eye Scope, Stereo-Orthoptor, Rotoscope, Controlled Prism Reader, and Stereo-Projector were all popular in their day. Although they proved highly effective, most are no longer manufactured, having been replaced by vision therapy techniques incorporated in computer programs connected to video or liquid crystal display screens.

When using prisms as part of binocular vision therapy, the patient may be either stationary or moving while viewing an object that is stationary or moving. Prisms with their bases in opposite directions (vergence prisms), or with their bases in the same direction (yoked prisms), may be used. For example, a Marsden ball may be swung in different directions while prisms of differing power are placed before the patient's eyes, the objective being to have the patient maintain single binocular vision in all positions of gaze. The patient may also be requested to bunt the ball with a rolling pin held in both hands, or to hit the ball with one hand and then the other. This same technique may be used while the patient walks forward and backward and sideways on a walking rail or balances on one or the other foot either on or off a balance board. This type of therapy has been implemented, mainly by behavioral optometrists,[9] to address postural deficits of the body, head, and eyes and to develop and restore more normal intersensory and perceptuomotor functions. The rationale has been based on the classical experiments of Stratton[19] and Kohler.[20]

The Wayne saccadic fixator (a computerized electronic display of depressible light-emitting diode buttons arranged in concentric circles) also provides opportunities for prism training leading to improved fusional reflexes and hand-eye coordination, using vergence or yoked prisms.

Prisms and reading ability

Vision therapy and the development of fusional vergence reserves through the use of prisms, lenses, and stereograms, along with the Controlled Prism Reader, have all been shown to make reading more comfortable and efficient. Designed especially to reduce visual discomfort and asthenopia, they help persons avoid those types of diplopia that affect the separation of small symbols at near. Taylor and Solan[21] have devoted a book to the value of visual training with the Prism Reader in which they describe the successful effects of dynamic fusional reserve training coordinated with the cognitive act of reading.

Ocular posture related to perceptual and thinking functions

There have been both speculation and experimentation attempting to relate the different positions of ocular gaze with perceptual brain function. Figure 10-4 illustrates the various gaze postures supposedly related to visual construction, memory of smell, visual memory, auditory construction, sensory synthesis, auditory memory recall, body sensation recall, memory of taste, and emotional memory.[22]

According to Sutton,[22] the oculomotor nuclei originate in the reticular system of the midbrain and act either involuntarily or voluntarily "to send a beam or impulse to the brain to stimulate a particular sensory memory recall." If the oculomotor system operates in this fashion, there appears to be some justification for prescribing yoked prisms that would place the eyes in various positions of gaze to develop and stimulate the different perceptual memory recall systems.

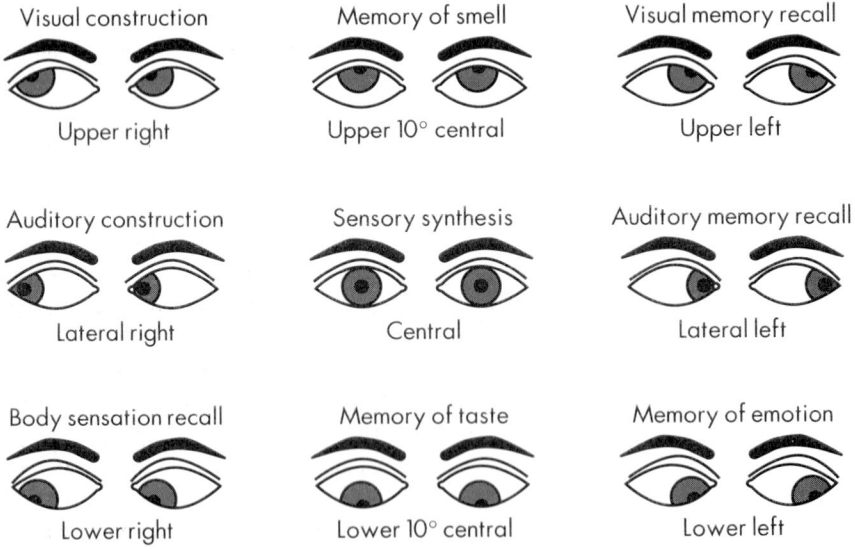

FIGURE 10-4 Ocular postures related to perceptual memory recall.

Conclusions

The usefulness of prisms in vision therapy may be seen in their application to improving the monocular, biocular, and binocular vision skills of a patient. In strabismus, particularly, they play a part in breaking down suppressions and disrupting anomalous correspondence. When normal binocular vision is present, prisms help to expand fusional vergence ability and raise the efficiency levels of binocular vision and stereopsis. They can also play a profound role in helping to correct spatial disorientations and address a patient's postural and perceptuomotor anomalies. The purpose of such prism therapy has been directed toward improving sensorimotor and perceptual spatial/temporal integration. Much of what has been written in this chapter applies to therapy concerned with the posturing of eyes as part of the basic orienting perceptual system and what may be done through the use of prisms to help regulate this system. Prisms should also be considered for the effect they have on the auditory/ vestibular and haptic/kinesthetic systems as well as on the comfort and homeostatic perceptual systems. In the final analysis, it must be recognized that the judicious and scientific use of prisms forms an integral part of comprehensive vision care and therapy.

Addendum

In preparing for the writing of this chapter, besides referring to the major classical works on prisms, I did a literature search on the subject spanning the 3 years 1989 to 1991. Fifty-seven papers were found concerning prisms. However, most of these bore no reference to prisms used in orthoptics or vision therapy. (Many referred to the prism shape of teeth in dentistry.) However, there has been much expounded, mainly by Optometric Extension Program proponents and behavioral optometrists, over the past 60 or so years recommending the use of prisms in vision therapy. In their *Guide to Vision Therapy,* Richman and Cron[23] provide an abundance of diagnostic and therapeutic interventions that incorporate the use of prisms. It would seem as if the vision care professions regard the old and established thoughts on the use of prism as being adequate for treatment purposes. That this should be so is surprising, because the use of prisms is in many respects still contentious. The advent of advanced technologies and new discoveries in neuroscience, particularly concerning brain and visual function, should stimulate new ideas and treatment regimens expanding the use of prisms in vision therapy.

References

1. Welch RB, Warren DH: A comparison of intersensory bias and prism adaptation (Chapter 18). In Spillmann L, Wooten BR (eds): *Sensory experience, adaptation, and perception,* London, 1984, Lawrence Erlbaum.
2. Craske B: Adaptation to prisms: change in internally registered eye position, *Br J Psychiatry* 58:329-335, 1967.
3. Choe CS, Welch RB: Variables affecting the intermanual transfer and decay of prism adaptation, *J Exp Psychiatry* 102:1076-1084, 1974.
4. Welch RB: *Perceptual modification: adapting to altered sensory environments,* New York, 1978, Academic Press.
5. Welch RB, Harrington J, Warren DH: An examination of the relationship between visual capture and prism adaptation, *Perception Psychophysiol* 25:126-132, 1979.
6. Ebenholtz SM: Perceptual coding and adaptations of the oculomotor systems (Chapter 19). In Spillmann L, Wooten BR (eds): *Sensory experience, adaptation, and perception,* London, 1984, Lawrence Erlbaum, pp 335-344.
7. Gibson JJ: *The senses considered as perceptual systems,* New York, 1966, Houghton Mifflin.
8. Bartley SH: Some misconceptions concerning perception, *Am J Optom Physiol Opt* 47:259-266, 1970.
9. Sutton AA: Spatial characteristics of lenses and prisms, *OEP Curr II* 57:25-29, 1985.
10. Julesz B: *Foundations of cyclopean perception,* Chicago, 1971, University of Chicago Press.
11. Worth C: *Squint: its causes, pathology, and treatment,* London, 1903, Bale & Danielsson.
12. Borish IM: *Clinical refraction,* ed 3, Chicago, 1970, Professional Press, p 1297.
13. Flax N: Prism saccadic training, *Opt J Rev Optom* 100:31-33, 1963.
14. Greenwald I: *Effective strabismus therapy,* Duncan, Okla, 1979, Optometric Extension Program Foundation (a, pp 15-19; b, pp 87-93).
15. Savage GC: *Ophthalmic myology: systemic treatise on ocular muscles,* ed 2, Nashville, 1911, published privately.
16. Sheard C: *Selected writings in visual and ophthalmic optics,* Philadelphia, 1967, Chilton, pp 26-27.
17. Kaplan M: Consolidating spatial stability, *OEP Curr II* 60:11-14, 1987.
18. Kaplan M: Vertical yoked prisms, *OEP Curr II,* Duncan, Okla, 1979.
19. Stratton GM: Vision without inversion of the retinal image, *Psychol Rev* 4:341-360, 1897.
20. Kohler I: The formation and transformation of the visual world, *Psychol Issues* 4:38-46, 116-123, 1964.
21. Taylor EA, Solan HA: *Visual training with the Prism Reader,* ed 2, New York, 1964, Educational Development Laboratories, p 15.
22. Sutton AA: Selective attention: the heart of the mental process, *OEP Curr II* 61:82-85, 1989.
23. Richman JE, Cron M: *Guide to vision therapy,* South Bend Ind, 1988, Bernell.

Self-Assessment Questions

1. Prisms cause the image of a white object
    a. to be displaced towards its apex
    b. to bow toward its base
    c. to have a red fringe towards its base and an indigo fringe towards its apex
    d. all of the above

2. Base-down and base-in prisms
    a. expand the apparent space volume
    b. reduce the apparent space volume
    c. displace the visual space inward
    d. tend to increase the tonicity of the back and neck muscles
    e. compensate for palsies of the lateral and medial rectus muscles

3. Yoked base-up prisms make one feel that
    a. the ground slopes down and viewed objects are further away
    b. the ground slopes down and viewed objects are nearer
    c. the ground slopes upward and viewed objects are nearer
    d. the ground slopes upward and viewed objects are further away

4. A person's orientation (Where am I?) is altered by the effects of
    a. binocular base-in prisms
    b. binocular base-out prisms
    c. binocular yoked prisms and prism placed in front of one eye under monocular conditions
    d. all of the above

5. Overcorrecting prism therapy utilizes
    a. the most amount of prism (base in the same direction as the strabismus) that exceeds the fusional vergence reserve
    b. the most amount of prism (base in the opposite direction to the strabismus) that exceeds the fusional vergence reserve
    c. the least amount of prism (base in the opposite direction to the strabismus) that exceeds the fusional vergence reserve
    d. the least amount of prism (base in the same direction of the strabismus) that exceeds the fusional vergence reserve
    e. any amount of prism worn over the refractive correction

---

Answers: 1. d.   2. a.   3. b.   4. c.   5. d.

11

Uses of Prism in Low Vision

Norman J. Weiss
William L. Brown

Key Terms

low vision	glaucoma	cerebrovascular
visual field	Fresnel prism	accident
enhancement	yoked prism	central scotoma
homonymous	coloboma	macular
hemianopia	traumatic brain	degeneration
prism jump	injury	nystagmus
retinitis pigmentosa		

For low vision patients, ophthalmic prisms are used not only for the usual correction and enhancement of binocular vision but also for visual field enhancement, prism relocation, and other special purposes. These applications will be explored in this chapter.

Peripherally Placed Sector Prisms for Field Enhancement

Some patients with binocular peripheral visual field defects learn to use scanning eye movements to aim the remaining useful area of their visual field in the direction of the blind areas. Others, however, find the exaggerated head and eye movements to be very difficult. For instance, a patient with a right homonymous hemianopia must move the eyes and head to the extreme right to see objects on the blind right side. Visual field enhancement enables him/her to view the unseen visual field with less effort. It may involve the use of an optical device, such as a prism, to shift the blind field closer to the line of sight.

Historical Review

The earliest reference to a prismatic correction for field enhancement is by Sir Stewart Duke-Elder,[1] who described a prism cemented to a spectacle correction to reduce the effects of hemianopia (see Fig. 11-1). His brief account proposed that the prism be used in a manner similar to that found in the earliest contemporary publications with regard to field enhancement.

The contemporary concepts of field enhancement began about 25 years ago with adaptations to the hemianopic mirror.[2] This mirror system, designed specifically for temporal hemianopia, was placed on the nasal part of the spectacle frame (Fig. 11-2). The patient was required to look toward the nose to be able to view objects in the blind temporal area by reflection. The shifting of gaze toward the nose to see something in the temporal field, however, caused confusion.

Weiss[3] modified the hemianopic mirror to reduce the patient's confusion. Realizing that the natural tendency is to move the eye temporally when one wants to view the temporal field, he moved the

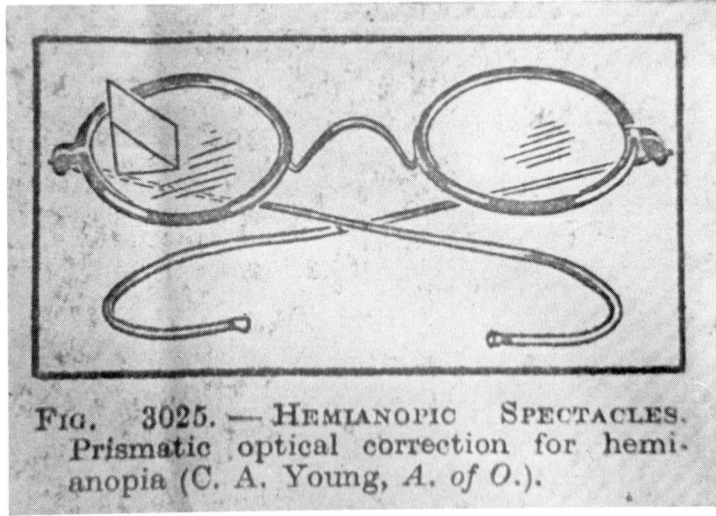

FIG. 3025. — HEMIANOPIC SPECTACLES. Prismatic optical correction for hemianopia (C. A. Young, A. of O.).

FIGURE 11-1 Early concept of cemented prism for hemianopia as described by Duke-Elder. (From Duke-Elder S, Abrams D: Ophthalmic optics and refraction, vol V. In Duke-Elder S (ed): *System of Ophthalmology*, St Louis, 1970, Mosby, p 705.)

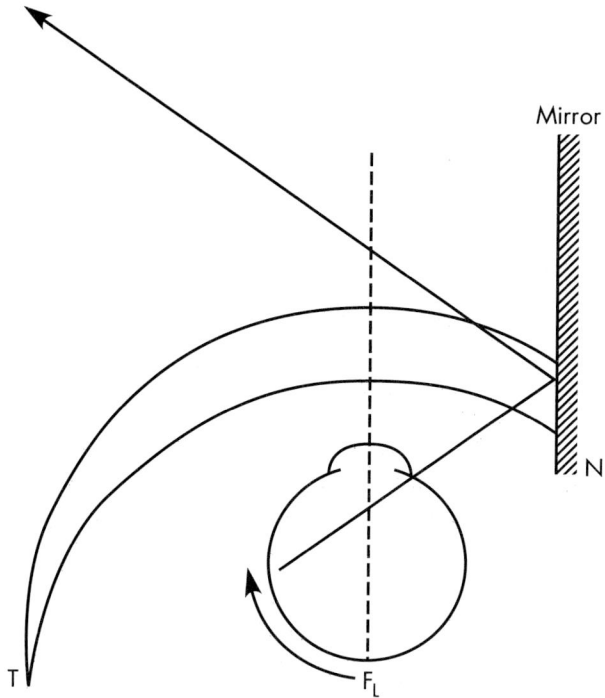

FIGURE 11-2 A hemianopic mirror as originally designed for the nasal portion of the frame. Note the change of gaze required to shift from viewing centrally to viewing the temporal area. *T*, temporal; *N*, nasal; F_L, fovea OS.

mirror from the nasal edge of the frame and mounted it on the spectacle lens itself at the edge of the field defect. The patient would then shift gaze temporally to view objects in the temporal field through the mirror (Fig. 11-3). The mirror was half-silvered so that some of the light from the temporal field was reflected while some from objects behind the mirror was transmitted through it. As a result the reflected image of the peripheral field was superimposed on the transmitted image of the field behind the mirror. This afforded more natural continuity between the two fields than could be achieved by a nasally placed mirror.

Although the half-silvered mirror at the edge of the field defect was an improvement over the traditional hemianopic mirror, the thin glass used for the mirror was easily broken. To give the system more stability, a right-angle reflecting prism was substituted for the mirror. However, a prism comparable in size to the mirror was bulky and heavy. Reducing the prism to the size originally suggested by Duke-Elder[1] to decrease its weight and bulk unfortunately reduced the field of view and limited field enhancement and patient mobility.

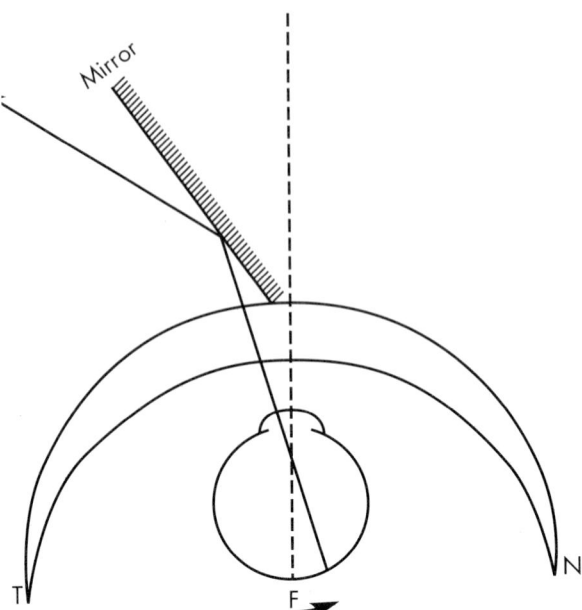

FIGURE 11-3 Adaptation of the hemianopic mirror mounted on the spectacle lens at the edge of the visual field defect. *T*, temporal; *N*, nasal; *F*, fovea.

Weiss[3] found that refracting prisms improved the stability significantly, although the range of peripheral awareness was reduced. Although mirrored surfaces continue to be used for field enhancement,[4,5] we will not explore this subject further.

Characteristics and Definitions

Plano prisms, with the refracting medium bounded by two intersecting planes (see Chapter 1), are used for field enhancement. All prisms have distortion (because of differences in magnification) and "jump" (because of image displacement as the line of sight passes across the prism apex). When the prism is scanned from base to apex, its displacement and magnification increase in the base-apex meridian (Chapter 1). The angle of deviation in degrees is approximately half the angle in prism diopters (Δ).

In field enhancement the prism moves the image of an object in the blind area closer to the useful field of view. As a result, the patient does not have to look as far to the side to see it and the required amount of version eye movement is less. Consequently, a patient with a hemianopia would not have to use as much eye movement to see an object in the blind field. Viewing toward the blind field through a 15 Δ prism with its base toward the blind field, he/she would appreciate an increase of approximately 7.5° in the visual field with smaller versions required (Fig. 11-4).

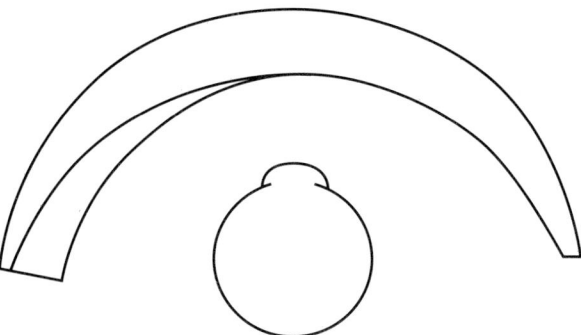

FIGURE 11-4 Base-left prism cemented on the rear surface of the lens to assist with a left homonymous hemianopia.

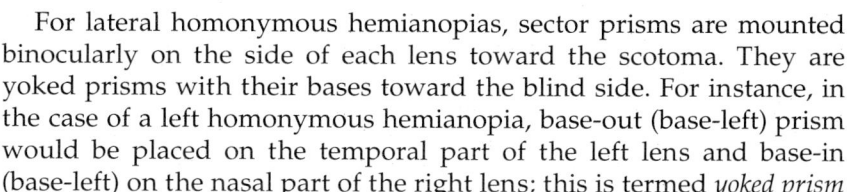

CLINICAL PEARL

In field enhancement the prism moves the image of an object in the blind area closer to the useful field of view. As a result, the patient does not have to look as far to the side to see it and the amount of version eye movement decreases.

For lateral homonymous hemianopias, sector prisms are mounted binocularly on the side of each lens toward the scotoma. They are yoked prisms with their bases toward the blind side. For instance, in the case of a left homonymous hemianopia, base-out (base-left) prism would be placed on the temporal part of the left lens and base-in (base-left) on the nasal part of the right lens; this is termed *yoked prism base-left.*

CLINICAL PEARL

For patients with a lateral homonymous hemianopia, yoked sector prisms are mounted with their bases toward the scotoma.

A major difficulty with using prisms binocularly stems from the sudden image displacement (prism jump) that occurs as the eye crosses the apex of the prism. This results in a prism-induced scotoma at the apex of each prism that leaves some objects unseen through either the carrier lens or the prism. To compensate for the induced scotoma, the patient must move his/her head side to side slightly. Most patients can learn to do this. The alternative—mounting prism on one lens only—has the greater disadvantage of diplopia.

For general peripheral binocular field constrictions, such as those caused by retinitis pigmentosa or glaucoma, prism can be placed base-up in the upper part of the lens and base-down in the lower part, as well as base-out temporally and base-in nasally. However, the patient will often feel "closed in" with this arrangement and may prefer the horizontal prism only or the vertical prism only or may reject prisms entirely in favor of scanning.

It has been our experience that prism correction has limited success with severe peripheral field constrictions (such as those caused by retinitis pigmentosa and glaucoma). It is much more useful for hemianopic or altitudinal visual field deficits.

> **CLINICAL PEARL**
>
> *Prisms for visual field enhancement are more useful in hemianopic or altitudinal visual field deficits than in severe peripheral field constrictions (such as those caused by retinitis pigmentosa and glaucoma).*

Weiss[9] has described a case in which lateral cemented prisms were placed with their apices abutting and no space between them for a case of peripheral field construction. The patient was unable to distinguish viewing through the carrier from viewing through the prism (see Fig. 11-5). This is an exceptional situation, however, since most patients function better with the prism set peripherally so it does not interfere with normal straight-ahead viewing.

Clinical Procedures for Homonymous Hemianopia

When applied to the ophthalmic lens of a patient with homonymous hemianopia, the prism should not cover the entire lens or obstruct the patient's line of sight under normal viewing conditions. It should cover the blind field and be used only when a willful version movement is made into it specifically to investigate the blind area. The position of the prism and the method used to determine this position

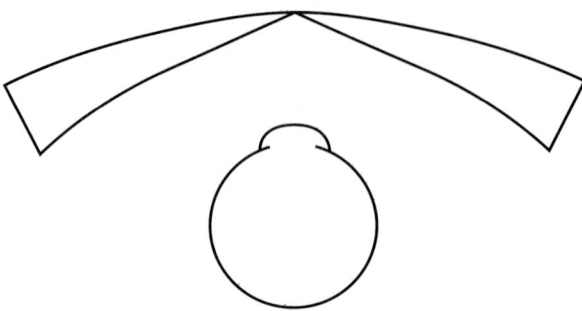

FIGURE 11-5 Prism correction with apices abutted.

have been the subject of some controversy.[3,6,8] In general, however, the edge of the blind visual field is marked on the spectacle lens and the prism is placed in the blind area with its base toward the blind area and its apex close to the edge of the blind field.

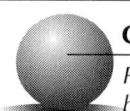

CLINICAL PEARL

Prism for homonymous hemianopia should be placed with its base toward the blind area and positioned on the lens so that it is only in the blind field. This way, it will be used only when a willful version movement is made specifically to investigate the blind area.

Following is a description of a useful method for determining the placement of Fresnel prisms on the spectacle lenses of a patient with a hemianopic field defect:

1. Seat the patient comfortably in a chair with the spectacle correction in place and the headrest properly adjusted so the patient's eyes are in primary gaze.
2. Instruct the patient with regard to the nature of the prism, its intent, and effect. Demonstrate the effect by occluding one eye and placing a loose prism in the blind field. Hold a small light or object and instruct the patient to look at it through the prism. Then quickly remove the prism. The patient should report that the object disappears and an eye movement is required to see it again. Repeat this demonstration until the patient understands the effect of the prism and its use in allowing him/her to see more peripheral objects.
3. If the patient responds positively, then proceed by having the patient view a small target placed straight ahead and at eye level on an uncluttered uniformly illuminated wall.
4. While instructing the patient to hold his/her head motionless in the headrest, move a strip of adhesive tape from the blind area toward the seeing area, and ask the patient when the leading edge of the tape is seen.
5. Repeat this several times to find the edge of the seeing field accurately. Place the tape on the spectacle lens with its leading edge marking the edge of the seeing field of view (Fig. 11-6).
6. Repeat Steps 1 to 5 for the other eye if the correction is to be binocular.
7. Remove the occluder and ask the patient to look toward the tape. If one eye sees the tape before the other, move the tape more peripherally to match the position for the other eye so both eyes see the leading edge at the same time.
8. Determine the position for the leading edge of the prism (that is, the prism apex). Place the prism 1.5 to 2 mm peripheral to the leading edge of the tape. The initial placement of the leading

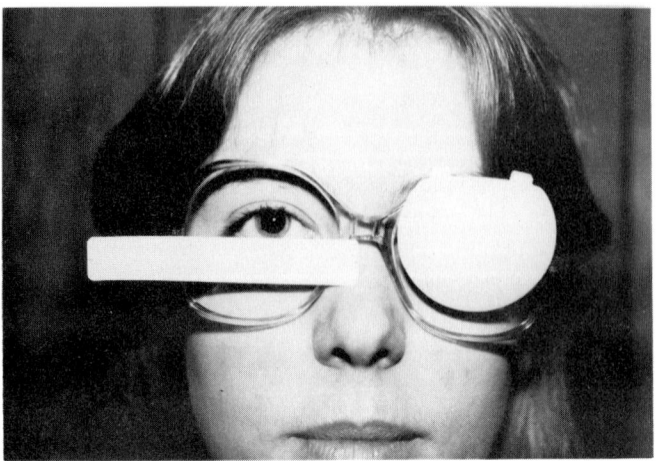

FIGURE 11-6 Tape outlining the limits of the inferior field for an altitudinal defect.

edge of the prism has been the subject of debate. Weiss[3] indicates that it should be 1.5 to 2 mm from the edge of the seeing field as marked on the spectacle correction. Jose[6] states that it can be more peripheral. Perlin[8] prefers that it subtend 20° from primary gaze.

Regardless of the method used to place the prism, its position must be tested to determine if the patient appreciates the improved peripheral awareness with short eye excursions into the prism area. In addition, to prevent diplopia as the eyes enter the prisms, each eye should be tested so that it reaches the leading edge of its prism at the same time as the other eye (Fig. 11-7).

Fresnel Prism Application

In our experience the most effective prism power to use for visual field enhancement is 15 Δ. Patients seem to be more intolerant of prism aberrations when the power is greater than 15 Δ. Some situations, however, will warrant using a different power—larger magnitudes can be used for patients who are tolerant of prism distortion, smaller magnitudes for patients who are less tolerant. Fresnel membrane prisms are used initially because they are relatively inexpensive, lightweight, and thin; they are also convenient to place and modify. Once the practitioner is satisfied that the Fresnel prisms are placed and used properly, they can be replaced with cemented prisms if desired.

The procedure for applying a Fresnel prism to the ocular surface of a spectacle lens is outlined in Chapter 3. However, those instructions assume that the prism is to cover the entire lens. For homonymous

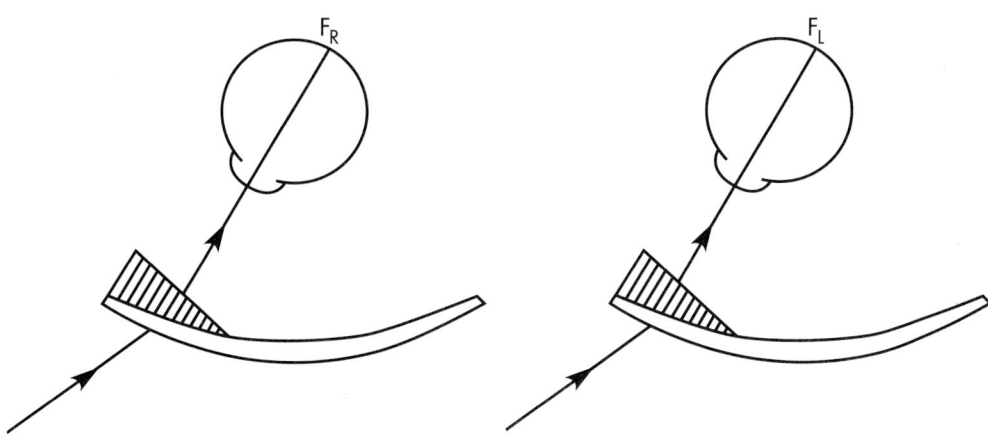

FIGURE 11-7 Proper placement of prisms for field enhancement in patients with a right homonymous hemianopia. The prisms are yoked with their bases toward the blindside. Note that the visual axes reach the prisms at the same time. F_R, fovea OD; F_L, fovea OS.

hemianopia the prism is placed only on part of each lens. It is usually possible to cut the prism for both lenses from a single Fresnel membrane; therefore, this procedure is described. To start, a vertical line is marked on the front surface of each lens at the spot determined for the leading edge of the prism. A strip of transparent tape is then placed on each mark to protect it from liquids used during the application process. The lenses are removed from the frame and the Fresnel prism is placed smooth side against the ocular surface of the lens requiring prism on its temporal aspect. (This should be larger than the nasal prism needed for the other lens and is therefore cut first.) The prism is positioned with its base in the proper direction and aligned over the temporal aspect of the lens so its edge barely covers the temporal edge of the lens (to conserve as much of the remaining prism as possible for the other lens). The nasal edge of the prism is marked at the vertical line drawn earlier on the front of the lens. With a straight edge and sharp knife, the Fresnel prism is divided at this mark, the cut being made parallel to the prism grooves. (The extra piece is set aside for nasal placement on the other lens.) The straight edge of the measured piece is then aligned with the vertical line on the lens, and the outline of the temporal aspect of the lens is traced on the prism. Using long smooth cuts, the prism is cut with a sharp scissors and set aside for application. Now the other piece is placed on the nasal aspect of the ocular surface of the other lens with its straight edge toward the nasal edge of the lens, its curved edge toward the vertical line, and its grooves aligned vertically. This orients the prism base properly (base-nasal). The prism is then adjusted so it covers the entire nasal aspect of the lens (from the vertical line to the nasal edge) and its temporal edge is marked at the vertical line. With the straight edge and knife, a straight vertical cut is made through the mark on the prism, and the prism is returned to the ocular surface of the lens. Its straight edge should now align with the vertical line on the lens, and its nasal aspect is traced on the prism. Finally, it is cut in a smooth curve.

Before mounting the prisms permanently (in the prescribed way, using a liquid), place them on the ocular surfaces of the lenses (they will adhere temporarily by surface tension) and allow the patient to walk about to determine if they are properly positioned. Modify the prism placement as necessary and then apply them carefully to the ocular surfaces of the lenses. After cleaning the lens surfaces and prisms, pour a small amount of alcohol on the rear surface of each lens. Alcohol evaporates quickly, so the prisms will quickly become less movable. Apply them as described in Chapter 3. Surface tension will hold them in place once the liquid dries, but they can easily slide out of place until then, so the patient should be cautioned not to touch them or clean the lenses for 24 hours. Once dry, the lenses can be cleaned in the prescribed manner, using soap and water, care being taken not to catch an edge under a fingernail.

Training and Evaluation

When prism is prescribed for visual field enhancement, a training period is essential. The patient must be taught to localize objects properly while viewing through the prism.

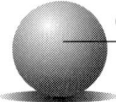

CLINICAL PEARL

When prism is prescribed for visual field enhancement, a training period is essential. The patient must learn to localize objects properly while viewing through the prism.

The training begins with the patient making simple observations of objects while seated. It needs to be determined if he/she is capable of distinguishing between times when the prism is being used and times when it is not. Then instruction can progress to viewing a moving object while stationary, such as looking at a doorway from the blind side when someone is coming through. Eventually instruction can progress to the patient walking. This should be done only when the patient looks through the carrier lens. Patients should not walk when looking through the prisms.

Once these simpler tasks have been successfully accomplished, the patient is ready to attempt more complex activities, such as walking through an obstacle course of chairs, tables, stools, etc. The services of a mobility instructor may be utilized to help in this phase, and the patient can progress to more realistic situations such as sidewalks and shopping malls. For altitudinal defects, stair climbing and the use of escalators are particularly important tasks.

After the patient has successfully adapted to the prisms and reports using them successfully, their effectiveness must be reconfirmed. If they are removed or reversed and there is a noticeable decrease in performance, it is reasonable to conclude that the prisms are being used correctly. If they are accepted in the incorrect position, it is likely that the patient is not using them properly and retraining will be necessary.

Once the prisms have been properly placed, their power determined, and their effectiveness verified, documentation of correct positioning on the lenses can be made by photocopying the front of the spectacle frame with the prisms in place. This placement can be duplicated for almost any frame by placing the bridge of the new glasses over the bridge of the photocopy and marking the new lenses.

CLINICAL PEARL

Successful prism placement can be documented by making a photocopy of the front of the spectacle frame with the Fresnel prisms in place. This placement can be duplicated for almost any frame by positioning the bridge of the new glasses over the bridge of the photocopy and marking the new lenses.

After the success of Fresnel prisms is determined, the option of replacing them with cemented sphero-prisms should be considered. This will reduce the blur inherent with Fresnel prisms and make the correction more cosmetically acceptable since the grooves are no longer present. The thickness and weight of sphero-prisms, though greater than that of Fresnel prisms, can be reduced by using high index lenses.

Applications of Full-Diameter Yoked Prisms

Yoked prisms are prisms of equal power with their bases in the same direction in each lens. Full-diameter prisms cover the entire surface of each lens. Although visual field enhancement of homonymous hemianopias can be done using yoked prisms that cover only part of the lenses, some low vision situations are better treated with full-diameter yoked prisms.

Coloboma

Field enhancement is most commonly used for hemianopic field constrictions, but any binocular field constriction is potentially amenable to prismatic treatment. Colobomas usually occur inferiorly and produce a superior altitudinal visual field defect. To allow more vision superiorly, the patient may use an upward head turn or eye rotation. Placing prism whose base is in the direction of the field defect (base-up) will often reduce or eliminate the necessity for the anomalous head position or eye rotation. While 15 Δ may be the typical amount, the least prism that achieves the desired effect should be used.

Prisms used to treat visual field defects due to colobomas provide two major advantages: (1) Retinal images are shifted from blind areas of the retina toward seeing areas, with images in the superior field shifted toward the inferior field; (2) An adjustment of anomalous head posture closer to the primary gaze position is possible.

The initial evaluation should be performed using the trial frame. When prescribing for a coloboma patient who has fusion, it is best to use full-diameter yoked prisms binocularly. Begin with Fresnel prisms and, if these are successful, use cemented prisms for greater clarity.

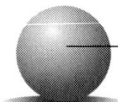

CLINICAL PEARL

When prescribing for a coloboma patient who has fusion, it is best to use full-diameter yoked prisms binocularly.

Traumatic Brain Injury/Cerebrovascular Accident

Full-diameter yoked prisms have been used for the relief of disabling body positions often associated with traumatic brain injury (TBI) and cerebrovascular accidents (CVA).[10,11] The problems commonly found with sitting, standing, or walking erect may be caused by a distorted concept of the midline. For example, a right-side weakness in a TBI patient causes a shift in body weight to the left side when the person is seated. An object in the midline will be reported as centered when it is located in front of the left eye. The concept of midline is also distorted, the apparent midline being shifted in the direction of the stronger side. Padula[10,11] advocates using yoked prisms with their bases toward the weak side to reposition a distorted midline. This presumably will permit the patient to accept the weight transferred to the weak side and cause his/her posture to become more erect.

Similarly, vertical yoked prisms may be used on a patient whose body is bent forward. Yoked base-down prisms move the images upward and cause the gaze to be shifted upward, which can sometimes cause the weight to be shifted backward and result in a more erect posture.

Reading with Left Homonymous Hemianopia

A common problem for patients with left homonymous hemianopia and sparing of the macula is not being able to see the beginning of the line on the printed page. Many of these patients consistently miss the first word or two of every line because they underestimate the distance to the beginning of the next line. Among the solutions proposed for this problem are having the patient look for a black border held at the left side of the page or holding the reading material at a 45° angle. Before either of these approaches is used, however, small amounts of base-left prism (4 to 6 Δ) should be evaluated to see if that helps locate the beginning of the line more easily. Prism in this direction displaces the image from the blind left field toward the seeing right.

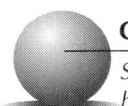

CLINICAL PEARL

Small amounts of yoked base-left prism (4 to 6 Δ) may help a patient with left homonymous hemianopia locate the beginning of a line of type more easily.

Less prism is needed for reading than for mobility. The patient should be evaluated initially with 4 to 6 Δ of yoked prisms in the trial frame. The amount is then modified depending upon the patient's subjective response. The patient should be able to report greater ease in finding the beginning of the lines and more fluidity in reading continuous text.

When prism is prescribed, it is recommended that the ground-in type in spectacle lenses be used rather than the Fresnel type, since the blurred image caused by Fresnel prisms detracts from the patient's ability see clearly.

Image Displacement/Relocation with Central Scotomas

The use of prisms to displace or relocate the retinal image from the affected macula in cases of macular degeneration has been suggested by Romayananda et al.[12] Presumably, the prism moves the image out of the central scotoma and into the adjacent seeing visual field.

The procedure is summarized as follows:
1. Seat the patient with head and eyes in the primary position and direct the patient to maintain this position throughout the testing.
2. Place the distance refractive correction and add in the trial frame, with the cylindrical correction in the rear stationary cell and the spheres in the rotating cells. Occlude one eye.
3. Instruct the patient to view the smallest readable line on the near acuity chart with the most suitable illumination.

4. Place a 6 Δ trial prism in the rotating cell of the trial frame and slowly turn it while the patient looks straight ahead at the near chart. Ask whether any position improves the ability to read letters on the chart.
5. If the answer is yes, first refine the base-apex direction by using a bracketing technique to find the two limiting positions where the patient first notices diminished acuity. Orient the prism base midway between these two positions, increasing and decreasing the power of prism to find the power that gives maximum acuity.
6. Repeat this method for the other eye, even if there is a significant difference in the visual acuities.
7. Place yoked prism in both lenses with the power and base-apex direction corresponding to those of the eye that shows the greatest improvement in vision.

There are several valid questions regarding the fundamental assumptions of this prism displacement technique:

The first is whether the patient can hold fixation in the primary position and abandon any eccentric viewing while the prism is rotated before the eye. Eccentric viewing often becomes very natural and almost involuntary for patients with a central field defect. Even if it can be eliminated from the testing procedure, it then needs to be eliminated from habitual use after the lens corrections have been prescribed so the improved vision will be maintained.

A second question is whether duplicating or even approaching the successes reported by Romayananda et al.[12] is possible. We have noted only occasionally an improvement in the *quality* of vision, and more rarely an improvement in visual acuity of but a few letters. Sometimes a patient is disappointed in his/her visual performance after the prism glasses have been tried for a few days; the new glasses fall short of expectations.

A third question is the lack of consistency. Once the prism specifications have been determined, rechecking the amount and axis of the prism often indicates improvement in another base-apex direction or no improvement at all.

Finally, why doesn't eccentric viewing of the same amount and direction as the prism improve the vision as well as the prism does? Prism displacement may help some patients who have difficulty mastering eccentric viewing; however, it is our experience that it does not work for every patient with a macular scotoma.

Nystagmus

Nystagmus is a condition in which the eyes undergo involuntary, rhythmic oscillations. For some patients the intensity and frequency of eye movements are reduced when the eyes are in a particular position, the *null point*. A patient's habitual head posture often reflects the null point position. For example, if the patient's chin is depressed (thereby rotating the eyes upward), the null point is likely to be in superior gaze. When the null point is away from primary gaze, yoked prisms will sometimes help reduce the nystagmus by moving the eyes to the null point. For example, if the nystagmus is noticeably diminished in far right gaze, base-left prism (BO OS, BI OD) will shift the images so the eyes move right. If on evaluation one notes that the nystagmus decreases with a head turn to a certain position (thereby moving the eyes in the opposite direction), a yoked prism prescription should be considered.

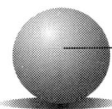

CLINICAL PEARL

Yoked prisms may help reduce a nystagmus by moving the patient's eyes to the null point.

The nystagmus is evaluated by having the patient follow a muscle light to various positions of gaze—including right, left, up, down, and oblique. The effect of convergence should also be evaluated by moving the fixation light along the midline toward the patient, since convergence sometimes reduces nystagmus. If no reduction in nystagmus is found in any position of gaze, prism will not be useful. If a position with reduced nystagmoid movement is found, however, yoked prisms of equal powers should be evaluated. The prisms are oriented with their bases opposite the null point so the eyes will shift toward the null point. Testing begins with about 6 Δ and the amount of prism is modified to find the power that produces the largest reduction in nystagmus, as noted either by the examiner objectively or by the patient subjectively. If convergence quiets the nystagmus, binocular base-out prisms are prescribed (as long as they do not disrupt fusion).

The amount of prism may be modified according to the patient's ability to accept prism distortion and blur. Before ordering prism, it is prudent to have the patient read, walk, climb stairs, and reach for objects while wearing the prism in a trial frame. If this effect is intolerable, the prism can be reduced even though some control of nystagmus is sacrificed. If the smallest prism power necessary to produce a minimal decrease in nystagmus cannot be tolerated, prism is discontinued. Prism is ordered either ground into or cemented onto the lenses. Fresnel prisms are usually not used since the increased aberrations and reflections may reduce visual acuity further and contribute to intolerance. Tints, edge coatings, and antireflection coatings should be considered to make the spectacles more acceptable cosmetically.

The base directions are ordered using the meridians noted in the trial frame—OD, base-out and down @ 60; OS, base-in and down @ 60. It is not necessary to calculate the horizontal and vertical components of the prisms, although including a diagram of the base directions with the prescription will help the laboratory.

Adaptation to the prism correction begins with a careful check of the position and amount of prism when it is received from the laboratory as well as a precise adjustment of the frame. Training with the yoked prism correction should be gradual. Some patients will feel comfortable using the prisms all their waking hours. Some will prefer using the prisms for 1 or 2 hours at first and gradually increasing the wearing time. All patients should be seen periodically during this process so the doctor can follow and document improvement.

Full Prism for Monocular Hemianopia

A hemianopia with sparing of the macula in one eye when the other eye is blind may be accompanied by a turn of the seeing eye to center the remaining visual field around the normal straight-ahead direction; in other words, the eye is turned to aim the macula in the direction of the eye's blind half field so that the seeing half field will be centered more equally horizontally. Many of these patients prefer such an adaptation to having the macula directed straight ahead, with resulting field asymmetry (Fig. 11-8).

By using a full-diameter prism the patient can appreciate some centering of the functional visual field without as much eye turn (see Fig. 11-9).

The proper amount of prism is determined by beginning with 6 Δ and gradually increasing the amount until the best result is achieved. While larger amounts of prism may achieve better centering of the visual field, the patient may not tolerate the distortion. The final prism power should represent a balance between the centering of the field and the amount of prism distortion tolerated.

Once the prism correction has been determined, Fresnel prism may be used or prism ground into or cemented to the lens may be considered to provide the clearest vision.

Prisms with High Plus Reading Corrections

When a reading-only prescription is designed for a fully sighted person to read at 40 cm, decentering the lenses to the near pupillary distance (taken for 40 cm) causes the lines of sight to pass through the optical centers of the lenses. No prism is induced through the lenses,

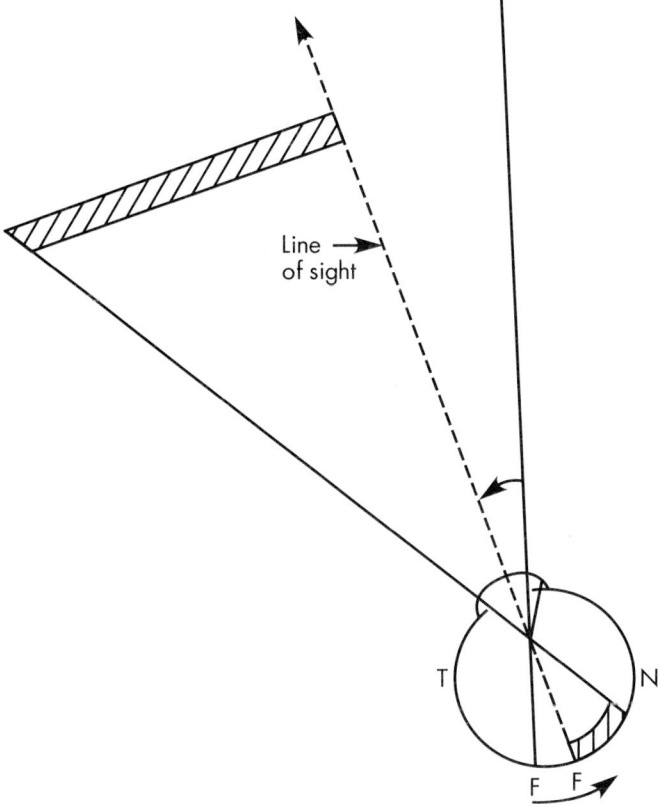

FIGURE 11-8 Centering the hemianopic field by turning the eye.

and the patient is comfortable as long as the phoria is well compensated by fusional vergence. For most partially sighted patients, however, the adds for reading are higher than the normal +2.50 D limit and the working distances are therefore less than the customary 40 cm.

These shorter working distances cause a greater convergence demand for the patient with binocular vision. For example, with a 60 mm pupillary distance the convergence demand using a +2.50 D add at 40 cm is (6 cm)(2.5 D) or 15 Δ, with the optical centers of the lenses placed at the near pupillary distance; for a +8.00 D add, however, the convergence demand is (6 cm) (8 D) or 48 Δ, even if the optical centers are moved in farther to the pupillary distance at the 12.5 cm working distance.

If the add is greater than +12.00 D (working distance less than 8 cm), it is generally nonproductive to try to maintain binocularity since the convergence demand is so great. If the acuity is significantly different between the two eyes, as is often the case in partially sighted patients, the poorer-seeing eye usually contributes little to the reading

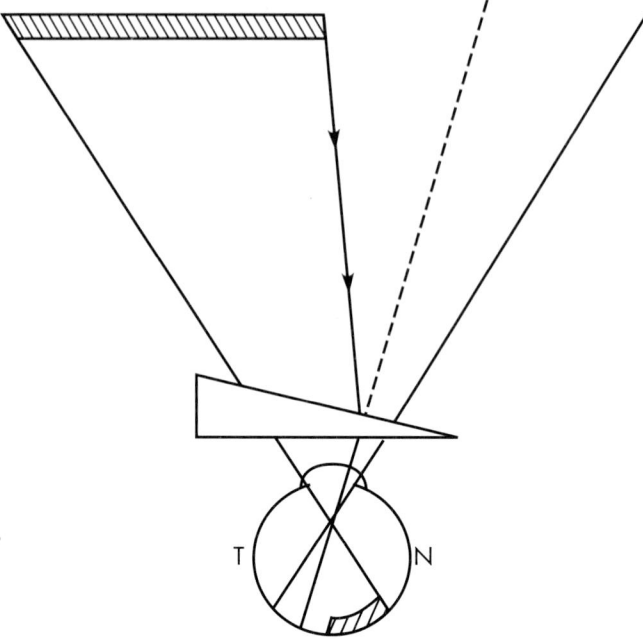

FIGURE 11-9 Shift of the eye with a full prism.

process and in fact often detracts from the performance of the better eye. If gross fusion is not demonstrated at distance or near, binocularity will not be obtained through the high add. In these cases, suppression or occlusion of the poorer eye is more useful than trying to obtain binocularity through prisms. Sometimes a *biocular* (similiar to monovision contact lens) correction is used, with the two lenses focused for different distances. For example, one eye may be focused for distance and the other for close reading; or one lens may be focused at a 40 cm reading distance for large print and the other at a much closer range for smaller print.

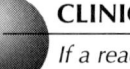

CLINICAL PEARL

If a reading add is greater than +12.00 D (working distance less than 8 cm), it is generally nonproductive to try to maintain binocularity since the convergence demand is so great.

The subjective measurement for prism with high adds begins with an assessment of the phoria at the working distance. The simple technique is outlined as follows:

1. Prepare the trial frame with the patient's full distance refraction and reading add and set the pupillary distance for the interpupillary distance at the working distance.
2. Measure the phoria at the working distance.
   a. Dissociate fusion using a Maddox rod (orientated to measure a horizontal deviation) in one lens cell.
   b. With the patient viewing a muscle light at the working distance, introduce base-in prism until superimposition of the Maddox rod and light occurs.
   c. Check for a vertical deviation as well.
3. Remove the Maddox rod and divide the prism equally between the two eyes.
4. Evaluate the fusion responses using appropriate reading material and refine the amount of prism to suit the patient's subjective reaction to fusing.
   a. The correction should be used for an extended period to determine the patient's comfort level.
   b. The practical limit for a binocular add is +12.00 D.[13]
5. When the glasses are about to be fabricated, consider the following:
   a. Full-diameter versus half-eye correction
   b. Antireflection coatings
   c. Tinted correction for glare sensitivity and possible edge coating
   d. Fresnel prisms are usually not used because they reduce image clarity.

Reading corrections in stock half-eye or full-diameter styles are available in 2 D increments up to +12.00 D with standard amounts of prism. The prismatic power is 2 Δ more than the dioptric power of the lens (that is, each +8.00 D lens has 10 Δ BI, and each +10.00 D lens 12 Δ BI). Often this type of correction is adequate, particularly if the patient has very little distance refraction or is not sensitive to a distance cylindrical correction for reading.

CLINICAL PEARL

Reading corrections in stock half-eye or full-diameter styles are available in 2 D increments up to +12.00 D with standard amounts of prism. They are often adequate if the patient has a minor distance refraction or is not sensitive to a distance cylindrical correction for reading.

Summary

The use of prisms for low vision patients is a special application that addresses very particular goals and needs. The practitioner must be prepared not only to evaluate the patient and prescribe the prism appropriately, but also to select patients whose needs will allow the best acceptance of this type of treatment. Prism can be very useful for enhancing the visual field of patients with a hemianopic or altitudinal defect and for shifting the eyes of a patient with nystagmus toward the null point. They are also useful for preserving binocular vision in partially sighted patients who must use a high plus add to read and for helping patients with a left homonymous hemianopia locate the beginning of the line when reading. Prism use in low vision rehabilitation can challenge the practitioner, but positive results are highly rewarding.

References

1. Duke-Elder S, Abrams D: Ophthalmic optics and refraction, vol V. In Duke-Elder S (ed): *System of Ophthalmology*, St Louis, 1970, Mosby.
2. Weiss NJ: Management of the low vision patient with peripheral field loss, *J Am Optom Assoc* 40:830-832, 1969.
3. Weiss NJ: An application of cemented prisms with severe field loss, *Am J Optom Physiol Opt* 49:261-264, 1972.
4. Goodlaw E: Rehabilitation of the patient with homonymous hemianopia, *J Vis Rehab* 7:13-16, 1993.
5. Nerenberg B: A new mirror design for hemianopia, *Am J Optom Physiol Opt* 57:183-186, 1980.
6. Jose RJ, Smith AJ: Increasing peripheral field awareness with Fresnel prisms, *Rev Optom* 113:33-37, 1976.
7. Bailey IL: Prismatic treatment for field defects, *Optom Monthly* 69:1073-1078, 1978.
8. Perlin RR, Dziadul J: Fresnel prisms for field enhancement of patients with constricted or hemianopic visual fields, *J Am Optom Assoc* 62:58-64, 1991.
9. Weiss NJ: An unusual application of prisms for field enhancement, *J Am Optom Assoc* 61:291-293, 1990.
10. Padula WV: Neuro-optometric rehabilitation for persons with a TBI or CVA, *J Optom Vis Dev* 23:4-8, 1992.
11. Padula WV, Shapiro JB, Jasin P: Head injury causing post trauma vision syndrome, *N Engl J Optom*, 41(2):16-21, 1988.
12. Romayananda N, Wong SW, Elzeneiny IH, Chan GH: Prismatic scanning method for improving visual acuity in patients with low vision, *Am Acad Ophthalmol* 89:937-945, 1982.
13. Faye EE: *Clinical low vision*, ed 2, Boston, 1984, Little, Brown.

Self-Assessment Questions

1. Which of the following statements concerning peripherally placed prisms for visual field enhancement is false?
   a. The prism moves the image of the object in the blind visual area closer to the useful field of view.
   b. The amount of version eye movement required to see objects in the blind field becomes less.
   c. A prism-induced scotoma leaves some objects unseen through either the carrier lens or the prism when this type of prism is used binocularly.
   d. Equal success is found when using this method for peripheral field constrictions resulting from glaucoma and for hemianopic field defects.

2. Which of the following prism prescriptions is appropriate for a patient with bilateral inferior colobomas that have resulted in superior altitudinal visual field defects?
   a. BUOD, BUOS
   b. BDOD, BDOS
   c. BUOD, BDOS
   d. BDOS, BUOD

3. Full-diameter yoked prism can be useful for patients with all of the following conditions except:
   a. Nystagmus with a null position in right gaze
   b. Colobomas
   c. Left homonymous hemianopia with difficulty locating the beginning of a line of type
   d. Right homonymous hemianopia with mobility difficulty
   e. A disabling body position from traumatic brain injury or a cerebrovascular attack

4. Which of the following prism prescriptions would be appropriate for a patient with a left homonymous hemianopia?
   a. BI prism on the nasal part of the OS lens
      BO prism on the temporal part of the OD lens
   b. BO prism on the temporal part of the OS lens
      BI prism on the nasal part of the OD lens
   c. BI prism on the temporal part of the OS lens
      BO prism on the nasal part of the OD lens
   d. BO prism on the nasal part of the OS lens
      BI prism on the temporal part of the OD lens

Answers: 1. d.   2. a.   3. d.   4. b.

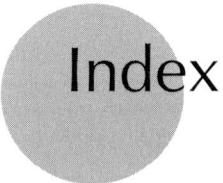

Index

Page numbers in *italics* indicate illustrations. Page numbers followed by t refer to tables.